TRANSPLANTATION
ETHICS

D0223270

TRANSPLANTATION ETHICS

ROBERT M. VEATCH

GEORGETOWN UNIVERSITY PRESS
WASHINGTON, D.C.

Georgetown University Press, Washington, D.C.
© 2000 by Georgetown University Press. All rights reserved.
Printed in the United States of America

10 9 8 7 6 5 4 3 2 1   2000

This volume is printed on acid-free offset book paper.

Library of Congress Cataloging-in-Publication Data

Veatch, Robert M.
        Transplantation ethics / Robert M. Veatch
            p.   cm.
        Includes bibliographical references.
        ISBN 0-87840-811-8 (cloth : alk. paper)
        1. Transplantation of organs, tissues, etc.—Moral and ethical aspects. I. Title.

    RD120.7   .V43   2000
    174'.25—dc21
                                                                00-026843

❖ CONTENTS

PART TWO | PROCURING ORGANS

❖ Acknowledgments

Introductory Chapters

Chapter 1 is based in part on testimony before the Subcommittee on Investigations and Oversight of the Committee on Science and Technology, U.S. House of Representatives, 98th Congress, April 13, 14, 27, 1983 (Washington, DC: U.S. Government Printing Office, 1983), pp. 336–50. That testimony is greatly expanded and supplemented with information on non-Western traditions for this work.

Chapter 2 was written for this volume.

Part One

Chapter 3 is based in part on "Brain Death: Welcome Definition or Dangerous Judgment?" *Hastings Center Report* 2 (5, Nov. 1972): 10–13.

Chapter 4 is based in part on chapters 1 and 2 of *Death, Dying, and the Biological Revolution* (New Haven, CT: Yale University Press, 1989), and on the adaptation of those chapters that has appeared as "The Definition of Death: Problems for Public Policy," in *Dying: Facing the Facts*, ed. Hannelore Wass and Robert A. Neimeyer (Washington, DC: Taylor & Francis, 1995), pp. 405–32. Used by permission.

Chapter 5 is based in part on "The Whole-Brain-Oriented Concept of Death: An Outmoded Philosophical Formulation," *Journal of Thanatology* 3 (1975): 13–30. Copyright 1975 John Wiley & Sons, Inc.

Chapters 6 and 8 are based in part on "The Impending Collapse of the Whole-Brain Definition of Death," *Hastings Center Report* 23 (4, July–Aug. 1993): 18–24.

Chapter 7 is based in part on "The Conscience Clause: How Much Individual Choice in Defining Death Can Our Society Tolerate?" in *The Definition of Death: Contemporary Controversies*, ed. Stuart J. Youngner, Robert M. Arnold, and Renie Schapiro (Baltimore: Johns Hopkins University Press, 1999), pp. 137–60. Copyright 1999, Johns Hopkins University Press.

Part Two

Chapter 9 was written for this volume.

Chapter 10 is based in part on *Transplantation Proceedings* 27, Robert M. Veatch and Jonathan Pitt, "The Myth of Presumed Consent: Ethical Problems in New Organ Procurement Strategies," 1888–1892. Copyright 1995, with permission from Elsevier Science.

Chapter 11 is based in part on "Routine Inquiry about Organ Donation—An Alternative to Presumed Consent," *New England Journal of Medicine* 325 (17, Oct. 1991): 1246–49.

This chapter first appeared in a slightly different form in the NEJM. Copyright 1991, Mass. Medical Society, all rights reserved.

Chapter 12 was written for this volume.

Chapter 13 is based in part on "Consent for Perfusion and Other Dilemmas with Organ Procurement from Non–Heart-Beating Cadavers," in *Procuring Organs for Transplant: The Debate over Non–Heart-Beating Cadaver Protocols*, ed. Robert M. Arnold, Stuart J. Young-ner, Renie Schapiro, and Carol Mason Spicer (Baltimore: Johns Hopkins University Press, 1995), pp. 195–206. Copyright 1995, The Johns Hopkins University Presss, and *Transplantation Proceedings* 29, Robert M. Veatch "Non–Heart-Beating Cadaver (NHBC) Organ Procurement: Two Remaining Issues," 3339–40. Copyright 1997, with permission from Elsevier Science.

The beginning of Chapter 14 is the report of the Anencephaly Task Force of the Washing-ton Regional Transplant Consortium, which I chaired and for which I wrote the original draft. It has not been published previously. It also includes a brief addendum that has also not been published previously. The addendum should not be attributed to the Anencephaly Task Force.

Chapters 15 and 16 were written for this volume.

Chapter 17 is based in part on "From Fae to Schroeder: The Ethics of Allocating High Technology," *Spectrum: Journal of the Association of Adventist Forums* 16 (1, April 1985): 15–18, and *Transplantation Proceedings* 18, Robert M. Veatch, "The Ethics of Xenografts," 3, 93–97. Copyright 1986, with permission from Elsevier Science.

PART THREE

Chapter 18 is based in part on "Who Empowers Medical Doctors to Make Allocative Decisions for Dialysis and Organ Transplantation?" in *Organ Replacement Therapy: Ethics, Justice and Commerce*, ed. W. Land and J. B. Dossetor (Berlin: Springer-Verlag, 1991), pp. 331–36.

Chapters 19, 20, and 21 were written for this volume.

Chapter 22 incorporates material from a lecture at the International Symposium on Senescence and Kidney Transplantation, Zürs, Austria, which has not been previously published, as well as "Equality, Justice, and Rightness in Allocating Health Care: A Response to James Childress," in *A Time to Be Born and a Time to Die*, ed. Barry S. Kogan (New York: Aldine De Gruyter, 1991), pp. 205–16.

Chapters 23 and 24 were written for this volume.

Chapter 25 is based in part on "Egalitarian and Maximin Theories of Justice: Directed Donation of Organs for Transplant," vol. 23, no. 5, pp. 456–76. Copyright 1998 by *The Journal of Medicine and Philosophy*, Inc. Reprinted by permission.

❖ PREFACE

THE ETHICS OF organ transplantation naturally divides itself into three general topics: deciding when human beings are dead, deciding when it is ethical to procure organs, and deciding how to allocate organs once they are procured. These three topics provide the overall framework for this book. After two introductory chapters, one summarizing major religious and cultural views on transplant and one sketching an overarching ethical framework, Part One addresses the definition of death, Part Two addresses procuring organs, and Part Three addresses allocating them.

I have written this book primarily for those interested in a broad and systematic overview of the ethics of transplantation—for transplant professionals, physicians, nurses, social workers, and those participating in the public policy process, including members of organ procurement organizations and government officials involved in the regulation of transplantation. I hope it will also be useful to students of bioethics who are seeking a systematic study of one area of applied ethics. I have tried to write the book assuming no special preparation of the reader in either the science of transplantation or the science of ethical analysis. When medical facts or ethical theory are needed, I attempt to provide enough information so that the reader not previously familiar with the literature should be able to follow the discussion. Nevertheless, several of the chapters carry quite far into either transplantation science or ethical theory. Particularly the chapters on the conscience clause (Chapter 7), required response (Chapter 11), and socially directed donation (Chapter 25) are meant to press the discussion to the cutting edge, introducing in the socially directed donation chapter, for instance, the idea that transplant policy has the potential to challenge the currently dominant theory of justice in philosophy. Chapters 1 and 2 provide an orientation into the views of various cultures on the key issues of this volume and the ethical framework that will be used. Those not feeling a need for that orientation should feel free to move directly to one of the three main parts of the book as their interest dictates.

The definition of death debate is historically linked intimately with transplantation. The Harvard Committee that put forward a brain-based definition of death was completing its work at the same time heart transplantation hurled itself onto the world scene. The first heart transplant took place in South Africa in December of 1967 and the Harvard Committee reported in May of 1968, having worked for many months before that. Part One of the book starts with a case study I was marginally involved in that received considerable publicity at the time. A heart was taken from a man in Richmond, Virginia, without any advance permission or even a clear agreement that he was dead. I wrote an early "exposé" of how problematic this procurement was. That article becomes the basis of Chapter 3. Then Chapter 4 sets out the core philosophical and public policy issues in the definition of death debate, introducing the three major alternative definitions now recognized in Western culture (heart, whole-brain, and higher-brain definitions). Chapter 5 is a revised version of an early paper I wrote in 1973 (and published in 1975). I intentionally have left this chapter intact, adding only slight editing to correct for the now-appropriate gender-neutral usage and making the chapter flow as part of the present book project. It was, as far as I know, the first effort to point out that the view that defining death based on loss of all functions of the entire brain may well be "too conservative" a view. It claims that rather than seeing "brain death" as a liberal alternative to heart-based definitions, it should be seen as a mere waystation toward an even more liberal "higher-brain-oriented" definition. Although this "three-alternatives" view became the framework for the debate in the 1970s, by the time another decade had passed it had become clear to me that there were actually many variations in the definition of death, so that it had become appropriate to speak of the "impending collapse" of the whole-brain view, while recognizing that no single alternative definition was likely to be seen as correct by any more than a minority. This view is set out in Chapter 6 and leads directly to the suggestion, which I have been promoting since the early 1970s, that individuals should be allowed, within limits, to pick their own definition of death, relying on what I call a "conscience clause" to record their dissent from some societally adopted default definition. This view, together with a discussion of what seems like the obvious problems it would create, is the focus of Chapter 7. The discussion of the need for a new definition of death is concluded in Chapter 8, where a proposal for a new definition of death incorporating these ideas is set out.

The reader who is less interested in the definition of death than the explicit ethical issues of organ procurement and allocation may wish to turn, after the two introductory chapters, directly to Part Two, keeping in mind that those chapters presume that some understanding of what it means to be dead has already been accomplished.

Part Two addresses the ethics of procurement. Chapter 9 sets out the core ethical controversy for procurement of organs: whether they can be "routinely salvaged" without individual consent or whether they must be "donated," either in advance by the deceased or by some surrogate. The alternatives of salvaging and donating organs represent two polar options I refer to as "taking" and "giving" organs. This chapter also sets the stage for certain more subtle variants on these polar alternatives: markets in organs, rewarded gifting, routine salvaging with opting-out, presumed consent, required request of next of kin, and required response of persons while competent.

The next two chapters examine some of these options in greater detail. Chapter 10 discusses "presumed consent" and Chapter 11 explores "required or routine response." Next, in Chapter 12 I turn to the only alternative to procuring organs from dead bodies: procuring them from living donors—people willing to volunteer to give one of their kidneys to a relative, a friend, or potentially even to a stranger. This chapter also includes consideration of several types of donors who are at the margins of life who most consider still alive but some might consider deceased. These include anencephalic and persistently vegetative individuals. The chapter also introduces discussion of some new kinds of living donor arrangements: paired donor exchanges and live donor–cadaver "swaps" (in which a living donor supplies an organ to the cadaver donor pool in exchange for his or her loved one getting first priority for a cadaver organ).

Chapter 13 returns to potential donors who are dead—but not dead based on brain criteria. It considers procurement of organs from two groups who are "non–heart-beating cadaver donors," people who die (by old-fashioned heart criteria) unexpectedly in emergency rooms following medical emergencies and those with critical or terminal illnesses who die following a planned decision to forgo life support.

Chapter 14 returns to the special problem of anencephalic sources and what it would take to obtain organs from this tragic group of seriously afflicted newborns. In Chapter 15 the role of age in procuring organs is examined: whether some people are too old or too young to donate organs or have their organs donated by someone on their behalf.

Chapter 16 considers another group of individuals who are not presently considered appropriate sources for organs: people who die from infectious diseases such as HIV or who show no evidence of infection but who live such high-risk lifestyles that surgeons fear they may be harboring infections in ways that do not yet manifest themselves. The problem is not only HIV but cancer, hepatitis, and some conditions of lesser concern such as cytomegalovirus. I will refer to these organs collectively as "tainted organs" and press for a more careful look at the logic of automatically excluding all such organs.

In Chapter 17 I take up what could turn out to be the true solution to the organ shortage. However, it could also lead to a world-shaking catastrophe. Xenografts are transplants from one species to another. We are particularly interested in taking organs from nonhuman animals for use in humans. At first we considered the use of primates, but they are not only scarce and expensive, they also raise particularly acute questions about the rights of these rather close relatives to the human. People increasingly are thinking in terms of using pigs or other vertebrates, but even in these cases we shall see there is enormous potential for controversy as well as danger.

Once we have examined the nuances of procuring organs, we can turn to deciding how to allocate them. Part Three begins with Chapter 18, which calls into question the assumption that doctors have difficult choices to make in allocating organs. We shall see that, in fact, if there are difficult choices, they will not have to be made by physicians at the bedside because the choices are not the physician's to make. They are the responsibility of all of us as members of society; such decisions are rightly made by national and state governments, by courts, and by local organ-procurement organizations governed by diverse groups.

After making sure we understand the nature of the decisions to be made, in Chapter 19 I set out a general, overall theory of organ allocation, noting that, although most transplant surgeons were nurtured on the Hippocratic ethic of doing as much good for their patients as possible, it is not at all obvious that we want to allocate organs to be maximally efficient in benefiting patients. The law, in fact, requires that the allocation system consider not only efficiency but equity as well. Seeing how to integrate these two moral mandates is the project of this chapter.

Chapter 20 introduces the third major moral criterion for an allocation policy: respect for the autonomy or freedom of choice of potential recipients. The issue is not limited to granting transplant candidates the right to decline the offer of an organ. The real problem at issue is whether voluntary lifestyle choices have led some people to have a need for an organ—a liver for an alcoholic, for instance. If we believe that there are voluntary behavioral choices that cause people eventually to need transplants, should those choices be relevant in deciding who gets an organ? If so, in just what way ought they to be relevant? This is the troublesome subject of this chapter.

Increasingly, as grafts are rejected, some recipients are coming back for second, third, and even fourth transplants. And as we get better at managing transplants, people are stepping forward to receive more than one organ at a time: a kidney and a pancreas, a heart and lungs, or, in one case we shall consider, no fewer than four different organs. Inevitably, someone perceives these repeat and multiple transplants as consuming more than one's fair share of the scarce resource. Chapter 21 takes on this problem and argues that not all of these "high-consumer" cases are unjustified.

Then, in Chapter 22 I press an increasingly contentious problem of whether some people are too old or too young to receive organs and what role age ought to have in deciding priorities in allocation. I suggest a formula that will, for the first time, take age into account in deciding organ allocation. This will be followed by Chapter 23 on the role of fame or status in allocation. For instance, it is widely believed that Mickey Mantle got special consideration when, even though there were more than 4,000 people waiting for a liver, he received one a few hours after being listed. I will argue that there are insurmountable moral problems with granting queue-jumping privileges on the basis of status, but that, contrary to widely held beliefs, there is little evidence that once a famous person like Mantle gets listed he gets any special consideration based on his status.

Chapter 24 takes up a newer and even more contentious issue: whether the present allocation formula that gives priority to people in the same local area in which an organ is procured is causing gross inequities. The case for some version of a national allocation list will be explored and defended against the dominant consensus within current leadership of the United Network for Organ Sharing (UNOS).

Finally, in Chapter 25 I will analyze the most controversial proposal yet to surface. Some people contemplating donation of their own organs or those of their loved ones consider making a gift with strings attached, giving in such a way that the organs can be used only for members of a certain race, religion, gender, or other sociological group. This "socially directed donation" became controversial after a dramatic case emerged that is presented at the beginning of the chapter. We shall see that, carefully analyzed, this very practical public policy problem not only raises critical questions for transplantation but also presents a challenge to philosophical theorists who are developing more abstract theories of the just allocation of resources.

Although many of these chapters had their origins in articles or chapters for journals in transplantation, bioethics, or medical journals and books, several (including most of both introductory chapters, Chapters 10, 12, 15, and 16 of Part Two and Chapters 19, 20, 21, 22, and 24 of Part Three) were written specifically for this volume. All those that had their origins in previously published material have been updated and revised to attempt to make the presentation consistent and current. Two chapters have a special status. Chapter 11, the chapter claiming that there are, in fact, no "presumed consent" laws outside of Latin America anyplace in the world, was originally developed with Jonathan Pitt while he was an intern at the Kennedy Institute of Ethics. His research on the laws regarding organ procurement made that chapter possible and he eventually became a collaborator in the writing of the article for *Transplantation Proceedings* on which this chapter is based. I am grateful to him for his permission to include this chapter.

In 1989–1990 I chaired the Anencephaly Task Force of the Washington Regional Transplant Consortium (WRTC), charged with the responsibility of developing a policy for this organ procurement organization with regard to the use of organs from anencephalic infants. Chapter 14 is the report of that task force. I wrote the original draft and, although the final document does not say everything exactly the way I would have said it, I support the general conclusions so firmly that I saw no point in writing a new chapter on the subject for this volume. I have, however, added a well-identified addendum that in no way can be assumed to represent the views of the WRTC. I am grateful to Keith Ghezzi, the president of the WRTC, and Lori Brigham, its executive director, for their permission to let me include the task force report in this book.

My debt to them and to the other dedicated staff and board of the WRTC is much greater. I have served for more than a decade on the WRTC board and all of that time also as a member of its Medical Advisory Committee. It is through the patience of its members and staff that I have attempted to learn the esoteric details of tissue typing, cold-ischemia time, and immunosuppression regimens. It is also with them that I have debated very concrete moral and policy issues that, I hope, bring a sense of nitty-gritty reality to this ethicist's ruminations on these matters. Over these years I have also served three terms on the national UNOS Ethics Committee, which has given me an exposure to the cutting-edge debate on the moral and policy issues as they emerge on the national scene. The various chairpersons, members, and staff have been enormously helpful and tolerant when I either failed to understand or pressed certain concerns too aggressively. I am particularly grateful to James F. Burdick and Jeremiah G. Turcotte, each of whom served as chairs of the committee and who eventually became coauthors with me of the report of the subcommittee I chaired on allocation of organs when that report was published in *Transplantation Proceedings*.

I have had long-term involvement in at least five other transplantation-related settings for which I must express appreciation. I served as a member of the National Data Safety and Monitoring Committee for the NIH/National Eye Institute Multi-Center Collaborative Cornea Transplant Study from 1986 to 1992. This study, which was working at the frontiers of tissue-typing research, provided an ideal lab for on-the-job training in immunology, tissue-typing, and immunosuppression science. I am grateful to Richard Thoft (chair of the committee), Maureen G. Maguire (director of the coordinating center), and Walter Stark (study cochair) for the wonderful collegial relationship that emerged over those years. In the world of privately funded research I served on the Data Safety Monitoring Board of the Syntex Development Research study of the immunosuppressive drug mycophenolate mofetil, an agent for preventing acute rejection in cardiac transplantation. Also, over the past decade I have been involved in the transplant programs of Georgetown University Medical Center, working on occasion with its living donor kidney transplant program and serving on its Organ and Tissue Donation Committee. I served a three-year term as the ethics consultant to the North American Transplant Coordinators Organization, during which time I assisted on a number of issues, particularly some related to xenotransplantation. Finally, in the years when the definition of death debate was in its infancy, I had the privilege of falling under the wing of and then working with the chair of the Harvard Ad Hoc Committee, Henry Beecher, as well as several of its committee members, especially my mentor Ralph Potter, first while I was a graduate student at Harvard and then for many years when I served as the staff director of the Hastings Center's Research Group on Death and Dying. These two people as well as the other members of that research group provided the ideal context for collaboration and stimulation of ideas, with some of the most creative and controversial minds in the definition of death debate. It was there that I developed and nurtured my analysis that fills the first part of this book. I mention these relationships to reveal any unintentional interests but primarily to acknowledge the great support and collegiality they have provided.

To literally hundreds of transplant professionals, bioethics colleagues working in transplantation, transplant recipients, and donor families, I express my gratitude for the insights, shared experiences, and stimulation over the many years that I have pursued the issues of this volume. It is often when we have fought most intensely that I have learned the most. The ones with whom I have done intellectual battle will be only to happy to confirm that they are not responsible for views expressed here, but at the same time I am grateful to the many people whose ideas I have borrowed and transformed into the product now appearing.

During the 1998–1999 academic year I was privileged to have two research assistants cooperating with my research activities. Liat Wexler devoted the entire year to research on this volume, providing crucial support, tracking philosophical, legal, religious, and public policy information, and identifying and confirming much of the data presented. She and Brendan Howe both helped in the editing and rewriting of chapters. Julie Eddinger has served ably as my administrative assistant during the course of the writing of this volume and receives my acknowledgment of great appreciation. Finally, I am grateful to John Samples, the director of Georgetown University Press, whom I have known and admired as an editor, academic, and lover of books for many years, for the opportunity to place this volume in the press's bioethics series.

Robert M. Veatch
Washington, D.C.

ONE

INTRODUCTION: RELIGIOUS AND CULTURAL PERSPECTIVES ON ORGAN TRANSPLANTATION

THE BIOETHICAL DEBATE over organ procurement does not go back much further than the first kidney transplant in 1954—only a moment in time in the history of the world's religions and cultures. The current generation of controversy, however, is even more recent. It can be dated from December 3, 1967, when Christiaan Bernard transplanted the first human heart into the chest of Louis Washkansky. It is safe to say that the great religious and philosophical leaders of history could scarcely have imagined the enterprise of moving human organs from one body to another. It is thus necessarily difficult to determine what the great historical religious and cultural traditions might have thought about such a project.

We can imagine someone seeing such an enterprise as tampering with God's creation. On the other hand, Judeo–Christianity has long taught that human beings were created with the command to have dominion over the earth and subdue it—to use the God-given faculties of reason and observation to overcome illness and heal the afflicted. Although some sectarian religions might see all of modern medical science as a lack of adequate faith, the mainstream Western religious traditions have supported the use of medical science. They have run hospitals, trained physicians and nurses, and contributed countless sums of money to overcome disease.

Before pursuing the more specific issues of the ethics of transplant, however, I want to look at the positions of the major religious and cultural traditions over the past 30 years to see how they incorporate this very new issue into their ancient ethical frameworks.

The contemporary bioethical debate over organ transplantation contains two issues I shall label as *preliminary* and two issues that I shall label as *central*

1

or *core*. The ethics of the definition of *death*, which is the focus of Part One of this volume, and potential controversy over intervening in a dead body for the removal of cadaver organs I take to be preliminary. The donation versus salvaging controversy, which is the subject of Part Two, and the ethics of fairness in organ distribution, which will be explored in Part Three, I take to be central.

Defining Death and Desecrating the Corpse: Two Preliminary Issues

Turning first to what I have called the preliminary issues, I will summarize what the major religious and cultural traditions have had to say about the definition of death and then turn to whether they have raised objections to the medical manipulation of the human corpse in order to serve the interests of others who remain alive.

Defining Death

All major religious groups reveal some differences of opinion over a shift to the use of a brain-oriented definition of death, a shift important if organ procurement is to be facilitated.

JUDAISM

Within Judaism there has been the greatest resistance to shifting to a brain-oriented definition of death. Rabbi David Bleich, philosopher at Yeshiva University, for example, opposes any shift, saying that "the patient cannot be pronounced dead other than upon the irreversible cessation of both cardiac and respiratory activity."[1] On the other hand, other Rabbis from Conservative and Reformed traditions have endorsed the use of brain criteria for death pronouncement.[2]

ROMAN CATHOLICISM

Pope Pius XII opened the door among Catholics for a shift in the definition of death in 1957, saying, "It remains for the doctor, and especially the anesthesiologist, to give a clear and precise definition of death and the moment of death of a patient who passes away in a state of unconsciousness."[3] There have never been any principled theological objections to a brain-oriented definition of death among Catholics, although occasionally conservative Catholics, often those most militantly associated with right-to-life positions, have expressed fear that endorsing the view that an individual is dead when the brain is dead might indirectly lessen respect for those who are still living.[4]

PROTESTANTISM

Protestant theologians and Protestant groups, when they have spoken on the subject, have almost uniformly favored some brain-oriented definition of death, whether they represent more conservative (Paul Ramsey[5]) or liberal (Joseph Fletcher[6]) perspectives. Major Protestant communions support the use of such a definition, including Anglican,[7] Lutheran,[8] Methodist,[9] and the Reformed traditions.[10] The same can be said for Eastern Orthodox groups.[11] Thus although there is some concern about the use of a brain-oriented definition of death, at least some responsible members of all major Judeo–Christian religious traditions accept it theologically and find it appropriate as a basis for procuring cadaver organs. Most have not pursued the more recent distinction made in Part One of this book between whole-brain and higher-brain views, although some in both the Catholic and Protestant communities have moved on to endorse the higher-brain view.

Most of the other major religions of the world also have members who have come to accept death pronouncement based on brain criteria.

ISLAM

The 1981 *Islamic Code of Medical Ethics of the International Organization of Islamic Medicine* is vague on the subject. In language reminiscent of Pius XII, this document reads, "To declare a person dead is a grave responsibility that ultimately rests with the Doctor."[12] It says nothing against the use of brain criteria for death pronouncement but does not explicitly endorse them either. Initially there were reservations among Muslims about death defined as lack of brain activity rather than the conventional definition of respiratory and cardiac arrest. These issues were discussed at a seminar titled, "Human Life: Its Inception and Its End as Viewed by Islam."[13] The report that was published as a result of this meeting concluded that the Quran does not define death. The participants came to the conclusion that when the area of the brain responsible for vital body functions, which they identified as the brain stem,[14] is lifeless, the patient can be said to have died. They concluded that while the brain stem is still alive, all efforts must be made to revive the person. If the brain stem is dead, even when signs of activity are still visible in the bodily organs and if there is no hope of reviving the patient, then the patient is "considered to have withdrawn from life," and behaviors associated with the dead—including procuring of organs—are permitted.[15] A similar conclusion was reached at the Third International Conference of Islamic Jurists meeting in Amman, Jordan, in October of 1986, at which attendees endorsed the view that a person may be declared dead either based on heart criteria or if there is "complete stoppage of all the vital functions of the brain, and the doctors decide it is irreversible, and the brain has started to degenerate."[16] Some Islamic countries, such as Turkey, have explicit law defining death in terms of irreversible loss of brain function.[17]

HINDUISM

Traditionally, Hindu texts associated death with respiratory failure. Physician Prakash Desai, who is a specialist on Indian medical ethics, claims, however, to see a basis for support of brain death in the notion from folklore that at death the *prana* (breath) may escape from the brain.[18] Suffice to say that there appears to be no formal resistance to death pronouncement based on brain-function criteria in Hinduism.

CONFUCIANISM/TAOISM

In China traditional religious and cultural systems of thought are still influential, although it is often hard to draw direct links between traditional views and contemporary biomedical practices. Because brain death was not explicitly recognized in ancient times and traditional Chinese religious thought has not received much attention in contemporary Marxist China until very recently, it is hard to know exactly what the major Chinese systems of belief and value would think about it. There is nothing explicit to which one can point to identify resistance to brain-based concepts of death in either Confucian or Taoist thought, but there are reports that there is "lack of widespread acceptance of 'brain death' criteria in China."[19]

BUDDHISM AND SHINTOISM

In addition to the traditions already mentioned, India and China—as well as many other Asian countries—are influenced by Buddhism. Buddhism is decidedly ambivalent about organ transplantation and especially efforts to redefine death that are linked to facilitating transplant. As with the other major religious traditions, Buddhism comes in many different varieties, and its expression varies from one country and group to the next.

Japan is particularly well known for its resistance to brain-oriented definitions of death, and that resistance is often attributed either to Buddhist influences or to the indigenous Japanese belief system Westerners call Shintoism. Buddhism does not directly oppose brain-oriented definitions of death but has sometimes suggested skepticism. A 1990 report from the Japanese Association of Indian and Buddhist Studies could only state the opinion that "Buddhists should resolve the issue of brain death and organ transplantation," expressing the confusion found in Pope Pius XII and other Western thinkers that this is a question for physicians to resolve: "We Buddhists ask the medical world to make a consensus among medical doctors."[20]

Some Buddhist scholars find a brain-based concept of death compatible with their traditional concept of death. The Buddhist concept of *prana*, variously translated as "breath" or "life," is associated with brain-stem functioning by the Thai monk Bhikkhu Mettananda.[21] This conclusion is shared by other Buddhist scholars, even though they would clearly reject a higher-brain view.[22] One Western analyst goes further, associating death in Buddhist thought with loss of consciousness.[23] In 1995 Soka Gakkai, Japan's largest lay Buddhist organization, endorsed support of brain-based criteria for death pronouncement once the medical community supports such efforts.[24]

Nevertheless, some Buddhist scholars find themes in Buddhism that lead them to conclude that pronouncing death based on brain criteria requires viewing the body as an "assemblage of organs." As Masao Fujii, a professor of religious studies at Taisho University (a private Buddhist university located in Nishi-Sugamo, northwest Tokyo), puts it,

> Brain death . . . seems unequivocally opposed to Buddhist ideals. For brain death regards the body simply as an assemblage of organs, of which the brain is the critical one. Thus, if the brain dies, one is to disregard the fact that other organs are still functioning, and declare the whole body and the whole person dead. In this respect, the cycle of birth and death is broken; one is permitted to explant particular organs whose cells are alive from a body whole brain is death. This way of thinking is incompatible with the Buddhist ideal of the "oneness of birth and death."[25]

The same Western analyst who associates Buddhist notions of death with loss of consciousness suggests that Buddhists will not localize that consciousness in the brain and also notes that this consciousness may reside within the body for up to a week after the dying process would be considered by Westerners to be completed. He ends up concluding that Buddhism actually opposes brain-based concepts of death.[26] The most reasonable conclusion seems to be that there is sufficient ambiguity within Buddhist thought that brain-based definitions of death can be both defended and opposed.[27]

It is possible that the uniquely Japanese resistance to brain-based definitions of death should be traced more to indigenous religious beliefs called Shintoism. Two themes are particularly important. First, Shinto thought resists a rigid separation of the body and the soul, making the association of death with a particular organ difficult. One wise Japanese medical professional once told me, "You Westerners believe that the soul resides in the brain. We Japanese think the soul exists throughout the body." In this observation, she was reflecting a classical

Shinto insight. Second, Shinto thinkers have held unique beliefs about the newly dead body, maintaining that there is a period of some 49 days when the soul is considered polluted by death in which the person is considered not yet fully dead.[28]

Given these reservations based on traditional religious views, it is not surprising that Japan has been one of the last countries of the developed world to adopt a brain-oriented definition of death. After a decades-long national debate, in 1997 Japan adopted a very narrowly focused law authorizing death pronouncement based on brain criteria, but only if the intent is to procure organs and then only if the deceased has consented in advance to both organ procurement and the use of brain-based criteria and if the family also agrees.[29] Even so, many Japanese continue to resist brain-based death pronouncement.

Desecrating the Corpse

JUDEO–CHRISTIANITY

Perhaps more significant, there is substantial ethical agreement on the second preliminary ethical question, the ethics of intervening into the dead body to remove organs. There has in general been no objection among either the secular or religious bioethical communities to the removal of organs for lifesaving purposes from human bodies of persons once it is established those persons are dead.

Catholic and Protestant Groups. Protestants and Catholics have raised no serious questions about cadaver organ removal provided appropriate respect is shown for the deceased and appropriate permissions are obtained.[30] In fact, these groups have generally endorsed such lifesaving gift-giving as a noble act. They have also tended to support xenotransplantation of organs from nonhuman animals. These views are related to the religious view of creation that places the human in a privileged position, considering the "lower animals" to have a subordinate status over which humans should have dominion.

Judaism. Jewish thought poses a more serious question, because in Judaism there are religious obligations to bury the dead with organs intact.[31] However, this obligation is superseded when a cadaver organ can be removed for the purpose of saving a life of another identified person in need. Thus the dominant American religious traditions accept the legitimacy of removing cadaver organs for lifesaving transplantation. Some may insist on more conservative heart-and-lung-oriented criteria for death, and some, especially Orthodox Jews, may object to organ removal for research or educational purposes, but the two preliminary ethical problems pose no insurmountable obstacles for cadaver organ procurement. In fact, Judaism,[32] Catholicism,[33] and the major Protestant[34] denominations all place a high value on the saving of human life, so that although the state may not be authorized to salvage organs routinely, individuals bear at least a moral obligation to facilitate organ procurement for lifesaving purposes.

Fundamentalist Protestantism. One religious doctrine potentially poses a problem for members of more fundamentalist Protestant groups. Christianity is a religion that affirms a bodily resurrection. For certain fundamentalist groups, this doctrine plays a very central role. The resurrection in bodily form is a vivid hope for the oppressed and the near-constant source of solace for those who have been separated from loved ones. This is an otherworldly spiritualism that takes the Biblical vision of a new heavenly life quite literally. To such believers the thought of a resurrection without some of their vital organs must be quite horrifying, and such an image has undoubtedly produced some resistance to organ donation.

This turns out, however, to be a fear only for the theologically unsophisticated Fundamentalist. Their more theologically astute brethren know that worry about a disease or damaged physical body has been a concern of Christian theologians since the Middle Ages. After all, deaths have always occurred with painful, debilitating disease, and deaths involving immolation in fires or in body-crushing accidents would have always posed a serious concern for believers in a bodily resurrection. A sophisticated understanding of church teaching, however, reveals that the medieval theologians held the doctrine of the "new" or "perfect" body. They held that the saved would regain life in bodily form but the body would be in a new and perfected form. Such a perfect body would have the same physical appearance as one's earthly body but without any of its flaws, diseases, or damage. Medieval theologians had seen skeletal remains of deceased humans and knew that flesh deteriorates but formulated early on a theological solution to this problem. The idea of the new body is well known in contemporary fundamentalist Christianity. Consider, for example, the very popular gospel song, "I'll Have a New Body," recorded by Hank Williams, Sr.:

> When 'ol Gabriel blows his trumpet and we walk the streets of gold
> I'll have a new body, praise the Lord I'll have a new life
> No more pain, worry, sorrow in this wicked world of sin
> I'll have a new body praise the Lord I'll have a new life!

Never let it be said that those country singers didn't know their medieval theology. Thus fundamentalist Christians who really understand their church's doctrine should not have a problem with organ donation as far as belief in a resurrection of the body is concerned.

African American Christianity. African American culture is heavily influenced by the Black church, which is often Protestant. Its power cannot be overemphasized. As with the more fundamentalist White Protestant churches, which were often historically the source of Black denominations, concern about the body and its resurrected condition has often been great. Much attention has been given to the reasons why African Americans are statistically less inclined to donate organs for transplant. This is a particular problem, because hypertension rates are much higher among Blacks and therefore kidney failure is a significant problem generating the need for organs that are histocompatible with Black recipients.

Clive Callender, director of the Transplant Center at Howard University, has conducted research attempting to determine the reasons for the low donation rate among Blacks. He has identified eight reasons, including a perception among Blacks that organs are inequitably distributed, distrust of the White-dominated health care system, and fear that signing donor cards will lead to premature declaration of death. He also lists suboptimal use of the community as a change agent, inadequate involvement of the community in decision making, lack of transplant awareness, and inadequate emphasis on behavior modification toward health promotion and disease prevention as social and educational reasons. In addition, one of the reasons he identifies is "religious myths and misperceptions."[35]

As one member of the clergy put it, "On their great getting-up morning, blacks don't want to go to the pearly gates without organs . . . they want to go to Jesus whole."[36] A very insightful and sensitive analysis of the relationship between the African American church and organ donation is provided by Howard Divinity School professor Cheryl Sanders.[37] She acknowledges that the Black church has sometimes endorsed views about the resurrection that have made African Americans resistant to donation but is critical of those who would simply ridicule these beliefs as superstition and "myth" (in the pejorative sense). She, however, "revisits" the religious considerations in an effective attempt to show that Black theology can provide a basis for supporting organ donation. She reviews the arguments leading to the conclusion that the resurrection of the body cannot be contingent on the condition of the bodily remains,[38] pointing to the effect on the corpse of embalming practices that remove blood as potentially posing similar problems for those concerned about a resurrected body that was damaged during earthly life. She concludes that "it may well be that the individual whose body has been mutilated as a result of a decision to donate based upon the practice of [the Christian virtues of] faith, hope, and love will fare much better in the final judgment than the one whose body parts remained intact because of a refusal to take steps to provide the gift of life for someone else."[39]

Sanders suggests, based on a Doctor of Ministry dissertation of Father George Ehusani, an African who is a Roman Catholic priest,[40] that African American religious concerns about preservation of the body intact may have roots that are deeper than the fundamentalist Protestant theology taught by Caucasians. Ehusani, describing the beliefs of his own Ebira of Nigeria, indicates that African culture attributes sacredness to the entire human body, viewing each part or organ as a microcosm of the whole person, leading to the practice of carefully disposing of hair and nail clippings because of the spiritual power associated with any human body parts. Sanders observes that "a people who discern spirit identity in hair and nail cuttings would necessarily be skeptical of the practice of removing and transplanting vital bodily organs such as the kidney and the heart."[41] Thus African American resistance to organ donation may reflect lingering hints of a deeply embedded belief system that will have to be considered by programs designed to promote organ donation in this community.

OTHER MAJOR RELIGIONS

The other major religious traditions all have doctrines or traditions that pertain to handling of the dead body. Some of them seem to have implications relevant to organ procurement.

Islam. Muslims hold that the body is sacred—entrusted to one's care on earth. They maintain that harm must not be done to it in life or in death. Arab countries generally agree with organ procurement, whereas Muslims of the Indian subcontinent usually do not. For example, it is reported that many Muslim jurists in Pakistan have concluded that organ donation is not acceptable.[42] Although the general population tends to feel positively toward donation,[43] guidelines set limits, including that transplants occur only when no other treatment is available, that the procedure has a good chance of success, that voluntary consent is obtained from either the donor or the next of kin to procure the organs, and that death has accurately been pronounced. Live organ donation is considered to be a risk to the body and is only permitted when it is a life-saving procedure. But as part of a collective society, it is a Muslim's duty to aid others through donation if life is at stake.[44]

Although there has been considerable debate within various Islamic societies, procurement by donation has been considered acceptable to many Muslims. In fact, in ways similar to Judaism, the donation of organs in Islam is seen as a duty to one's fellow human beings. According to the Islamic Code of Medical Ethics,

> The individual patient is the collective responsibility of Society, that has to ensure his health needs by any means inflicting no harm on others. This comprises the donation of body fluids or organs such as blood transfusion to the bleeding or a kidney transplant to the patient with bilateral irreparable

renal damage. This is another "Fardh Kifaya," a duty that donors fulfill on behalf of society.[45]

Physician–medical ethicist Hassan Hathout further explicates, citing other authoritative meetings within the Islamic community. He cites two juridical rules: that "necessities overrule prohibitions" and that "the choice of the lesser of two evils" is morally preferred,[46] both of which are interpreted as supporting organ procurement.

Hinduism. It is reported that cadaveric organ transplantation is rare in India.[47] But the evidence of any religiously based objection is complex. The fact that organs are regularly procured from living sources (donor is not the right word, as we shall see later in the chapter) suggests there is no principled objection either to organ procurement or transplantation itself. The great expense of transplantation and the relatively small numbers of people that it benefits suggests that India may simply have other priorities.

Wendy Doniger points out that the Hindu religious imperative to reduce the body to ashes and the belief that a dead body is literally untouchable may account for Hindus' disinclination to donate their organs.[48] On the other hand, she traces Hindu as well as Buddhist myth that treats the giving of eyes and other body parts as virtuous behavior.[49] Desai cites these myths as a basis for his claim that organ transplants are well received when they are available.[50] That these myths involve living donors is probably not irrelevant to current live-donor and live-vendor practices in India (which will be discussed later).

Doniger also sees significance in the Hindu doctrine of karma, which holds that the action one engages in in this world affects how one will be reborn. This creates what she calls a "boundary" problem.[51] Karma can be transferred in intimate exchanges with others. This affects Hindu understanding of the sharing of food and sexual relations. It surely would also have bearing on organ exchanges. Depending on whether good or bad karma is being transferred, a Hindu may be more or less inclined to donate or receive organs of others. Citing the work of E. Valentine Daniell, Doniger summarizes, "The fluidity of bodies in India makes you more, rather than less, nervous about sharing body parts."[52]

Relatively little information is available about the medical-ethical views of the Sikhs, a modern movement with roots in Hinduism that is monotheistic and rejects the Hindu caste system. Black, however, reports that Sikhs also accept organ transplant.[53]

Confucianism/Taoism. As noted earlier, there is relatively little information available in the West regarding Chinese ethical views on transplantation.[54] Aside from the reported resistance to the use of brain criteria for death pronouncement, I have found no principled objection to organ procurement for transplantation. Kidney transplantation has been performed in China for many years. The main resistance seems to be one of economic priority. There is a clear preference for using scarce resources for prevention and early-stage treatment. Ren-Zong Qiu, the leading biomedical ethicist in China today, says, "The emphasis should be put on prevention, early treatment, treatment of pre-end-stage renal diseases, and non-dialysis treatment."[55]

These attitudes seem compatible with traditional Confucian views that are more accepting of the inevitability of death than Western religious traditions.[56] On the other hand, Taoism has tended toward more aggressive pursuit of the prolongation of life, an attitude that could fuel support for organ transplantation.[57]

Buddhism. Buddhism, the other great religious tradition of Asia, is somewhat more ambivalent about transplantation. One scholar noted that by his writing in 1988 the Sangha, the organization of Buddhist followers, has taken no absolute position on organ transplantation.[58] Buddhist scholars generally praise donation of organs as a compassionate and praiseworthy gesture. Scholars of Buddhism writing about transplantation point to the teaching of Buddha encouraging dedication to the benefit of others through giving, including admiration of self-immolation, which is seen as relevant to donation of body parts.[59] In fact, they give this generosity such prominence that they are not always greatly concerned about whether death has been firmly established before organs are procured.[60] Moreover, Buddhism deemphasizes the importance of the body, and its embrace of cremation is taken by Buddhist scholars as evidence that the body is unimportant for any future life.

On the other hand, although there is no direct proscription on transplant in Buddhism, there are tenets within the tradition that might discourage it. For one, Buddhism opposes an "unseemly attachment to life as well as disruption of the dying process."[61] This leads Maseo Fujii to conclude that "Buddhism affirms the idea of giving one's internal organ to others, but the idea that a recipient would receive an organ with the desire to prolong his own life is not supported."[62] Any uncertainty about whether the still-respiring body is really dead could be exacerbated by these concerns. According to anthropologist Margaret Lock, most Japanese remain aware that in Buddhism "the process of dying is not complete until services held on the seventh and forty-ninth days are performed."[63] This surely could create an environment in which a family would be reluctant to support procurement of organs from the body.

Nolan, after considering the claim that Japanese resistance to organ transplant can be traced to Buddhist beliefs about reincarnation, concludes that "concerns about survival in the afterlife and bodily reincarnation actually fit more closely with Confucian and Shinto beliefs about the unity of body and spirit than with Buddhist notions of rebirth."[64]

Shintoism. In addition to the indigenous Japanese religious beliefs about the unity of body and spirit, Shintoism traditionally has considered all contact with the dead body ritually polluting.[65] Moreover, Shintoism centers on the religious significance of the spirits of the ancestors. Not only does this lead to skepticism about the use of brain criteria for pronouncing death, but also to pervasive doubt that procuring organs is an appropriate way to show respect for one's future ancestors.[66] Helen Hardacre, in a review of Buddhist and Shinto views on brain death and organ transplantation, concludes that Shinto writers are either clearly opposed to organ transplant or extremely cautious.[67]

The Two Central Ethical Issues

This brings us to the critical and controversial core ethical issues that will become the focus of this book: the controversies over donation versus routine salvaging of organs and over allocating organs once they are procured.

Routine Salvaging versus Donation

It has been recognized for years that there are two basic alternatives for organ procurement: donation and salvaging. A more detailed examination of these two major alternative models for organ procurement will be given in Chapter 9. At this point it is simply important to see how the major religious and cultural traditions approach this central choice.

Under salvaging schemes, such as that proposed by lawyer Jesse Dukeminier and physician David Sanders in 1968, cadaver organs would be routinely "salvaged"—that is, taken without any formal consent when they are needed as a social resource.[68] The dead body would simply be presumed to be the property of the state when the body could serve a useful purpose. Normally, advocates of salvaging would permit individuals to object in writing while living or even permit relatives to object in cases in which the individual has not expressed his or her wishes to the contrary.

The other alternative relies on donation. The assumption is that an individual has rights over and against the state, including the right to bodily integrity. Holders of this view insist that these rights do not cease at death. Although the state possesses certain rights to protect society from infectious disease and to perform autopsy when foul play is suspected, it does not automatically have the right to appropriate body parts. Under this approach, the deceased retains some right of control over how his or her body is treated, even after death. The relatives acquire a limited right to make certain decisions about disposition (within the framework of the deceased's own wishes). They have what is sometimes referred to as a quasi-property right. But that right entails duties as well—including the duty to dispose of the bodily remains respectfully and properly. Thus they acquire a right to make the decision whether to permit organs to be procured (within the constraints of the deceased's own wishes).

JUDEO-CHRISTIANITY

It is the second alternative of donation that has been favored by virtually every writer within the Judeo-Christian tradition and by every religious group speaking on the subject.[69] The reason is that according to the Judeo-Christian tradition, respect for the individual and the rights associated with that individual do not cease at death. Obligations of respect—for the wishes of the deceased and the integrity of his or her earthly remains—must continue. In the Judeo-Christian tradition, as opposed to much pagan Greek thought, the body is affirmed to be a central part of the total spiritual being. Any scheme that abandons the mode of donation in favor of viewing the cadaver as a social resource to be mined for worthwhile social purposes will directly violate central tenets of Christian thought and create serious problems for Jews as well, especially in a state not based on Jewish law. It will predictably produce vociferous, agitated opposition. Although I cannot predict street riots comparable to those sparked in Israel after the passing of autopsy laws permitting routine violation of the corpse,[70] it is safe to say there would be sustained and vocal opposition.

At the same time there is uniform support in all major traditions not only for the ethical acceptability of donation, but for the actual moral obligation to take organ donation seriously. In fact, Judaism has been interpreted as imposing a positive duty to provide organs for transplant if an identifiable life can be saved. This suggests that although Judeo-Christianity would oppose routine salvaging by the state, these traditions would look favorably on public policies to make donation as easy as possible. Given the fact that these religious traditions all support organ donation in at least some circumstances and in fact consider it a morally weighty obligation, they would favor public policies making it as easy as possible to express a willingness to donate organs for lifesaving purposes.

The public policy implication is that the correct solution to the donation versus salvaging controversy is maximum encouragement to facilitate donation, provided this does not subtly coerce those unwilling to donate and does not trick them into donating unintentionally. The schemes to indicate willingness to donate on state drivers' licenses, for example, would seem reasonable. In addition, questions on federal documents, especially those already computerized for easy retrieval such as income tax or Social Security records, would also seem appropriate. This is a proposal I shall make more formally in Chapter 11.

ISLAM

Islamic documents stress that organ procurement must be by voluntary donation either from the deceased, through an advance gift, or from the family. According to the Islamic Code of Medical Ethics, "Organ donation shall never be the outcome of compulsion, family embarrassment, social or other pressure or exploitation of financial need."[71] There is also a stricture that the donation "not entail the exposure of the donor to harm,"[72] a requirement easily met in the case of cadaver donation but presumably difficult to satisfy in the case of living donation. However, because the code speaks clearly of developing regulations for live donation of organs, some level of harm greater than that of live-donor organ procurement must be implied. Even in the face of the commitment that saving another's life is morally imperative, still, according to Islamic scholars, no organ should be taken by coercion or even pressure. Markets in human organs are proscribed by key Fatwas (legal rulings), although some opening to markets may be implied by the maxim that necessity makes prohibited behavior acceptable.[73]

HINDUISM

Although many cultures debate the differences between donation and routine salvaging, some theoreticians propose organ markets in which those needing organs who are able and willing to pay can buy a kidney from someone who would rather have the money than the organ.[74] The one culture in which such markets are known to exist is India.[75] A surgeon, K. C. Reddy, brokers transactions in which those desperate for money sell one of their kidneys to those willing to pay.[76] The relationship with Hinduism is difficult to establish. Prakash Desai,[77] a respected physician–interpreter of bioethics in India, and C. M. Francis,[78] the director of St. Martha's Hospital in Bangalore, condemn the practice. Nevertheless, even though there are many critics, something in Indian culture makes a market in organs thinkable in a way that it is not in other societies. Some of those reasons are undoubtedly socioeconomic. The poverty of large masses in India makes their situation desperate. Even modest payments from wealthy elites from India or elsewhere provide multiples of yearly incomes for the destitute. It is very hard for people from other cultures to understand the economic pressures and even harder to be critical of a mother who decides to sell her kidney to feed her children.

The tougher question is whether there is something in Indian culture—perhaps in Hinduism—that contributes to this complex and tragic situation. The

Hindu doctrine of karma suggests that people are reborn into this world into positions determined by their previous lives. Those who are born into lower socioeconomic strata (reflecting a traditional caste system grounded in Indian religion and culture) may be said to deserve what they get. Perhaps that contributes to an indifference that helps make a market in organs possible.[79]

CONFUCIANISM/TAOISM

Traditional Confucian ideals isolate the practice of medicine from the business of medicine. In fact, in ancient orthodox Confucianism the norm was to strive to practice medicine within the family rather than having to make do with a "mere professional" physician.[80] There are still signals of moral preference for donation of organs and opposition to commercialization.[81] Nevertheless, recent reports out of China suggest compromises, first with what appears to be a widespread practice of organ procurement from condemned prisoners (albeit with the formal requirement of consent), and second with reports of markets in organs.[82]

BUDDHISM AND SHINTOISM

Buddhism also places great emphasis on organs being donated freely. Nolan quotes the Tibetan meditation master Sogyal Rinpoche:

> Masters whom I have asked . . . agree that organ donation is an extremely positive action, since it stems from a genuine compassionate wish to benefit others. So, as long as it is truly the wish of the dying person, it will not harm in any way the consciousness that is leaving the body. On the contrary, this final act of generosity accumulates good karma.[83]

In Japan explicit consent of both the donor and the donor's family is required by the new transplantation law, a policy that has been grounded in Buddhist affirmation of giving.[84] Routine salvaging seems unlikely, and buying and selling organs is illegal.[85] If organs were obtained by any intervention other than one based on donation, the act would manifest "little or no virtuous benefit."[86] In 1992, presumably relying on the traditional cardiac definition of death, a physician who is also a Buddhist priest turned off the respirator of a comatose woman and removed the kidneys and corneas. He did so based on the specific request of the donor and the consent of the family.[87] On the other hand, Japanese culture includes patterns that would make obtaining such a donation difficult. Asking for the gift is something physicians are reluctant to do. Moreover, gift-giving ritual in Japan is extremely complex and normally requires reciprocity, something the organ recipient would not be able to provide to the deceased. Finally, although markets in organs are prohibited, it is a common practice for Japanese people to give gifts to their physicians and surgeons. This could potentially lead to associating reward to surgeons with the provision of the transplant, which could leave the borders between gift-giving and payment ambiguous.[88]

Fairness in the Distribution of Organs

This brings us to the other critical issue, that of fairness in the distribution of organs once they are procured. This will be the topic of Part Three of this book, but a preliminary summary of the views of the major religious traditions is appropriate. Parts of this chapter grew out of the congressional hearing held in 1983 before the U.S. House Subcommittee for Investigations and Oversight of the Committee on Science and Technology, chaired by then-Representative Al Gore. Representative Gore, in his communication to me about those hearings, indicated that the subcommittee was particularly interested in looking at approaches to promote efficient distribution of organs to transplant recipients. Although those standing within the religious traditions I am attempting to summarize would encourage efficient distribution, I emphasized to him that the religious traditions would place at least equal emphasis on the problems of fair distribution—which sometimes can be inefficient. It is striking that the National Organ Transplant Act of 1984 called for both efficiency and equity in organ allocation.[89]

I pointed out that there have from time to time been casual references to the use of market mechanisms to promote efficient transfer of organs to recipients (a topic that will be discussed further in Part Two). For example, a Detroit newspaper some years ago carried an ad with an offer to buy a kidney for $3,000.[90] Markets in organs might turn out to be efficient, but I am convinced they would be opposed vigorously by the mainstream of these religious and secular cultural traditions. They would be opposed because the allocation, though perhaps efficient in maximizing the number of organs transplanted, would be grossly discriminatory against those unable to pay.

JUDEO-CHRISTIANITY

The Judeo–Christian tradition is deeply committed to distribution on the basis of need. The single dominant theme of both Jewish and Christian ethics has been the responsibility to those in need—the lame, the halt, the blind, and those in need of organs. Any allocation scheme that permits other variables such as ability to pay or judgment about how socially useful a recipient will be has been uniformly opposed by all commentators working from within these traditions.

Some unfair allocation schemes may not be as blatant as direct-market mechanisms to buy organs. In the early years of transplant, Medicare policy prohibited funding of heart transplants under government health insurance, a policy that had a similar impact of discriminating against needy individuals. It is my sense that spokespeople for religious groups and theologians writing within these traditions are realists. They recognize that the government cannot make a commitment to pay for all possible medical care. They do, however, share with the members of the President's Commission for the Study of Ethical Problems in Medicine and Biomedical and Behavioral Research the conviction that there should be some base level of health care under which no one ought to fall. In the allocation of scarce organs for transplant, at least in cases such as hearts, kidneys, or livers, in which the organs are literally life-saving, allocation is simply unfair if it is based on ability to pay. If anyone has access, all should have an equal chance, by some lottery system; random assignment of organs to those in equal need or by the randomness of having each wait in line for needed organs. That is the conclusion reached by virtually every theologian writing out of the Judeo–Christian tradition, and, I am convinced, the only one they can reach and be consistent with that tradition's commitment to equal treatment based on need. No one should get an organ for transplant until there is a fair, nondiscriminatory allocation system in place that gives everyone in equal need for lifesaving organs an equal opportunity of access.

Islam

Little is said in Islamic medical ethical literature about the specific principles of allocation of organs for transplant, but the implications of more general statements about the duty of the society to protect the individual seem clear. In the section quoted previously of the Islamic Code of Medical Ethics dealing with modern biomedical advances (primarily about organ transplant) the collective responsibility of the community is stated directly: "The individual patient is the collective responsibility of the Society."[91] Although this literature offers no explicit injunction to allocate scarce organs equitably, that conclusion seems evident from the emphasis on collective responsibility. If one member suffers an ailment, all others "rally in response." In a section focusing on equitable access to health care, Gamal Serour emphasizes that the ethical principle of justice in Islam implies that all people should have equitable access.[92] Nevertheless, at least one source suggests that when it comes to a Muslim accepting an organ, it should come from a non-Muslim only if none is available from a Muslim.[93]

Hinduism

Traditional Hinduism is well known to have embraced a caste system that places socioeconomic status on a deep-seated religious basis. The idea that one's future lives will be affected via the doctrine of karma by the life one is presently leading permeates a Hindu sense that people "get what they deserve." This is reflected in medicine and attitudes about the allocation of medical resources. For example, the Caraca Samhita, the most well-known ancient code of ethical conduct for physicians from the Vedic scriptures, contains the following:

> No persons, who are hated by the king or who are haters of the king or who are hated by the public or who are haters of the public, shall receive treatment. Similarly, those who are extremely abnormal, wicked, and of miserable character and conduct, those who have not vindicated their honor, those who are on the point of death, and similarly women who are unattended by their husbands or guardians shall not receive treatment.[94]

Of course, not all modern Hindus subscribe rigidly to this ancient doctrine, but such a stance cannot help but provide a background for contemporary theories of allocation of organs. One suspects that this ancient religious doctrine shapes both the enormous differences in income levels in modern India and the willingness of many of its people to tolerate such practices as markets in organs. If the poor and wealthy are in their position because of their own past actions, toleration of great inequities is easier. That karma may be exchanged in the process of transplant provides even further reason why there may be tendencies to want to match castes when organs are transplanted. Similar inclinations have been reported in the case of semen donation.[95]

CONFUCIANISM/TAOISM

Traditional Confucian thought was concerned about equality of treatment in its medical ethics. The late-sixteenth-century Confucian scholar, Chu Hui-ming, said, "In antiquity it was said: 'There are no two kinds of drugs for the lofty and the common: the poor and the rich receive the same medicine.' "[96] This egalitarianism is a common theme in Confucian medical ethics. By contrast, Ren-Zong Qiu sees a much more social utilitarian view in contemporary China. He says the watchword is *profit*, a term interconnected in Chinese with *benefit* and *utility*. He reflects contemporary attitudes about organ allocation, giving emphasis to those whose lives can be considerably improved and who "will probably make potential contributions to society and/or mankind."[97] He suggests that although these may often be people "in higher rank cadres or on the higher grade on the wage scale," this will not necessarily be the case. He specifically rejects choosing patients for transplantation by first-come, first-served rankings, or by lottery, seeing this approach only as a secondary principle if other conditions are the same for two patients. He asks, rhetorically, "Is this unjust to those patients who are barred from dialysis or transplantation for financial reasons or shortage of machines or organs?" His response is, "Yes, in the sense that their condition dictates treatment . . . but under the present conditions we cannot avoid all unfortunate events, and sometimes we have to choose the lesser of two evils."[98] Apparently, both the traditional Confucian ideal and the ideology of Marxism are tempered by the contemporary reality.

BUDDHISM AND SHINTOISM

Because Buddhism and Shintoism have been so ambivalent about organ transplant and thrive in countries that for either economic or cultural reasons have not pursued transplant, they have had little opportunity to develop an explicit ethical position on how organs should be allocated among potential recipients. Live donation has taken place primarily among family members, foreclosing the problem of deciding who among a long list of potential recipients has the first claim on organs.

That forces us to examine more general works on Buddhist and Shinto ethics to glean some hint of how Buddhists and Shinto scholars would allocate organs. In particular, we would like to know how these traditions would respond if a society must choose between an allocation to the one who predictably will get the most benefit and to the one who has the greatest need.

Unfortunately, these are not major themes in the more general ethical writings of these traditions either.[99] For example, no discussion of justice or resource allocation occurs in Damien Keown's book-length treatment of *Buddhism & Bioethics*.[100] Fujii suggests that Theravada Buddhism (the branch of Buddhism dominant in Sri Lanka, Myanmar, Thailand, Laos, and Cambodia) has borrowed its social ethics from the Brahmanic tradition of Hinduism—a tradition that is notoriously hierarchical and not inclined toward concerns about justice for the most needy. On the other hand, Mahayana Buddhism, which is more influential in Tibet, Mongolia, China, Vietnam, Korea, and Japan, is not as closely tied to Hinduism. However, the available literature from these countries does not provide much guidance on the ethics of the allocation of resources either.

Conclusion

No major religious or cultural group provides outright opposition to organ transplantation. They all have resources within them that endorse brain-based criteria for death pronouncement—although some, such as Shinto and Buddhist beliefs, provide considerable resistance. None offer explicit, principled objection to cutting on the corpse when it can be lifesaving to do so. Some, such as Judaism, actually view transplantation as an affirmative moral duty when it will save life. Other traditions, including some Buddhists and Hindus as well as Native Americans, hold beliefs that can arouse suspicion about the value of merely extending biological existence in this world, but at least some within these traditions support organ transplant. Some forces within the Black American and fundamentalist Protestant culture are skeptical not only about theological matters related to a belief in the bodily resurrection but also about the underlying fairness of the transplant system. Nevertheless, all of these groups participate in organ transplant, sometimes enthusiastically, and none offers formal objection to it. Worldwide the preference is for the "donation" model of procuring organs. Although, as we shall see, in some cultures, particularly those that stress community solidarity, that have accepted laws that procure without explicit consent, even those tend to favor the right of individuals who record their opposition to opt out of procurement of their organs. This tension between donation and salvaging useful body parts without explicit consent is the focus of Part Two of this book. Finally, all the major religious and cultural traditions reveal strong commitments to allocating organs in ways that stress justice or equity. The tension between maximizing the benefits of the transplant program and distributing organs equitably is the focus of Part Three.

ENDNOTES

1. J. David Bleich, "Neurological Death and Time of Death Statutes," *Jewish Bioethics*, ed. Fred Rosner and J. David Bleich (New York: Sanhedrin Press, 1979), p. 310.

2. Fred Rosner, "Organ Transplants: The Jewish Viewpoint," *Journal of Thanatology* 3 (1975): 233–41.

3. Pius XII, "The Prolongation of Life" (An Address to an International Congress of Anesthesiologists, Nov. 24, 1957). *The Pope Speaks* 4 (Spring 1958): 396.

4. Paul A. Byrne, Sean O'Reilly, and Paul M. Quay, "Brain Death—An Opposing Viewpoint," *Journal of the American Medical Association* 242 (Nov. 2, 1979): 1985–90.

5. Paul Ramsey, "On Updating Procedures for Stating that a Man Has Died," *The Patient as Person* (New Haven, CT: Yale University Press, 1970), pp. 59–112.

6. Joseph Fletcher, "Cerebration," *Humanhood: Essays in Biomedical Ethics* (Buffalo, NY: Prometheus Books, 1979), pp. 159–65.

7. Judith A. Granbois and David H. Smith, "The Anglican Communion and Bioethics," in *Bioethics Yearbook, Volume 5: Theological Developments in Bioethics: 1992–1994*, ed. B. Andrew Lustig (Dordrecht: Kluwer Academic, 1997), pp. 93–119.

8. Paul Nelson, "Lutheran Perspectives on Bioethics," in *Bioethics Yearbook: Volume 3: Theological Developments in Bioethics: 1990–1992*, ed. Baruch A. Brody, B. Andrew Lustig, H. Tristram Engelhardt, and Laurence B. McCullough (Dordrecht: Kluwer Academic, 1993), pp. 178–80.

9. Robert L. Shelton, "Biomedical Ethics in Methodist Traditions," *Bioethics Yearbook, Volume 3: Theological Developments in Bioethics: 1990–1992*, ed. Baruch A.

Brody, B. Andrew Lustig, H. Tristram Engelhardt, and Laurence B. McCullough (Dordrecht: Kluwer Academic, 1993), pp. 228–29.

10. Kenneth L. Vaux, *Health and Medicine in the Reformed Tradition: Promise, Providence, and Care* (New York: Crossroad, 1984), p. 38.

11. Stanley Samuel Harakas, "Eastern Orthodox Bioethics," in *Bioethics Yearbook: Volume 3: Theological Developments in Bioethics: 1990–1992*, ed. Baruch A. Brody, B. Andrew Lustig, H. Tristram Engelhardt, and Laurence B. McCullough (Dordrecht: Kluwer Academic, 1993), pp. 119–20.

12. International Organization of Islamic Medicine, *Islamic Code of Medical Ethics* (International Organization of Islamic Medicine, 1981), p. 67.

13. K. Mazkur et al. (eds.), *Human Life: Its Inception and Its End as Viewed by Islam*, trans. M. M. S. Asbahi, IOMS (Islamic Organization for Medical Sciences) and KFAS (Kuwaiti Foundation for the Advancement of Science, Kuwait), as summarized in Hassan Hathout, "Islamic Concepts and Bioethics," in *Bioethics Yearbook, Volume 1: Theological Developments in Bioethics: 1988–1990*, ed. Thomas J. Bole (Dordrecht: Kluwer Academic, 1991), pp. 112–14.

14. This is also the position of many in Britain and in the British Commonwealth countries. Because the death of the brain stem is closely associated with the death of the entire brain, the significance of the difference between brain stem death and whole-brain death is minimal. In a later review Hathout actually refers to this position as "total brain death," implying he does not see a significant difference between the two. See Hassan Hathout, "Bioethical Developments in Islam," in *Bioethics Yearbook, Volume 3: Theological Developments in Bioethics: 1990–1992*, ed. B. Andrew Lustig, Baruch A. Brody, H. Tristram Engelhardt, and Laurence B. McCullough (Dordrecht: Kluwer Academic, 1993), pp. 133–48.

15. Hassan Hathout, "Islamic Concepts and Bioethics," in *Bioethics Yearbook, Volume 1: Theological Developments in Bioethics: 1988–1990*, ed. Thomas J. Bole (Dordrecht: Kluwer Academic, 1991), pp. 103–18; for a similar conclusion see V. Rispler-Chaim, "Islamic Medical Ethics in the 20th Century," *Journal of Medical Ethics* 15 (1989): 203.

16. Cited in Abdullah S. Daar, "Islam," in *Organ and Tissue Donation for Transplantation*, ed. Jeremy R. Chapman, Mark Deiehoi, and Celia Wight (New York: Oxford University Press; 1997), p. 32.

17. For a somewhat more cautious account including descriptions of scholars continuing to support cardiovascular definitions of death, see Gamal I. Serour, "Islamic Developments in Bioethics," in *Bioethics Yearbook, Volume 5: Theological Developments in Bioethics: 1992–1994*, ed. B. Andrew Lustig (Dordrecht: Kluwer Academic, 1997), pp. 171–88.

18. Prakash Desai, "Medical Ethics in India," *Journal of Medicine and Philosophy* 13 (1988): 240.

19. Ren-Zong Qiu and Da-Jie Jin, "Bioethics in China: 1989–1991," in *Bioethics Year-book, Volume 2: Regional Developments in Bioethics, 1989–1991*, ed. B. Andrew Lustig, Baruch A. Brody, H. Tristram Engelhardt, and Laurence B. McCullough (Boston: Kluwer Academic, 1992), pp. 355–77; and Ren-Zong Qiu, "Ethical Problems in Renal Dialysis and Transplantation: Chinese Perspective," in *Ethical Problems in Dialysis and Transplantation*, ed. Carl M. Kjellstrand and John B. Dosseter (Boston: Kluwer Academic, 1992), pp. 227–28.

20. Japanese Association of Indian and Buddhist Studies Committee for Inquiry on Brain Death and Organ Transplantation, September 1990. Text reprinted in Masao Fujii, "Buddhist Bioethics and Organ Transplantation," *Okurayama Bunka-kaigi Kenkyunenop* 3 (2, 1991): 1–11.

21. Bhikkhu Mettananda, "Buddhist Ethics in the Practice of Medicine," in *Buddhist Ethics and Modern Society: An International Symposium*, ed. Charles Wei-hsun Fu and Sandra A. Wawrytho (New York: Greenwood Press), pp. 195–213.

22. D. Ikeda, "Thoughts on the Problem of Brain Death (1): From the Viewpoint of the Buddhism of Nichiren Daishonin," *Journal of Oriental Studies* 26 (1987): 193–216; Damien Keown, *Buddhism & Bioethics* (London: St. Martin's Press, 1995), p. 153–58.

23. Phillip A. Lecso, "The Bodhisattva Ideal and Organ Transplantation," *Journal of Religion and Health* 30 (1; 1991 Spring): 39.

24. Catrien Ross, "Towards Acceptance of Organ Transplantation: Tokyo Perspective. [News]," *Lancet* 346 (8966; 1995 July 1): 41.

25. Masao Fujii, "Buddhism and Bioethics," in *Bioethics Yearbook, Volume 1: Theological Developments in Bioethics, 1988–1990*, ed. B. Andrew Lustig, Baruch A. Brody, H. Tristram Engelhardt, and Laurence B. McCullough (Boston: Kluwer Academic, 1991), p. 67.

26. Lecso, "The Bodhisattva Ideal and Organ Transplantation," p. 39; see also Helen Hardacre, "Response of Buddhism and Shinto to the Issue of Brain Death and Organ Transplant," *Cambridge Quarterly of Healthcare Ethics* 3 (1994): 595.

27. Kathleen Nolan, "Buddhism, Zen, and Bioethics," *Bioethics Yearbook, Vol. 3: Theological Developments in Bioethics, 1990–1992*, ed. Andrew B. Lustig, Baruch A. Brody, H. Tristram Engelhardt, and Laurence B. McCullough (Dordrecht: Kluwer Academic, 1993), pp. 204–05.

28. Eric Feldman, "Defining Death: Organ Transplants, Tradition and Technology in Japan," *Social Science and Medicine* 27 (4; 1988): 341.

29. "The Law Concerning Human Organ Transplants" (The Law 104 in 1997). For accounts of the protracted controversy see Rihito Kimura, "Japan's Dilemma with the Definition of Death," *Kennedy Institute of Ethics Journal* 1 (1991): 123–31; Yoshio Watanabe, "Why Do I Stand against the Movement for Cardiac Transplantation in Japan?" *Japanese Heart Journal* 35 (6; Nov. 1994): 701–14; Eric A.

Feldman, "Culture, Conflict and Cost: Perspectives on Brain Death in Japan," *International Journal of Technology Assessment in Health Care* 10 (3; 1994 Summer): 447–63; Kazumasa Hoshino, "Legal Status of Brain Death in Japan: Why Many Japanese Do Not Accept " 'Brain Death" ' as a Definition of Death," *Bioethics* 7 (2/3; 1993 April): 234–38.

30. Paul Ramsey, "Giving or Taking Cadaver Organs for Transplant," *The Patient as Person*, esp. pp. 205–09; *Ethical and Religious Directives for Catholic Health Facilities*. Directive 30 (Washington, DC: Dept. of Health Affairs, United States Catholic Conference, 1971), p. 8; Benedict M. Ashley and Kevin D. O'Rourke, *Health Care Ethics: A Theological Analysis*, 2nd ed. (St. Louis, MO: Catholic Health Association of the United States, 1982), pp. 308–12.

31. Paul Freund, "Organ Transplants: Ethical and Legal Problems," *Proceedings of the American Philosophical Society* 15 (Aug. 1971): 276; Fred Rosner, "Organ Transplantation in Jewish Law," esp. p. 360.

32. Elliot N. Dorff, "Choosing Life: Aspects of Judaism Affecting Organ Transplantation" in *Organ Transplantation: Meanings and Realities*, ed. Stuart J. Youngner, Renée C. Fox, and Laurence J. O'Connell (Madison: University of Wisconsin Press, 1996), pp. 168–93.

33. Antonia G. Spagnolo, and Elio Sgreccia, "The Roman Catholic Church" in *Organ and Tissue Donation for Transplantation*, ed. Jeremy R. Chapman, Mark Deierhoi, and Celia Wight (New York: Oxford University Press, 1997), pp. 27–29.

34. For example, the Church of England (John Habgood, "The Church of England" in *Organ and Tissue Donation for Transplantation*, ed. Jeremy R. Chapman, Mark Deierhoi, and Celia Wight (New York: Oxford University Press, 1997), pp. 25–27.

35. Clive Callender, "Testimony of Group 13" (Testimony presented at the hearings, "Increasing Organ Donation Liver Allocation," Dec. 10, 11, 12, 1996, Natcher Center, National Institutes of Health, Bethesda, Maryland); See also C. O. Callender, "Organ Donation in Blacks: A Community Approach," *Transplantation Proceedings* 19 (1987): 1551–54, where Callender groups these into five categories, including religious reasons.

36. L. Abraham, "Surgeon Preaches Need for Organ Donation," *American Medical News* (Oct. 2, 1987), cited in Cheryl Sanders, "African Americans and Organ Donation: Reflections on Religion, Ethics, and Embodiment," in *Embodiment, Morality, and Medicine*, ed. Lisa Sowle Cahill and Margaret A Farley (Boston: Kluwer Academic, 1995), p. 145.

37. Cheryl Sanders, "African Americans and Organ Donation," pp. 141–53.

38. Ibid., p. 148.

39. Ibid.

40. G. E. Ehusani, *An Afro-Christian Vision* (Lanham, MD: University Press of America, 1991), cited in Cheryl Sanders, "African Americans and Organ Donation: Reflections on Religion, Ethics, and Embodiment," p. 146.

41. Cheryl Sanders, "African Americans and Organ Donation," p. 147.

42. A. R. Gatrad, "Muslim Customs Surrounding Death, Bereavement, Postmortem Examinations, and Organ Transplants," *British Medical Journal* 309 (1994): 523. It is probably because most Muslims living in Britain come from Asian countries such as Pakistan and Bangladesh that Black reports that transplantation is rarely permitted among them. John Black, "Broaden Your Mind about Death and Bereavement in Certain Groups in Britain [Hindus, Sikhs, Moslems]," *British Medical Journal* 295 (1987 Aug. 29): 538.

43. V. Rispler-Chaim, "Islamic Medical Ethics in the 20th Century," *Journal of Medical Ethics* 15 (1989): 203–08; Abdullah S. Daar, "Islam," in *Organ and Tissue Donation for Transplantation*, ed. Jeremy R. Chapman, Mark Deierhoi, and Celia Wight (New York: Oxford University Press, 1997), pp. 29–33.

44. A. R. Gatrad, "Muslim Customs Surrounding Death, Bereavement, Postmortem Examinations, and Organ Transplants," pp. 521–23.

45. International Organization of Islamic Medicine, *Islamic Code of Medical Ethics*, p. 81, *also see* p. 84.

46. Hassan Hathout, "Islamic Concepts and Bioethics," in *Bioethics Yearbook, Volume 1: Theological Developments in Bioethics: 1988–1990*, ed. Thomas J. Bole (Dordrecht: Kluwer Academic, 1991), p. 115. These are also taken from the Islamic Code of Medical Ethics.

47. C. M. Francis, "Ancient and Modern Medical Ethics in India," in *Transcultural Dimensions in Medical Ethics*, ed. Edmund D. Pellegrino, Patricia Mazzarella, and Pietro Corsi (Frederick, MD: University Publishing, 1992), p. 194.

48. Wendy Doniger, "Transplanting Myths of Organ Transplants," in *Organ Transplantation: Meanings and Realities*, ed. Stuart J. Youngner, Renée C. Fox, and Laurence J. O'Connell (Madison: University of Wisconsin Press, 1996), p. 200.

49. Ibid., pp. 200–202.

50. Prakash Desai, "Medical Ethics in India," *Journal of Medicine and Philosophy* 13 (1988): 245. Black reports a similar conclusion for Hindus in Britain. See John Black, "Broaden Your Mind about Death and Bereavement in Certain Groups in Britain [Hindus, Sikhs, Moslems]," p. 537.

51. Wendy Doniger, "Transplanting Myths of Organ Transplants," pp. 210–12.

52. Ibid., p. 212.

53. John Black, "Broaden Your Mind about Death and Bereavement in Certain Groups in Britain [Hindus, Sikhs, Moslems]," p. 537.

54. Ren-Zong Qiu and Da-Jie Jin, "Bioethics in China: 1989–1991," p. 366.

55. Ren-Zong Qiu, "Ethical Problems in Renal Dialysis and Transplantation: Chinese Perspective," p. 230.

56. See Robert M. Veatch, A *Theory of Medical Ethics* (New York: Basic Books, 1981), p. 66. Also see Ping-cheung Lo, "Confucian Views on Suicide" (Hong Kong: Centre for Applied Ethics, Hong Kong Baptist University Occasional Paper Series, 1997).

57. Norman J. Girardot, "Taoism." *The Encyclopedia of Bioethics Vol. 1* (New York: Free Press, 1978), pp. 1631–38, esp. 1636.

58. K. T. Tsuji, "The Buddhist View of the Body and Organ Transplantation," *Transplantation Proceedings* 20 (1 Suppl., Feb. 1988): 1076–78.

59. Masao Fujii, "Buddhist Bioethics and Organ Transplantation," p. 5; Lecso, "The Bodhisattva Ideal and Organ Transplantation," p. 37.

60. Kathleen Nolan, "Buddhism, Zen, and Bioethics," p. 206.

61. Ibid., p. 205; Phillip A. Lecso, "The Bodhisattva Ideal and Organ Transplantation," p. 36.

62. Masao Fujii, "Buddhist Bioethics and Organ Transplantation," p. 8; Fujii, "Buddhism and Bioethics," p. 66.

63. Margaret Lock, "Deadly Disputes: Ideologies and Brain Death in Japan," in *Organ Transplantation: Meanings and Realities*. ed. Stuart J. Youngner, Renée C. Fox, and Laurence J. O'Connell (Madison: University of Wisconsin Press, 1996), p. 157.

64. Kathleen Nolan, "Buddhism, Zen, and Bioethics," p. 205.

65. Margaret Lock, "Deadly Disputes: Ideologies and Brain Death in Japan," p. 157.

66. Eric A. Feldman, "Defining Death: Organ Transplants, Tradition and Technology in Japan," *Social Science and Medicine* 27 (4; 1988): 342.

67. Helen Hardacre, "Response of Buddhism and Shinto to the Issue of Brain Death and Organ Transplant," p. 598.

68. Jesse Dukeminier and David Sanders, "Organ Transplantation: A Proposal for Routine Salvaging of Cadaver Organs," *New England Journal of Medicine* 279 (1968): 413–19.

69. Robert M. Veatch, "A Policy for Obtaining Newly Dead Bodies and Body Organs," in *Death, Dying, and the Biological Revolution* (New Haven, CT: Yale University Press, 1976), pp. 266–76.

70. Fred Rosner, "Autopsy in Jewish Law and the Israeli Autopsy Controversy," in *Jewish Bioethics*, eds. Fred Rosner and J. David Bleich (New York: Sanhedrin Press), p. 343.

71. International Organization of Islamic Medicine. *Islamic Code of Medical Ethics*, p. 81.

72. Ibid.

73. Abdullah S. Daar, "Islam," p. 32.

74. David A. Peters, "Marketing Organs for Transplantation," *Dialysis & Transplantation* 13 (Jan. 1984): 40–41; Thomas G. Peters, "Financial Incentives in Organ Donation: Current Issues," *Dialysis & Transplantation* 21 (May 1992): 270–73; Thomas G. Peters, "Life or Death: The Issue of Payment in Cadaveric Organ Donation," *Journal of the American Medical Association* 265 (March 13, 1991): 1302–05; Cf. J. Harvey, "Paying Organ Donors," *Journal of Medical Ethics* 16 (1990): 117–19; American Medical Association, Council on Ethical and Judicial Affairs, "Financial Incentives for Organ Donation," *Archives of Internal Medicine* 155 (1995): 581–89.

75. There are reports of such practices in other countries such as the Philippines and Turkey, but they are not well documented. See M. K. Mani, "The Argument against the Unrelated Live Donor," in *Ethical Problems in Dialysis and Transplantation*, ed. Carl M. Kjellstrand and John B. Dosseter (Boston: Kluwer Academic, 1992), pp. 163–68; C. M. Francis, "Ancient and Modern Medical Ethics in India," in *Transcultural Dimensions in Medical Ethics*, ed. Edmund D. Pellegrino, Patricia Mazzarella, and Pietro Corsi (Frederick, MD: University Publishing, 1992), p. 193.

76. K. C. Reddy, "A Perspective on Reality," in *Ethical Problems in Dialysis and Transplantation*, ed. Carl M. Kjellstrand and John B. Dosseter (Boston: Kluwer Academic, 1992), pp. 155–61. See also C. M. Francis, "Ancient and Modern Medical Ethics in India," in *Transcultural Dimensions in Medical Ethics*, ed. Edmund D. Pellegrino, Patricia Mazzarella, and Pietro Corsi (Frederick, MD: University Publishing, 1992), p. 193; B. N. Colabawala, "Kidneys for a Price," *Indian Post*, Feb. 23, 1989; "The Organs Bazaar," *India Today*, July 31, 1990, both cited in Prakash Desai, "Hinduism and Bioethics in India: A Tradition in Transition," p. 55.

77. Prakash N. Desai, "Hinduism and Bioethics in India: A Tradition in Transition," p. 55.

78. C. M. Francis, "Ancient and Modern Medical Ethics in India," pp. 175–96.

79. For further discussion of Indian culture and the impact of its Hindu roots, see ibid., pp. 175–96; Desai, "Hinduism and Bioethics in India: A Tradition in Transition," pp. 41–60, and more general accounts of Hinduism such as R. C. Zaehner, *Hinduism* (London: Oxford University Press, 1962).

80. Paul U. Unschuld, "Confucianism," *Encyclopedia of Bioethics*, ed. Warren T. Reich (New York: Free Press, 1978), pp. 200–204.

81. Ren-Zong Qiu and Da-Jie Jin, "Bioethics in China: 1989–1991," p. 366.

82. D. J. Rothman, et al., "The Bellagio Task Force Report on Transplantation, Bodily Integrity, and the International Traffic in Organs," *Transplantation Proceedings* 29 (6, 1997): 2739–45; David J. Rothman, "Body Shop," *The Sciences* (Nov./

Dec. 1997): 17–21; Lena H. Sun, "China's Social Changes Spur More Execu-
tions: Families Don't See the Body, But They Pay for The Bullet," *Washington
Post*, March 27, 1994, pp. A1, A22.

83. S. Rinpoche, *The Tibetan Book of Living and Dying* (San Francisco: Harper,
1992), p. 376, cited in Nolan, "Buddhism, Zen, and Bioethics," p. 206.

84. Phillip A. Lecso, "The Bodhisattva Ideal and Organ Transplantation," p. 37.

85. Margaret Lock, "Deadly Disputes: Ideologies and Brain Death in Japan," p. 148.

86. Phillip A. Lecso, "The Bodhisattva Ideal and Organ Transplantation," p. 40.

87. "53 sai josei 'sengensho' ikasu" (Written declaration of 53-year-old woman
restores life), *Yomiuri Shinbun*, Oct. 18, 1992, cited in Lock, "Deadly Disputes:
Ideologies and Brain Death in Japan," p. 149.

88. Margaret Lock, "Deadly Disputes: Ideologies and Brain Death in Japan," p. 158.

89. National Organ Transplant Act, U.S. Public Law No. 98-507 (Oct. 19, 1984),
98 Stat. 2339.

90. "$3,000 Offer for Kidney Brings Man 100 Donors," *New York Times*, Sept. 12,
1974, p. 36.

91. International Organization of Islamic Medicine. *Islamic Code of Medical Ethics*,
p. 81. See also the emphasis on justice in Azim A. Nanji, "Medical Ethics and
the Islamic Tradition," *Journal of Medicine and Philosophy* 13 (1988): 257–75, esp.
pp. 268–69.

92. Gamal I. Serour, "Islamic Developments in Bioethics," p. 181.

93. A. R. Gatrad, "Muslim Customs Surrounding Death, Bereavement, Postmortem
Examinations, and Organ Transplants," *British Medical Journal* 309 (1994): 523.

94. A. Menon and H. F. Haberman, "Oath of Initiation" (from the *Caraka Samhita*).
Medical History 14 (1970): 295–96.

95. Prakash N. Desai, "Medical Ethics in India," p. 247.

96. Chu Hui-ming, *Tou-chen ch'uan-hsin lu*, ch. 16, pp. 1b–3b, 5a–5b, in Ch'eng
Yung-p'ei, *Liu-li chai I-shu shih-chung*, reprinted in English translation in Paul U.
Unschuld, *Medical Ethics in Imperial China: A Study in Historical Anthropology*
(Berkeley: University of California Press, 1979), p. 63.

97. Ren-Zong Qiu, "Ethical Problems in Renal Dialysis and Transplantation: Chinese Perspective," pp. 232–33.

98. Ibid., p. 233.

99. Kathleen Nolan, "Buddhism, Zen, and Bioethics," p. 203.

100. Damien Keown, *Buddhism & Bioethics*.

❖ Two

An Ethical Framework

A GENERAL, OVERALL ethical theory in which to ground an ethic for transplantation is needed. To know how to procure and allocate organs ethically, one needs to know first what it means to act ethically in the generic. The approach taken in this book is to first provide a brief sketch of what we know about general theories of normative ethics (this chapter) and then (in the rest of the book) spell out what these theories mean for organ procurement and allocation.

General Theories of Ethics

It stands to reason that a theory for the ethics of organ procurement and allocation would somehow be related to more general ethical theories. In fact, the position one takes on important transplant issues should be determined by one's position on the classical controversies in ethics. It is only reasonable that a Marxist will procure and allocate differently than one who subscribes to classical liberal political philosophy; a utilitarian differently than a Kantian. The proper way to resolve the efficiency versus equity debate in organ allocation must be dependent on how one resolves these conflicts more generally. Each major normative theory of ethics should have its own implications for organ procurement and allocation. In this sense, the ethics of medicine—or a branch of medicine—does not have its own ethic "internal to medicine."[1] Rather, ethics of medicine is dependent on broader, more fundamental foundations. There will be as many ethics for medicine as there are ethical systems in the world—one medical ethic per system of belief and value; one medical ethic per religious or philosophical worldview.

Religious Approaches

One major group of approaches to ethics are those of the major world religions. As we saw in Chapter 1, no major world religion actively opposes organ procurement. Each religion, however, has positions regarding ethical norms that would shape the way organs are procured and allocated. Judaism and Christianity, for example, are religions of social justice. Moreover, they have particular interpretations of what a just world would look like. They give priority to those among us who have the greatest need: the lame, the halt, the blind, and, presumably, those in most serious organ failure. On the other hand, some more otherworldly versions of Christianity are committed to recognizing the limits of human existence. Many Catholic theologians, for instance, have been critical of experimental multiorgan transplants for people who have such severe medical problems that survival is unlikely. They see such efforts as placing too much emphasis on survival in bodily form in this world and not enough on the "final ends" of human existence that are more otherworldly. Some interpretations of the Hindu doctrine of karma may imply that some people with severe, chronic organ failure may be reaping the rewards of evils in a previous life.

Anyone deeply committed to a religious perspective will draw on his or her own tradition's ethical framework in deciding how organs should be allocated. For purposes of public policy, however, particular religious ethics will have only indirect impact. The competing secular ethical theories will be more central to the public formulation of an allocation system.

Secular Ethical Approaches

Secular normative ethical theory has been a lively field in recent decades. Old debates have run their course; new theoretical approaches are emerging, some of which have very definite implications for organ allocation.

VIRTUE THEORIES

Several approaches to ethics historically focused on the virtues. Virtue theories focus on the character of people rather than the rightness or wrongness of their behavior. A virtue is a character trait or a "persistent disposition" to act in a certain way. Classical Greek ethics, particularly the ethics of Aristotle,[2] was an ethics of virtues.

Classical Virtue Theories. The classical Greek virtues were *wisdom, courage, temperance,* and *justice.* People were considered virtuous to the extent that they manifested these character traits in their daily lives. There has been a recent resurgence in virtue theory, particularly in medical ethics.[3] Virtue theory is unique in that it focuses on the character of actors rather than the morality of actions. The key question is, "Was the disposition of the actor in accord with certain key virtues?" rather than, "Was the behavior morally the right behavior?"

The implication for transplant, however, is remote. Although some have spoken of the "virtues" of institutions, almost all virtue theory focuses on the character of individual humans. Because the organ allocation system is a practice that is grounded in an institution, asking what the character traits of individuals *should* be may turn out to be a question of only secondary importance. Moreover, focusing on the character of actors tends to ignore or minimize the question of what the ethically proper allocation should be. An ethical system that tells us to be courageous or temperate does not directly tell us whether organs should go to the sickest recipient or to the one who is expected to have the longest graft survival. Virtue theory, no matter how important for shaping the character of individuals, is not promising as a basis for developing a theory of organ allocation.

Feminist Theories. Recent developments in biomedical ethics also include a major movement under the label of feminist theory.[4] There is a great deal of work going on in biomedical ethics, particularly nursing ethics, in what is called care theory, which is closely allied with feminist theory.[5] Some interpret this work as a kind of virtue theory.[6] To the extent that care is a virtue, it describes a character trait that many consider important in practicing good medicine or good nursing. It is closely related to the virtues of compassion, humaneness, and benevolence. Certainly, we would very much want our organ procurement, allocation, and implantation personnel to manifest these virtues. It is less clear, however, how these virtues would provide guidance for when organs should be procured or on what basis they should be allocated. This cluster of virtues is more often associated with the clinical professions rather than the institutional and administrative groups that are responsible for organ procurement and allocation. To say that one should be caring or compassionate or humane in procurement or allocation does not really tell us very much about whether it is acceptable to procure organs from an HIV-positive donor or from someone who insists the organs go only to members of a certain race. These virtues do not tell us whether we should allocate organs to those who will get the most benefit or to those who need the organs the most. In fact, these virtues manifest in clinical professionals, including transplant surgeons, nurses, and social workers, can easily lead to advocacy for one's own patients—a commitment that can only distort the perspective of those concerned with how to procure and allocate organs ethically.

Hippocratic Ethics. The clinical focus on care and other virtue theories is often in creative tension with the classical ethical system of the health professions: the Hippocratic ethic. Although some people have viewed the Hippocratic ethic as a kind of timeless, all-purpose ethic for physicians and other health professionals, in fact it is only one among many possible ethics for medicine.

Hippocratic ethics has its roots in one particular kind of Greek medicine, sometimes called the Hippocratic school. The ethics reflected in the Hippocratic Oath is closely related to Pythagoreanism.[7] The Hippocratic ethical tradition is, at least indirectly, the perspective into which many organ transplant personnel have been socialized. In theory, we could develop an allocation system that reflects the Hippocratic ethic. It is puzzling, however, why health professionals or the general public would want to run an allocation on a system of ethics from an ancient Greek cult that functioned on a set of values quite alien to our present ones.

The Hippocratic ethic includes a virtue element. The original oath included purity and holiness. For the Florence Nightingale Pledge for nurses, the equivalent is purity and faithfulness. These are virtues that do not resonate with many moderns. The contemporary equivalents in the American Medical Association principles of ethics are compassion and respect for human dignity.[8] The American Nurses Association refers to respect for human dignity and the uniqueness of the client. Although these virtues seem uncontroversial, the problem is that they really do not tell health personnel how to procure or allocate organs.

In addition to its virtue component, Hippocratic ethics includes some important normative commitments that are not necessarily friendly to or useful for organ allocation. The core ethical principle is that the physician pledges to "benefit the patient according to my ability and judgment." Logically, this would require every clinical professional to work the system for the best interests of his or her patient. That could mean each surgeon lobbying for organs for his or her patients. At its worst it would require "gaming" the system (for example, by stretching the facts of a diagnosis so that a patient who will eventually need a transplant can get listed sooner) so that one's own patients beat out others to get scarce organs. This Hippocratic principle has two characteristics that are particularly controversial: *individualism* and *consequentialism*.

(1) Individualism. Often in ethics there are conflicts between one's duties to an individual (such as a patient) and duties to society. This is a major problem in using human subjects for medical research. It is a problem in certain confidentiality cases. It is a critical problem when it comes to allocating scarce resources. Imagine that we could align all ethical systems along a continuum from those that focus more on the duties to the individual to those that focus on the duties to society. Marxism might be seen as being on the societal end. So would social utilitarianism. Adherents to these views hold it is morally necessary when there is a conflict to sacrifice the individual for the good of society. Others line up much more at the end of the spectrum at which the society's interests are subordinated to one's duties to the individual.

The Hippocratic ethic is at the extreme individualist end of the spectrum. The physician's exclusive loyalty is to the individual patient. Taken literally, the Hippocratic ethic would never accept a physician using his or her patients for so-called nontherapeutic research. In such research, the purpose is to gain knowledge for the benefit of society. Even though the risk to the subject may be very small, what is done is not for the patient's benefit. A purely Hippocratic physician could not participate because he or she would not be working solely for the benefit of the patient.

Any ethic of resource allocation must look beyond the good of the individual patient. For these reasons, I claim in Chapter 18 that Hippocratic clinicians would make particularly bad allocators of organs. They would feel duty-bound to do what was necessary to benefit their patient at the expense of others.

(2) Consequentialism. The second characteristic of the Hippocratic ethic is that it focuses exclusively on consequences. The duty of the physician is expressed in terms of benefiting the patient and protecting him or her from harm. By contrast other ethics judge the rightness or wrongness of actions by considerations other than consequences. These ethics are sometimes called deontological. The term comes from the Greek word meaning "duty." The general idea is that there are certain behaviors that are simply one's duty regardless of the consequences. Anyone who believes it is wrong to tell a lie or break a promise—regardless of the consequences—understands that there can be more to ethics than merely calculating consequences. In bioethics, many people now hold that it is the physician's duty to respect the autonomous choices of their patients to refuse treatment—even if they know that the consequences would be better if the physician treated against the patient's wishes.

To see why simply striving to produce consequences that are as good as possible is ethically suspect, I will consider in Chapter 12 whether it would be wise for a group of people who each are near death from need of an organ (a heart, liver, lung, or pancreas, for example) to come together and sign a binding contract to hold a lottery in which the loser would be sacrificed (i.e., killed) so that his or her good organs could save the others. With such a lottery perhaps four or five people would live who would otherwise die, whereas without the lottery all would die. If ethics is nothing more than a matter of maximizing good consequences, it is hard to see why this lottery would not be ethically acceptable. On the other hand, if ethics involves something more—for example, an intrinsic duty not to kill—the lottery may pose serious problems.

Many of the most sophisticated ethical systems of the world insist that ethics is more than consequence-maximizing. These systems are deontological in character—that is, they include duties that go beyond consequences. The most well-known is the ethic of Immanuel Kant.[9] He held that ethics is a matter of doing one's duty independent of consequences.

Many twentieth-century ethical theories fall somewhere in the middle of the continuum between an exclusively consequence-oriented ethic and one that is totally nonconsequentialistic. W. D. Ross, for example, held a theory that includes both kinds of considerations.[10] Many doing contemporary work in bioethics position themselves similarly in the middle of this continuum. Some, for example Tom L. Beauchamp and James Childress in the *Principles of Biomedical Ethics*, claim that one must balance the concern about consequences with concerns about other principles, such as distributing goods fairly and respecting autonomy.[11] The point is that the Hippocratic ethic is exclusively consequentialistic. It has no principle of respecting autonomy and no notion of fairness or equity, as called for in the current American transplant policy. It looks only at benefits and harms, trying to maximize the benefit and minimize the harm.

Mainstream Theories of Right Action

Most modern normative moral theories that focus on the morality of actions rather than the morality of character can be described in terms of these two characteristics: the individualist–society dichotomy and the consequentialist–deontological dichotomy. Essentially no respectable ethical theory of today would do what the Hippocratic theory does: totally ignore duties unrelated to consequences and duties that are more social—allocation of resources, conflicts between the individual and society, and so forth. How one resolves the controversies over these matters of general theory could have a major influence on one's theory of organ procurement and allocation. Two major views have dominated.

SOCIAL UTILITARIANISM

The first view, called social or classical utilitarianism, is the view of philosophers such as Jeremy Bentham[12] and John Stuart Mill.[13] Social utilitarians hold that the only considerations that count in morality are consequences, but, unlike Hippocratic consequentialists, social utilitarians consider consequences for all affected parties. They hold that the course of action that produces the best net consequences is the morally right course, but they first determine the net of benefits minus harms for each individual and then add up the net benefits for each party to reach an aggregate sum. I will refer to social utilitarians as "*aggregate maximizers.*"

DEONTOLOGISTS

Deontologists, such as Kantians, by definition consider features of actions other than consequences to be relevant to deciding what the moral course of action is. They differ among themselves as to exactly which features are morally important. Deontologists vary in their emphasis on the individual and social dimensions of actions, as do consequentialists.

The Individual Level. The features of actions at the individual level that are sometimes included in the deontological view are respect for autonomy, fidelity (promise-keeping), veracity (truth-telling), and the duty to avoid killing.[14] Collectively these are sometimes referred to as "respect for persons." These deontologists insist that we show respect for persons by not infringing on choices made according to a substantially autonomous life plan (the principle of autonomy) and that we show respect by keeping promises made and avoiding lying. Finally, some deontologists believe that if we respect persons, we can never kill them (even when they are suffering so badly that a case could be made that the consequences would be better if they were dead). These are all principles that could be applied in one's actions toward a single individual. They all present alternatives to the Hippocratic way of treating an individual.

Most of the conflicts in medical ethics of the 1970s were conflicts at this individual level. Holders of these "respect-for-persons" views challenged traditional Hippocratic assumptions about how to treat the individual patient. The challengers said that we must respect autonomy, keep promises, avoid lying, and perhaps avoid killing as well, even though the results might be better for the patient if we were more Hippocratic. Almost everyone now believes that over the past 30 years the deontologists won this fight with the Hippocratists. At least the law requires that autonomy be respected. American law generally requires that promises—such as the promise of confidentiality—be kept even if the clinician believes the patient would be better off if these principles were rejected. The American Medical Association has revised its code of ethics, generally removing the Hippocratic paternalism in favor of more respect for patients, and as a result has a much more acceptable code because of it.[15]

The Social Level. Deontologists also differ from utilitarians at the social level. The key is understanding how each would handle the problem of distributing scarce resources. Whereas the social utilitarian will resolve conflicts among the interests of parties in a social setting by summing up net consequences of alternative courses of actions and opting for the choice that maximizes aggregate utility, deontologists may appeal to some other feature or features of the distribution. Thus, for example, if there are many more people waiting for livers than there are livers available, the social utilitarian will place the organs where they will do the most good. Those committed to the principle of justice, however, will recognize that the ones who need the organs the most may not be the same people who will predictably get the most benefit from them. For instance, those in greatest need may be so ill that the chance of a successful graft is less. Those committed to the principle of justice may focus on the potential recipients' need rather than the amount of good that will be done.

In general, those whose ethic of allocation concentrates on justice look at "patterned end-states"—that is, the pattern in the way that goods end up being distributed. For example, they may insist that people of all races have an equal chance at getting an organ, even though statistically, members of one racial group may be expected to do somewhat better (because they match the donor pool better or for some other reason). The morally correct pattern (in this case a pattern of equal access) is usually referred to as a *just distribution*. The principle that holds that the action is right that leads to a distribution matching this pattern is called the *principle of justice*. Because there are many different notions of exactly what the right pattern of distribution is, there are many different versions of the principle of justice.

Aristotle recognized that justice as a principle of distribution could have many different criteria. He considered distributing according to whether one was of "free birth," whether one was of "noble birth," or whether one was an aristocrat. These, apparently, were the only patterns of distribution that he could think of.

Modern justice theorists often are egalitarians. They are concerned about the pattern of distribution of the good, but the pattern that they consider to be right is one in which people have opportunities for equality. There is endless dispute among egalitarians over exactly what this means. Some seek end-state outcomes with the goal that people are equal in their welfare. Others have more sophisticated views. One of these views holds that what is really needed is a distribution in which there is equality of resources, leaving individuals to make decisions about what they want to do with their resources.[16] If, when considering resources, they include people's biological resources—their genetic makeup and their propensity for disease—giving people equality of resources could be the basis for an egalitarian health policy that focuses on getting those with poor health states opportunities to be normally healthy insofar as this is possible. This view of equality of resources combined with the right of people to choose how they use their resources will accept inequalities of outcomes provided the differences result from different choices that people make.

One important version of a justice theory is called the "maximin." It has been defended by the philosopher John Rawls.[17] Although it is a very complex, sophisticated theory, one of its features is that for a practice to be just it must redistribute goods so as to be to the maximum advantage of the worst-off persons or groups. (The allocation is designed to maximize the minimum good that persons have, hence "maximin.") This can differ from simply making everybody equal, a distinction that will prove important in our consideration of the ethics of directed donation in Chapter 25.

The one thing that these deontological justice theorists agree on is that distributing resources is not merely a matter of maximizing the aggregate good consequences. In *The Foundations of Justice* I argued that a patterned, end-state theory of justice has moral priority over the maximizing of aggregate net utility. Many other, but not all, theorists have reached the same conclusion. So do those who articulate the basic principles of liberal political traditions.

An ethic limited to maximizing good consequences has implications that are strongly counterintuitive. It would justify slavery—if only the sum of the consequences to the advantaged majority exceeded the burdens to the enslaved. It would justify compulsory conscription of a minority into dangerous medical research—if only the anticipated benefits to the population as a whole were large enough. It would even justify forced procurement of organs from some to benefit others—if only the benefit to the recipients exceeded the harm to the one whose organs were commandeered, an outcome easy to imagine if several could live for each person selected for death.

Consider a plan to pick a small group of people, perhaps those who are not very useful to society and who are mentally depressed to the point that they have only a slight preference for living. Killing one of them and taking the organs could save several lives of people desperate to live while generating only modest burden for the one person killed. It seems obvious that in such an instance the life-saving benefit multiplied by the number of people receiving the life-prolonging organs could easily exceed burden to the one person killed. Yet almost everyone would think it obvious that such a policy would be morally wrong, indeed an outrage. Why is such a policy so obviously wrong if the expected benefits seem large in comparison to the burdens?

The policy violates several of the basic principles we have identified. It violates respect for persons by violating the autonomy of the one selected to be killed. It violates that respect by treating the one who is killed as a mere means to the benefit of others. It violates such respect by intentionally killing. Finally, it distributes the benefits and burdens in a very unequal way. The benefits all go to one group, the harm entirely to someone else. Not only militant egalitarians but just about everyone recognizes the unfairness of such a foul distribution of the burdens and benefits. There is a sense that something is terribly wrong with assigning all the burdens to one and all the benefits to others. This moral sense, sometimes called a "sense of justice," appears commonly in our moral deliberations. It is not suppressed by the recognition that the aggregate social good would be greater, much greater, following only the principle of social utility-maximizing.

BALANCING COMPETING PRINCIPLES

Our public policies depend on how we compare the moral force of the principles of utility-maximizing and justice. I am convinced that striving for opportunities for equality of well being takes absolute priority over maximizing aggregate social utility and, at the level of the individual, the principles grouped under the rubric of respect for persons take precedence over net utility as well. I have argued that there is no clear priority among the deontological principles (between respecting autonomy and promoting justice, for example) so that when these principles conflict, the claims of each must be balanced to determine which is more weighty. On the other hand, once these deontological principles have been balanced against one another, the resulting moral imperative takes absolute precedence over considerations of consequences.[18] Considerations of utility, in this view, are not irrelevant, but they play a much smaller role than in utilitarian theory. Utility would merely break ties when two or more deontological principles are so evenly balanced that neither carries the day. Moreover, it is the nature of many of the deontological principles, especially those subsumed under the rubric of respect for persons, that they can often be fully satisfied rather easily. We can go through an entire day without lying, breaking a promise, or killing anybody. We can even go through the day without violating another's autonomy. When the requirements of the deontological principles are satisfied, then utility-maximizing takes its place on center stage as the guiding principle for both public policy and the individual moral life.

Conclusion

My analysis of organ procurement and allocation incorporates the view that these principles I have called deontological have priority over consequences. On the other hand, it is clear that there are some consequentialists (both Hippocratists and social utilitarians) in the policy discussion who are seriously committed to morally proper allocation.

It is in this context that we must understand the federal law mandating that United States organ allocation be based on both efficiency and equity. *Efficiency* is a term signaling concern about maximizing net benefits; *equity* requires that we pay attention to the patterns in the distribution—to the principle of justice. The law requiring both efficiency and equity in a national transplant program is, in effect, a law requiring that neither a purely utilitarian (consequence-maximizing) nor a purely deontological approach prevail.

The task for ethical analysis in public policy is to work out the implications of this mandate for organ procurement and allocation, keeping in mind that certain individuals will be committed to personal religious or secular ethics that focus exclusively on consequence-maximizing or on some deontological principle (such as respect for autonomy and self-determination or justice in allocating organs). My goal is to provide a moral framework for thinking about transplantation as a matter of public policy—that is, when both consequences (efficiency) and just allocation (equity) are taken into account.

ENDNOTES

1. For the contrasting view see Edmund D. Pellegrino and David C. Thomasma, *For the Patient's Good: The Restoration of Beneficence in Health Care* (New York: Oxford University Press, 1988), p. 115; Howard Brody and Franklin G. Miller, "The Internal Morality of Medicine; Explication and Application to Managed Care," *Journal of Medicine and Philosophy* 23 (1998): 384–410; and Edmund D. Pellegrino, "The Goals and Ends of Medicine: How are They to Be Defined?" in *The Goals of Medicine: The Forgotten Issue in Health Care Reform*, ed. Mark Hanson and Daniel Callahan (Washington, DC: Georgetown University Press, 1999).

2. Aristotle, *Nicomachean Ethics*, trans. Ostwald (Indianapolis: Bobbs-Merrill, 1962).

3. Alasdair MacIntyre, *After Virtue* (Notre Dame, IN: University of Notre Dame Press, 1981).

4. Helen Bequaert Holmes and Laura Purdy (eds.), *Feminist Perspectives in Medical Ethics* (Bloomington: Indiana University Press, 1992); Susan Sherwin, *No Longer Patient: Feminist Ethics and Health Care* (Philadelphia: Temple University Press, 1992); Margaret Olivia Little, *Feminist Perspectives on Bioethics Kennedy Institute of Ethics Journal* 6 (special issue; 1996): 1–103.

5. Nel Noddings, *Caring: A Feminine Approach to Ethics and Moral Education* (Berkeley: University of California Press, 1984); Anne H. Bishop and John R. Scudder, *Nursing Ethics: Therapeutic Caring Presence* (Boston: Jones and Bartlett, 1996); Alisa L. Carse, "The 'Voice of Care': Implications for Bioethical Education," *Journal of Medicine and Philosophy* 16 (1, 1991 Feb.): 5–28; Warren Thomas Reich, "Care: II. Historical Dimensions of an Ethic of Care in Health Care," in *Encyclopedia of Bioethics*, rev. ed., ed. Warren Thomas Reich (New York: Simon and Schuster Macmillan, 1995), pp. 331–36; Nancy S. Jecker and Warren Thomas Reich, "Care: III. Contemporary Ethics of Care," in *Encyclopedia of Bioethics*, rev. ed., ed. Warren Thomas Reich (New York: Simon and Schuster Macmillan, 1995), pp. 336–44; Virginia A. Sharpe, "Justice and Care: The Implications of the Kohlberg-Gilligan Debate for Medical Ethics," *Theoretical Medicine* 13 (4, 1992 Dec.): 295–318.

6. Virginia Knowlden, "The Virtue of Caring in Nursing," in *Ethical and Moral Dimensions of Care*, ed. Madeleine M. Leininger (Detroit, MI: Wayne State University Press, 1990), pp. 89–94; Pamela J. Salsberry, "Caring, Virtue Theory, and a Foundation for Nursing Ethics," *Scholarly Inquiry for Nursing Practice* 6 (2, 1992 Summer): 155–67; Howard J. Curzer, "Is Care a Virtue for Health Care Professionals?" *Journal of Medicine and Philosophy* 18 (1, 1993 Feb.): 51–69; Robert M.

Veatch, "The Place of Care in Ethical Theory," *Journal of Medicine and Philosophy: The Chaos of Care and Care Theory* 23 (2, 1998): 210–24.

7. Ludwig Edelstein, "The Hippocratic Oath: Text, Translation and Interpretation," in *Ancient Medicine: Selected Papers of Ludwig Edelstein*, ed. Owsei Temkin and C. Lilian Temkin (Baltimore: Johns Hopkins Press, 1967), pp. 3–64.

8. American Medical Association, Council on Ethical and Judicial Affairs, *Code of Medical Ethics: Current Opinions with Annotations, 1998–1999 Edition* (Chicago: Author, 1998).

9. Immanuel Kant, *Groundwork of the Metaphysic of Morals*, trans. H. J. Paton (New York: Harper and Row, 1964).

10. W. D. Ross, *The Right and the Good* (Oxford: Oxford University Press, 1930).

11. Tom L. Beauchamp and James F. Childress (eds.), *Principles of Biomedical Ethics*, 4th ed. (New York: Oxford University Press, 1994).

12. Jeremy Bentham, "An Introduction to the Principles of Morals and Legislation," in *Ethical Theories: A Book of Readings*, ed. A. I. Melden (Englewood Cliffs, NJ: Prentice-Hall, 1967), pp. 367–90.

13. John Stuart Mill, "Utilitarianism," in *Ethical Theories: A Book of Readings*, ed. A. I. Melden (Englewood Cliffs, NJ: Prentice-Hall, 1967), pp. 391–434.

14. For a much fuller discussion of these principles see Robert M. Veatch, *A Theory of Medical Ethics* (New York: Basic Books, 1981).

15. American Medical Association, Council on Ethical and Judicial Affairs, *Code of Medical Ethics: Current Opinions with Annotations, 1998–1999*.

16. Ronald Dworkin, "What Is Equality? Part 1: Equality of Welfare," *Philosophy and Public Affairs* 10 (Summer 1981): 185–246; Dworkin, "What is Equality? Part 2: Equality of Resources," *Philosophy and Public Affairs* 10 (Fall 1981): 283–345. For a fuller discussion see my book-length treatment of the issues in Robert M. Veatch, *The Foundations of Justice: Why the Retarded and the Rest of Us Have Claims to Equality* (New York: Oxford University Press, 1986).

17. John Rawls, *A Theory of Justice* (Cambridge, MA: Harvard University Press, 1971).

18. Robert M. Veatch, *A Theory of Medical Ethics* (New York: Basic Books, 1981); Robert M. Veatch, "Resolving Conflict Among Principles: Ranking, Balancing, and Specifying," *Kennedy Institute of Ethics Journal* 5 (Sept. 1995): 199–218.

PART ONE

DEFINING
DEATH

THREE

Brain Death: Welcome Definition or Dangerous Judgment?

ON MAY 25, 1968, at the beginning of the era of transplantation, Bruce Tucker was brought to the operating room of the hospital of the Medical College of Virginia. Tucker, a 56-year-old Black laborer, had suffered a massive brain injury the day before in a fall. He sustained a lateral basilar skull fracture on the right side, subdural hematoma on the left, and brain-stem contusion.

The following timetable is taken from the summary of the case by Judge A. Christian Compton, who eventually heard the case when it came to court:[1]

6:05 p.m. Admitted to the hospital

11:00 p.m. Emergency right temporoparietal craniotomy and right parietal burr hole.

2:05 a.m. Operation complete; patient fed intravenously and received "medication" each hour.

11:30 a.m. Placed on respirator, which kept him "mechanically alive."

11:45 a.m. Treating physician noted "prognosis for recovery is nil and death imminent."

1:00 p.m. Neurologist called to obtain an EEG with the results showing "flat lines with occasional artifact. He found no clinical evidence of viability and no evidence of cortical activity."

2:45 p.m. Tucker taken to the operating room. From this time until 4:30 p.m. "he maintained vital signs of life, that is, he maintained, for the most part, normal body temperature, normal pulse, normal blood pressure and normal rate of respiration."

3:30 p.m. Respirator cut off.

3:33 p.m. Incision made in Joseph Klett, heart recipient.

3:35 p.m. Patient [Tucker] pronounced dead.

4:25 p.m. Incision made to remove Tucker's heart.

4:42 p.m. Heart taken out.

4:33 p.m. Incision made to remove decedent's kidneys.

Tucker's heart and kidneys were removed by the surgical team. The heart was transplanted to Joseph G. Klett, who died about one week later. The case was to become the first widely publicized controversy about what it means to consider a person dead. Many interpret the case as establishing a brain-oriented death for the state of Virginia, but it could equally be viewed as the first case in which a ventilator was disconnected for the purpose of causing the death of the patient (by traditional heart criteria) to procure organs for transplant.

Tucker's brother, William E. Tucker, apparently saw it in this way. He sued for $100,000 damages, charging the transplant team was engaged in a "systematic and nefarious scheme to use Bruce Tucker's heart and hastened his death by shutting off the mechanical means of support."[2] William Tucker's attorney was a young Black Virginia state senator, L. Douglas Wilder, later to become governor and nationally known Democratic politician. According to the judge's summary:

> A close friend of the deceased was searching for him and made an inquiry at three of the hospital information desks, all without success. Tucker's brother, William, was at his place of business, located within 15 city blocks of the hospital, all day on May 25th until he left his business to go find his brother in the afternoon when he heard he had been injured. Among the personal effects turned over to the brother later was a business card which the decedent had in his wallet which showed the plaintiff's (brother's) name, business address and telephone number thereon.

The suit charged that the removal of organs was carried out with only minimal attempts to notify the victim's family and obtain permission for use of his organs.

In those early years of the definition-of-death debate and organ transplant controversy, this case was one of the most complicated and significant. Whether it should, in fact, be treated as a "brain death" case we shall consider later, but certainly that is the way the principals in the case and the press handled it. The Internal Medicine News Service headed their report, " 'Brain Death' Held Proof of Demise in Va. Jury Decision."[3] The New York Times' headline said, "Virginia Jury Rules That Death Occurs When Brain Dies."[4] Internal Medicine News, in one of the best stories covering the case, claimed—quite accurately—that "the landmark decision is not binding elsewhere but it is certain to be cited as precedent in related cases." In fact, not one news story with which I am familiar saw this as anything other than a brain-death case.

The surgeons who removed Tucker's heart evidently also interpreted it as a case of deciding when a patient is dead. Dr. David Hume, the assisting surgeon in the case, is quoted as saying that the court's decision in favor of the physicians "brings the law up to date with what medicine has known all along—that the only death is brain death." Most people assumed that when asked to decide whether the physicians were guilty of causing the death of the heart donor, the jury in the Tucker case was in effect being asked to make a public policy judgment about whether the irreversible loss of brain function is to be equated for moral, legal, and public policy purposes with the death of an individual. Because almost all organs for transplant come from the bodies of the newly deceased and getting those organs in a viable condition requires getting them as soon after death as possible, it is critical to get clear on exactly what it means for a human to be dead. Thus the first part of this book will focus on this question that is crucial to almost the entire organ transplant enterprise.

The task of defining death is not a trivial exercise in coining the meaning of a term. Rather, it is an attempt to reach an understanding of the philosophical nature of the human being and that which is essentially significant to humans that is lost at the time of death. When we say that an individual has died, there are appropriate behavioral changes: We go into mourning, perhaps cease certain kinds of medical treatment, initiate a funeral ritual, read a will, or, if the individual happens to be president of an organization, elevate the vice president to the presidency. According to many, including those who focus on the definition of death as crucial for the transplant debate, it is appropriate to remove vital, unimpaired organs after, but not before, death. This is what is usually called the "dead donor" rule. So there is a great deal at stake at the policy level in the definition of death.

Candidates for "Death"

As we shall see in greater detail in the next chapter, there are several plausible candidates for the concept of death. All are attempts to determine that which is so significant to a human being that its loss constitutes the change in the moral and legal status of the individual. The traditional religious and philosophical view in Western culture was that a human being died at the time when the soul left the body. This separation of body and soul is difficult to verify scientifically and is best left to the religious traditions, which in some cases still focus on the soul-departure concept of death.

Traditional secular thinkers have focused on the cessation of the flow of the vital body fluids—blood and breath; when the circulatory and respiratory functions cease, the individual is dead. This is a view of the nature of the human being that identifies the human essence with the flowing of fluids in the animal species.

There are also two new candidates. One of these is the complete loss of the body's integrating capacities, as signified by the activity of the central nervous system. This is the now popular concept frequently though inaccurately given the name "brain death." Most recently in the literature there are those who are beginning to question the adequacy of this notion of brain death, claiming that it already has become old fashioned. They ask why it is that one must identify the entire brain with death; is it not possible that we are really interested only in human consciousness: in the ability to think, reason, feel, experience, interact with others, and control body functions consciously? This is crucial in rare cases in which the lower brain function might be intact while the cortex, which controls consciousness, is utterly destroyed.

Moral, Not Technical

The public policy debate about the meaning of death involves a choice among these candidates for death and other variants that we shall encounter in succeeding chapters. The Harvard Ad Hoc Committee to Examine the Definition of Brain Death, a committee at Harvard Medical School made up of physicians, lawyers, theologians, and social scientists, established operational criteria for what it called *irreversible coma*, based on what was then taken to be sound scientific evidence. These four criteria are (1) unreceptivity and unresponsivity; (2) no movements or breathing; (3) no reflexes; and (4) flat electroencephalogram ("of great confirmatory value").

What the committee did not do, however, and what it was not capable of doing, was establishing that patients in irreversible coma are "dead"—in other words, that we should treat them as if they were no longer living human beings who possess the same human moral rights and obligations as other living humans. Although it may be the case that patients in irreversible coma, according to Harvard criteria, have shifted into that status where they are no longer to be considered living, the decision that they are "dead" cannot be derived from any amount of scientific investigation and demonstration. The choice among the many candidates for what is essential to the nature of the species and, therefore, the loss of which is to be called "death," is a philosophical or moral question, not a medical or scientific one.

This being the case, it is troubling, indeed, to hear physicians say, as Dr. Hume did, that the Virginia legal decision "brings the law up to date with what medicine has known all along—that the only death is brain death."[5] If some physicians have believed this (and certainly there is no consensus among medical professionals), they know it from their general belief system about what is valuable in life and not from their training as medical scientists. It is therefore distressing that "expert" witnesses, including Dr. William Sweet of Harvard Medical School, were called by the defense to testify before the jury. Dr. Sweet said, "Death is a state in which the brain is dead. The rest of the body exists in order to support the brain. The brain is the individual."[6] This may or may not be a sound moral philosophical position. It is certainly not a medical argument. And to ask a chief of neurosurgery at Massachusetts General Hospital to make the moral argument is certainly a kind of special pleading on the part of legal counsel for the defense. This led to the *New York Times'* story, which began, "A medical opinion that death occurs when the brain dies, even if the heart and other organs continue to function, has been reinforced by a jury here in a landmark heart transplant suit."[7] The claim that death occurs when the brain dies is opinion to be sure, but it is not, and by the very nature of the case cannot be, medical opinion. To leave such decision making in the hands of scientifically trained professionals is a dangerous, illegitimate, confused move.

Especially in such a fundamental matter as life and death itself, it is very difficult to see how the rest of society can shirk its responsibility in deciding what concept of death is to be used. To be sure, the scientific community can and should be asked to establish the criteria for measuring such things as irreversible coma, once the public, acting through its policy-making agencies in the legislature, has determined whether irreversible coma is to be equated with death. We shall see in the next chapter that one group (including both physicians and lay people) finds this answer too liberal. They would insist that people are not dead—and that therefore organs should not be taken—until the heart has irreversibly stopped beating. We shall also see that another group (also including both physicians and lay people) finds this answer too conservative. They would insist that some people may be dead for all legal and public policy purposes—including organ procurement—even though some portions of the brain continue to function.

The Origins of the Confusion in the Tucker Case

Let us return to the Tucker trial to see how this confusion between social and medical responsibilities developed. In the state of Virginia, according to the judge, there was a definition of death operative at the time of the events involving Tucker. That definition was that death is "the cessation of life; the ceasing to exist; a total stoppage of the circulation of the blood, and a cessation of the animal and vital functions consequent thereto such as respiration and pulsation."[8] On a motion for summary judgment for the surgeons, the judge ruled that the law-book definition of death must take precedence over medical opinion. In this opinion, Judge Compton directed that the court was bound by the legal definition of death in Virginia until it was changed by the state legislature.[9] Three days later, however, after considerable debate, Judge Compton may have backtracked on his commitment to the publicly established concept of death. He instructed the jury:

> In determining the time of death, as aforesaid . . . you may consider the following elements none of which should necessarily be considered controlling, although you may feel under the evidence that one or more of these conditions are controlling: the time of the total stoppage of the circulation of the blood; the time of the total cessation of the other vital functions consequent thereto, such as respiration and pulsation; the time of complete and irreversible loss of all functions of the brain; and whether or not the aforesaid functions were spontaneous or were being maintained artificially or mechanically.[10]

This instruction is ambiguous, to say the least. It could be that Judge Compton meant no innovation here. It could be that the "complete and irreversible loss of all function of the brain" might have been merely the "cause" of death traditionally defined—in other words, "a cessation of the animal and vital functions." Presumably if the head injury to Tucker led to the cessation of all brain function and thereby to the cessation of all other vital functions, death could have occurred in the traditional sense without or before the intervention of the surgeons. This almost certainly would have been the case if Tucker had received no medical attention. Then (traditional) death would have occurred and the "complete and irreversible loss of all function of the brain" would simply have been a relevant factor in causing Tucker's death. He would, under this interpretation, have died under Virginia law when his heart stopped beating.

But it also is possible to interpret the judge's instructions as authorizing the jury to use a new concept of death—one based directly on brain function—in determining when the patient died. If this is the case, it is a complete reversal of the judge's earlier statement and a major change in public policy. It would appear that this contradicts Judge Compton's earlier conclusion that "if such a radical change is to be made in the law of Virginia, the application should be made therefore not to the courts but to the legislature wherein the basic concept of our society relating to the preservation and extension of life could be examined and, if necessary, reevaluated."[11]

The legal case, in spite of the widespread assumption that it established a brain-based criterion of death in Virginia, leaves great ambiguity. No matter how outdated the old heart-and-lung basis for pronouncing death, the judge seems to get it right when he says that this is a matter for the people—the legislature—to decide, not individual physicians standing at the bedside and not judges.

Determining Who Should Have Made the Decision

The other candidates for a role in the decision in this case are obviously the patient and his or her relatives. Although it is the state's obligation to establish fundamental policy in this area, it would seem reasonable that it would oppose removing of any organs from an individual after death unless some authorization were given either by the individual patient, such as is now called for in the Uniform Anatomical Gift Act,[12] or by the patient's relatives, also as provided by that act. If the relatives of the patient were not consulted and sufficient time was not taken to establish that relatives were available, this would be a serious infringement on the rights of the patient and the patient's family.

The removal of organs in the rare situations in which relatives cannot be found raises a serious, if rather unusual, problem for those responsible for organ procurement. It would appear to be far wiser to avoid the risk of abuse in these cases, which will frequently involve indigent and isolated patients, by simply forbidding procurement of organs from this population. Certainly four hours (from the time Tucker was placed on a respirator until the respirator was turned off) was not sufficient time to seek permission from the next of kin.

Determining If This Was Really a Definition of Death Case

Up to this point, we have assumed that the defense, the prosecution, and the press were correct in interpreting Tucker's case as one focusing on the meaning and concept of death. Yet the case record, as presented to the court, leaves open some very serious questions. The medical team was operating with a definition of death that focused on the brain. Medical witnesses for the defense claimed that Tucker was "neurologically dead" several hours before the transplant operation. Yet according to the records presented of the case, at 11:45 A.M. Tucker's physician says prognosis is nil and death imminent. At 1:00 P.M. the neurologist took an EEG reading and found it "showing flat lines with occasional artifact" and he "reports no evidence of viability and no signs of cortical activity." Presumably Tucker was thought to be dead at that time by the surgeons, according to a brain-oriented concept of death.

This behavior is puzzling. First, if the neurologist took the EEG reading and found evidence of cortical activity lacking at 1:00 P.M., Tucker did not yet meet the Harvard criteria for being considered brain dead. The tests must be repeated over a 24-hour period and activity of the lower brain, not just the cerebral cortex, must be ruled out. Second, we are told the surgeons turned the respirator off at 3:30 P.M. One must ask what possible moral principle would justify turning off a respirator on a patient who was already dead? Presumably if one is dealing with a corpse, the moral imperative would be to preserve the organs for the benefit of the living in the best possible condition—by continuing the respiration process until the heart could be removed. We would find no moral problems with such behavior; in fact, it would be morally irresponsible to run the risk of damaging the tissue. Yet the respirator was turned off—from which one can only surmise that it must have been done to permit the heart and lungs to stop functioning. The only plausible reason for this would be that there was some lingering doubt about whether or not Tucker was dead. Of course, to introduce this dimension is to place doubt on the claim that the patient was dead at 1:00 P.M. when the EEG showed a flat tracing "with occasional artifact." If, however, the purpose was to turn the respirator off to allow the patient to die "all the way," the case is not one of a new definition of death at all; it is instead the common one of deciding to discontinue treatment on an irreversibly terminal patient. We have another Karen Quinlan case, one of foregoing life support on an inevitably dying (but not yet dead) patient.

The morality of ceasing treatment on such a terminal patient has been accepted widely in medical ethics.[13] Such procedures are practiced and accepted by Catholic, Protestant, and Jewish moral traditions alike. It could be, then, that this is really a case of deciding when it is morally acceptable to stop treatment on a dying patient rather than a case of deciding when a patient was dead. This seems to be the most plausible and morally acceptable reason for turning off the respirator under the law then existing in Virginia. Of course, the now-accepted practice of stopping life-sustaining treatment normally would require the consent of the patient or the approval of the next of kin, neither of which had been obtained in Tucker's case.

It is very important to note that the jury never announced that the brain-oriented concept of death was appropriate or that they themselves used such a concept. They were not asked or permitted to do this. They merely concluded that they found the defendants not guilty of wrongful death of the decedent. It may well be that at least some of them reasoned that the physicians did indeed hasten the dying process by turning off the respirator, but given the patient's condition, this was an acceptable way to behave—in other words, they may have considered that the physician could have justifiably decided to withdraw the mechanical means of support as "extraordinary for a patient in Tucker's irreversibly dying condition." We do not know this, of course, but we also do not know that the jury accepted brain-oriented concept of death.

At 3:35 P.M., five minutes after the respirator was turned off, the patient was pronounced dead. One would think this was because there had been cessation of heart beat and respiratory function and the death was pronounced according to the traditional heart–lung criteria. If this were the case, then the physicians would be operating under the traditional moral and legal requirements and the removal of organs for transplantation, presumably with the permission of the next of kin, would be an acceptable procedure. They would not be using the brain-oriented concept of death at all.

Determining If Tucker Was Neurologically Dead

There is one final problem that must be resolved. The summary of the proceedings raises some doubt about whether the patient was actually dead even according to the concept of death that focuses on the brain. The Harvard criteria call for the use of irreversible coma. But the Harvard report appeared in the *Journal of the American Medical Association*[14] dated August 5, 1968, and the surgeons at the Medical College of Virginia had to make their decision two months earlier, on May 25, 1968. Obviously they could not be expected to have followed the Harvard criteria precisely. Nevertheless, Tucker definitely could not have been declared dead according to the criteria since established by the Harvard committee and widely used as being the minimal tests for establishing irreversible coma. At the very least, the tests were not repeated 24 hours later. The patient was pronounced dead less than 2 hours and 35 minutes after the electroencephalogram reading.

To accept the jury's decision in this case as demonstrating that the physicians were justified in the use of brain evidence of death, one would have to accept four highly questionable premises. First is that the jury did indeed base its decision on a brain-oriented concept of death. Second is that individuals are really dead when they no longer have any capacity for brain activity. Third is that it was reasonable under 1968 conditions to conclude that the patient had irreversibly lost the capacity for any brain activity based on one EEG reading without repetition. Such a conclusion is premature even for the scientific evidence that exists today, some many years later. Fourth, one would have to accept that individual medical professionals should be vested with the authority to change public policy in areas as fundamental as whether one is alive or dead. This no one should be willing to tolerate.

This famous early case is still interesting some 30 years later. It not only shows how complex and confusing the links were between organ transplant and defining death in the early days of these activities, but it also reveals confusions that remain today. Many medical professionals still confuse the decision that someone is dead with the decision that the person is inevitably dying—that is, alive but terminal. Is it any wonder that lay people are similarly confused? Many medical professionals still confuse irreversible loss of the functions of the cerebral cortex with similar loss of the functions of the entire brain. They still talk about brain-dead persons being "terminally ill" as if they were not already dead.

The first critical task in creating an ethics of organ transplantation is getting completely clear on exactly when an individual dies. Chapter 4 attempts to establish a clear understanding of the definition of death.

ENDNOTES

1. *Tucker v. Lower*, No. 2831 (Richmond, Va. L. & Eq. Ct., May 23, 1972); also see Richmond Stanfield Frederick, "Medical Jurisprudence—Determining the Time of Death of the Heart Transplant Donor," *North Carolina Law Review* 51 (1972): 172–84.

2. *Tucker v. Lower*.

3. " 'Brain Death' Held Proof of Demise in Va. Jury Decision," *Internal Medicine News*, July 1, 1992, pp. 1, 19.

4. "Virginia July Rules That Death Occurs When Brain Dies," *New York Times*, May 27, 1972, p. 15.

5. " 'Brain Death' Held Proof of Demise in Va. Jury Decision."

6. Ibid.

7. "Virginia July Rules That Death Occurs When Brain Dies."

8. *Tucker v. Lower*, p. 7.

9. *Tucker v. Lower*, p. 10.

10. Judge A. Christian Compton, "Instruction No. 7," unpublished instruction to the jury in *Tucker v. Lower*.

11. *Tucker v. Lower*, p. 10.

12. A. M. Sadler, B. L. Sadler, and E. Blythe Stason, "The Uniform Anatomical Gift Act," *Journal of the American Medical Association* 206 (Dec. 9, 1968): 2501–06.

13. President's Commission for the Study of Ethical Problems in Medicine and Biomedical and Behavioral Research, *Deciding to Forego Life-Sustaining Treatment: Ethical, Medical, and Legal Issues in Treatment Decisions* (Washington, DC: U.S. Government Printing Office, 1983).

14. Harvard Medical School, "A Definition of Irreversible Coma. Report of the Ad Hoc Committee of the Harvard Medical School to Examine the Definition of Brain Death," *Journal of the American Medical Association* 205 (1968): 337–40.

FOUR

THE DEFINITION OF DEATH:
PROBLEMS FOR PUBLIC POLICY

AT 5:41 A.M. Sunday morning, November 10, 1985, Philadelphia Flyers' hockey star Pelle Lindbergh slammed his new Porsche into a cement wall of a Somerdale, New Jersey, elementary school. The headline on the story in the newspaper the next day read, "Flyers Goalie Is Declared Brain Dead." In spite of the claim that he was "brain dead" the story went on to say that Lindbergh was listed in "critical condition" in the intensive care unit of John F. Kennedy Hospital in Stratford.

Referring to his parents, who were called from Sweden to be at his side, Vicki Santoro, nursing supervisor at the hospital said, "They were just devastated." Flyers' team physician Edward Viner said that if Lindbergh's situation did not improve, the family would be left with a decision about how long to leave him on the respirator.

That was not the only decision they faced. If Lindbergh was dead even though some of his vital functions remained, he would be an ideal candidate to be an organ donor. His intact heart and kidneys could provide life-saving help for three other people. Possibly even his liver, lungs, pancreas, and corneas could benefit others. Suddenly it became a practical, lifesaving matter to figure out whether Pelle Lindbergh was dead or alive. The headline writer says he was "brain dead," but then the article went on to speak as if he was nevertheless still alive. The story referred to him as "near death."[1] We used to believe that persons with beating hearts were alive even though their brain function was lost irreversibly. Now we are not so sure. The way Pelle Lindbergh was treated, the decisions his parents had to make, the behavior of the physicians and nurses, and the fate of several desperately ill human beings all hinged on figuring out whether Lindbergh was already dead or rather was in the process of dying.

The public policy discussion of the definition of death began in earnest in the late 1960s, not long before surgeons were confronted by Bruce Tucker but almost 20 years before Pelle Lindbergh's accident. It began in the context of a world that had in the previous decade seen the first successful transplantation of an organ from one human being to another, including the initial 1967 transplant of a human heart. It cannot be denied that this sudden infatuation with the usefulness of human organs was the stimulus for the intense discussion of the real meaning of death. What many thought would be a rather short-lived problem, resolved by the combined wisdom of the health professionals and the nonscientists on the Harvard ad hoc committee, has lingered as an intractable morass of conflicting technical, legal, conceptual, and moral arguments. Much of this confusion can be avoided, however, by focusing exclusively on the problems for public policy.

Focusing on public policy means avoiding a full linguistic analysis of the term *death*. Although that may be an important philosophical enterprise, and many have undertaken it,[2] this analysis is only of indirect importance for public policy questions, including the organ transplant questions that are the subject of this book. Likewise, we need not provide a detailed theological account of the meaning of death. Those studies are numerous[3] but not of immediate concern in the formation of secular public policy. Nor are we concerned about the ontological question of when an entity ceases to be human. Some philosophers have tried to turn the definition of death debate into such a deep philosophical question.[4] Most significant, a scientific description of the biological events in the brain at the time of death will not be necessary. That is of crucial importance for the science of neurology, and a vast literature is available giving such an account.[5] The scientific, biological, and neurological description of precisely what takes place in the human body at the point of death is not a matter that need directly concern public policy makers.

The Public Policy Question

What we are interested in is the public policy question: When should we begin treating an individual the way we treat the newly dead? Is it possible to identify a point in the course of human events at which a new set of social behaviors becomes appropriate, at which, because we say the individual has died, we may justifiably begin to treat him or her in a way that was not previously appropriate, morally or legally? In short, what we are interested in is a social system of death behaviors.

Social and cultural changes take place when we label someone as dead. Some medical treatments may be stopped when an individual is considered dead that would not be stopped if the individual were alive—even if the living individual were merely terminally ill. This of course does not imply that there are no treatments that should be stopped at other times, either before or after the time when we label somebody as dead. Many treatments are stopped before death for technical reasons. According to many there are other treatments, including some that prolong life, that may justifiably be stopped before death because the treatments are no longer appropriate, either because they no longer serve a useful purpose or because they are too burdensome. In other cases, if the newly dead body is to be used for research, education, or transplant purposes, it is possible to continue certain interventions after death has been declared. Many have held that this is morally acceptable.[6] It appears, however, that, traditionally, at least, there have been some treatments that are stopped when and only when we decide that it is time to treat the individual as dead.

Other behaviors also have traditionally taken place at the time we consider the individual dead. We begin mourning in a pattern that is not appropriate in mere anticipatory grief.[7] We start several social processes that are not appropriately begun before the decision is made that death behavior is appropriate. We begin the process that will lead to reading a will, to burying or otherwise disposing of what we now take to be the "mortal remains." We assume new social roles—the role of widowhood, for example. If the individual who has been labeled as dead happens to have been the president of a country or an organization, normally labeling that individual as dead leads to the assumption of the role of president by the one who was formerly vice president. Finally, and perhaps of most immediate relevance to the concern that generated the definition of death discussion, we change the procedures and justifications for obtaining organs from the body. Before death, organs can only be removed in the interests of the individual, or, perhaps, in rare circumstances, with the consent of the individual or legal guardian.[8] (These issues involving "living donors" are the subject of Chapter 12.) At the moment we decide to treat someone as dead, an entirely different set of procedures is called for—the procedures designated in the Uniform Anatomical Gift Act drawn up in 1968. At that point, if one agreed to posthumous donation of organs while still alive, the organs may be removed according to the terms of the donation without further consideration of the interest of the former individual or the wishes of the family members. If the deceased has not so donated, and has not expressed opposition to donation, the next of kin or other legitimate guardian in possession of the body assumes both the right and the responsibility for the disposal of the remains and may donate the organs.

It is clear that at least in Anglo-American law the one with such a responsibility cannot merely dispose of the body capriciously in any way he or she sees fit, but bears a responsibility for treating the new corpse with respect and dignity.[9] This, however, has been taken both in law and in morality as permitting the donation of body parts by the one with this responsibility, except when there has been an explicit objection expressed by the deceased during the time of his or her life.[10] (The issues surrounding the "donation" model and the alternatives to donation will be explored in Part Two of this book.)

In short, traditionally there has been a radical shift in moral, social, and political standing when someone has been labeled as dead. Until the 1960s, there was not a great deal of controversy over exactly when such a label should be applied. There were deviant philosophical and theological positions and substantial concern about erroneous labeling of someone as dead, but very little real controversy about what it meant to be dead in this public policy sense.

Now perhaps for the first time there are matters of real public policy significance in deciding precisely what we mean when we label someone dead. In an earlier day all of the socially significant death-related behaviors were generated at the time of death pronouncement. Very little was at stake if we were not precise in sorting various indicators of the time when this behavior was appropriate. Virtually all of the plausible events related to death occurred in rapid succession, and none of the behaviors was really contingent on any greater precision.

Now matters have changed in two important ways. First, several technologies have greatly extended our capacity to prolong the dying process, making it possible to identify several different potential indicators of what we should take to be the death of the individual as a whole and making it possible to separate these points dramatically in time. Second, the usefulness of human organs and tissues for transplantation, research, and education makes precision morally imperative. In an earlier day, the most that was at stake was that an individual could for a few seconds or moments be falsely treated as alive when in fact he or she should have been treated as dead, or vice versa. Of course, it is important, out of our sense of respect for persons, that we not confuse living individuals with their corpses, so in theory it has always been important that we be clear about whether someone is dead or alive. Yet traditionally the very short time frame for the entire series of events meant that there was little at stake as a matter of public policy. We could pronounce death based on the rapid succession of an inevitably linked series of bodily events: heart stoppage, stoppage of respiration, or the death of the brain.

As we extend this period of time over which these events can occur, permitting much more precision in identifying what it is in the human body that signifies that it ought to be treated as dead, we must ask the question, Can we continue to identify a single definable point at which all the social behaviors associated with death should begin? It may turn out that as the dying process is extended, all of these behaviors will find their own niches and that it really will cease to be important to label someone as dead at a precise moment in time. Life-sustaining treatment could then be stopped at one moment, mourning begun at another, life insurance payoffs and funeral preparation at still others. Organ procurement could take place at it own special moment, independent of exactly when death is pronounced.[11] If so, death itself, as well as dying, may begin to be viewed as a process.[12]

However, it seems likely that this may not happen. Rather, we may want to continue to link at least many of these social events so that we shall continue to say there is a moment when it becomes appropriate to begin the entire series of death behaviors (or at least many of them). If so, then death of the individual as a whole will continue to be viewed as a single event rather than a process.[13] There are several plausible candidates for that critical point at which we can say the individual as a whole has died, including the time when circulatory function ceases, the time when all brain functions cease, or the time when certain important brain functions (such as mental function) cease.

The question is therefore not precisely the same as the one the philosopher asks when he or she asks the question of the endpoint of personhood or personal identity.[14] Analyses of the concept of personhood or personal identity suggest that there may be an identifiable endpoint at which we should stop thinking of a human organism as a person. That analysis by itself, however, never tells us whether it is morally appropriate to begin treating that human the way we have traditionally treated the dead unless personhood is simply defined with reference to death behavior, which it often is not. Under some formulations, such as those of Michael Green and Daniel Wikler,[15] for example, it is conceptually possible to talk about a living individual in cases in which the person no longer exists. (This would be true, for example, if we said that living humans were persons only when they possessed self-awareness or ability to distinguish themselves from others.) Some human individuals could then be alive but not persons. Logically, we would then be pressed to the moral and policy question of whether these living bodies that are no longer persons are to be treated differently from the way we are used to treating living persons.

Fortunately, for matters of public policy, if not for philosophical analysis, we need not take up the question of personhood but can confront directly the question of whether we can identify a point at which this series of death behaviors is appropriate. In this way death comes to mean, for public policy purposes, nothing more than the condition of some group of human beings for whom death behavior is appropriate. Can we identify this point? If we can, then, for purposes of law and public policy, we shall label that point as the moment of death. The laws reformulating the definition of death do not go so far as to say they are defining death for all purposes theological, philosophical, and personal. Some explicitly limit the scope, saying that the law defines death "for all legal purposes."

This policy-oriented formulation makes clear that when we talk about death, we are talking about death of the entity as a whole. It is with reference to the entire human organism that we want to determine appropriate behavior, not some particular body part.

Unfortunately, the term *brain death* has emerged in the debate. This is unfortunate in part because we are not interested in the death of brains; we are interested in the death of organisms as integrated entities subject to particular kinds of public behavior and control. In contrast, the term *brain death* is systematically ambiguous. It has two potential meanings. The first is not controversial at all; it simply means the destruction of the brain, leaving open the question of whether people with destroyed brains should be treated as dead people. It is better to substitute the phrase "destruction of the brain" for "brain death" in this sense. It makes clear that we are referring only to the complete biological collapse of the organ or organs we call the brain. Exactly how that is measured is largely a neurological question.

Unfortunately, brain death has also taken on a second, very different, and much more controversial, meaning. It can also mean the death of the individual as a whole, based on the fact that the brain has died. The problem is illustrated in the original report of the Harvard ad hoc committee,[16] which has become the most significant technical document in the American debate. The title of that 1968 document is "A Definition of Irreversible Coma." The article sets out to define "characteristics of irreversible coma" and produces a list of technical criteria that purport to predict that an individual is in a coma that is irreversible. The name of the committee, however, is the "Ad Hoc Committee of the Harvard Medical School to Examine the Definition of Brain Death." The presumption apparently was that irreversible coma and brain death were synonymous. We now realize that this is not precisely true. An individual can apparently be in irreversible coma and still not have a completely dead brain. In any case, the title of the report and the name of the committee, taken in context of what the committee did, imply that the objective of the committee was to describe the empirical measures of a destroyed brain.

The opening sentence of the report, however, says, "Our primary purpose is to define irreversible coma as a new criterion for death."[17] It does not claim to be defining the destruction (death) of the brain but *death simpliciter*, by which everyone, including the committee members, meant death of the individual for purposes of death behaviors, clinical practice, and public policy including, of course, transplantation. Yet the report contains no argument that the destruction of the brain (measured by the characteristics of irreversible coma) should be taken as a justification for treating the individual as a whole as dead. The members of the committee and many others believed that this should be so, possibly with good reason, but the reasons were not stated.

Because the term *brain death* has these two radically different meanings, there is often confusion in public and professional discussion of the issues. For instance, neurologists can claim that they have real expertise on brain death—meaning, of course, expertise in measuring the destruction of the brain. Others claim, however, that brain death is exclusively a matter for public policy consideration— meaning that the question of whether we should treat an individual as dead because the brain tissue is dead is really one outside the scope of neurological expertise. A far better course would be to abandon that language entirely, substituting precise and explicit language that either refers to the destruction of the brain or to the death of the individual as a whole based on brain criteria.

Preliminary Issues to Public Policy Discussion

Before turning to the substantive issues of the definition of death controversy, it is necessary to clarify two preliminary issues. We need to make sure we understand the importance of the difference between allowing a terminally ill patient to die and deciding that that person is in fact dead. Then we need to understand the difference between what I am calling the *criteria* for pronouncing death and the *concept* of death itself.

Allowing to Die versus Deciding that Someone Is Dead

In many cases the public fascination with the definition of death discussion may be misplaced. There have been several cases in which problems with the care of the critically ill have been addressed by trying to figure out whether the individual has died when the real issue is whether to let the still-living person die. For example, some people try to resolve the question of whether it is acceptable to stop providing life-supporting treatment by arguing that the individual is dead.

In the early phase of the discussion of the case of Karen Quinlan—the young woman in New Jersey who suffered irreversible brain damage and was sustained in a chronic vegetative state—the lawyer for her family, the judge, and many others initially cast their arguments in terms of the definition of death.[18] It was much later in the case that everyone became convinced that Quinlan was not dead according to any plausible definition but might be withdrawn from the respirator even though still alive. Likewise, when a Maryland nurse was prosecuted for disconnecting a respirator on a terminally ill cancer patient, her defense centered on the claim that her patient was dead according to brain criteria.[19] The jury was sufficiently confused over the definition of death that it was unable to reach a verdict, and charges were eventually dropped even though it was clear that a homicide took place because the patient was not dead by any definition; he was merely terminally ill.

Instead of insisting that we can resolve these problems of clinical care only by reformulating the definition of death, an alternative would be to recognize that it is possible that some living individuals are in such a condition that it would be appropriate to allow them to die. This of course raises moral questions of its own, but it does not force all of the complex problems of ethics concerning the terminally ill into the one potential solution of the redefinition of death. That prolonging life serves no purpose does not establish by itself that an individual has died.

There are several unfortunate and tragic situations in which a patient may be stabilized indefinitely and still be considered living for public policy and legal purposes. One of these might turn out to be the condition known as persistent vegetative state.[20] This is the condition in which Karen Quinlan lived for ten years.[21] It is crucial to realize that to justify a treatment-stopping decision in a case such as Quinlan's, it is not necessary to conclude that she is dead. It is logically quite possible to decide simply that she should be allowed to die because there is no longer any appropriate justification for continuing treatment.

The same argument applies even more forcefully to patients who are terminally ill while perhaps senile or in a semicomatose state but who nevertheless retain some limited capacities for mental activity. Society will at some point have to address the very difficult questions of public policy related to the care of such individuals. This is not, however, an appropriate matter for the definition of death discussion. The definition of death problem is one small subset of the moral and legal issues related to death and dying.

Criteria for Death versus the Concept of Death

One of the most crucial preliminary issues in public policy consideration of the definition of death grows out of the problem of the systematic ambiguity of the term *brain death*. Some of the questions related to the pronouncement of death based on brain-related criteria are clearly technical and scientific, whereas others are questions of morality, politics, and law. It is crucial that the two be kept separate and the public role in each of these kinds of questions be identified.[22]

CRITERIA OF DEATH: LARGELY A SCIENTIFIC MATTER

Virtually no one holds that every body structure and function must be destroyed for the individual as a whole to be considered dead for public policy purposes. That would mean that every cell in the body would have to be determined to be dead or at least every organ would have to be destroyed. We know, however, that certain cells—fingernails and hair, for example—continue to grow for hours after what we normally think of as death occurs.

It is also generally held that those with appropriate medical skills are capable of developing tests or procedures or criteria for predicting that a particular bodily function or structure is irreversibly destroyed. For example, if heart function is determined to be important in deciding when to treat people as dead, certain measures, such as feeling the pulse or taking an electrocardiogram, are available to diagnose and predict the future status of heart function. If lower brain functions are determined to be critical, then neurologists tell us that certain reflex pathways are good predictors of the status of the lower brain. If cerebral function is determined to be critical, different tests, based on the electroencephalogram and cerebral angiography, which measures blood flow, can be useful.

The tests or procedures or criteria for determining that critical bodily structures or functions have been lost must be established by those with scientific skills in biology or medicine—that is, those with the appropriate knowledge and skill.[23] These tests or procedures or criteria need not be incorporated into public policy or statutory law. In fact, because empirical measures of this sort are likely to change as the status of our scientific knowledge changes, many take the view that these tests should not be included in the statutory law. As a general rule, statutes that have been passed have not included any reference to any specific empirical measures or criteria.

Technically, it is not correct to treat even these criteria for measuring the death of the brain as purely scientific, completely lacking in evaluative or other public policy importance. For example, in testing to measure the destruction of the brain a judgment must be made about how often these tests are to be applied and for how long a period of time they must be satisfied before pronouncing death. Different sets of criteria propose different lengths of time. The Harvard criteria[24] call for 24 hours, the report of the medical consultants to the president's commission suggests 6 hours or 12 in the absence of confirmatory tests such as an EEG, and other groups have required 12 hours as the minimum time period to be satisfied.[25] If the tests are not applied over a long enough period, some individuals may be declared to have irreversibly lost brain function when, in fact, such function could return. On the other hand, if the tests are applied for too long a period of time, some individuals will be treated temporarily as if brain function has not irreversibly disappeared when, in fact, it has. Deciding on the correct length of time will depend on how one assesses the moral risks of falsely considering the brain to be dead and falsely considering it still to be alive. The best neurological science can do is tell us the probabilities of each kind of error after different time periods. It cannot tell us how to trade off the two kinds of errors. That is fundamentally a moral or policy issue.

If neurologists' intuitions about the relative moral risks of these two kinds of error were the same as others in the society, then little would be at stake in asking the neurologists to pick for the rest of us the balance between the errors. There is reason to doubt, however, that neurologists balance the two kinds of errors the same way that other people do. If they differed significantly—if, for example, they worried more than most people about falsely treating people as alive and less about falsely treating people as dead—then they would systematically recommend the wrong time period for repeating tests. Logically, deciding the mix of the two kinds of errors is not a scientific question; it is a policy question, which lay people ought to decide, even though most of us do not treat it that way.[26]

The Concept of Death: Essentially a Policy Matter

A more obvious policy question is just which structures or functions should be tested, which changes in the body should signal the time when death-related behavior is appropriate? Should it be loss of heart function or brain function? If it is the brain, just which functions are critical? We are attempting to determine when it is appropriate to treat the organism as a whole as dead. The loss of certain essential bodily structures or functions will almost certainly signal the time when such behavior is appropriate. These potential endpoints are normally called the *concepts* or *standards of death*. Picking among them, in principle, cannot be done scientifically. It is essentially a policy matter.

For example, some people take the position that the organism as a whole should be considered dead if there is irreversible cessation of spontaneous respiratory and circulatory functions. Other people take the position that the organism should be considered dead if there is irreversible loss of all spontaneous brain functions. Still others maintain that the organism should be considered dead if there is irreversible loss of certain spontaneous cerebral functions. Behind each of these formulations is some implicit view of what is essential in the human being's nature.

Although society might choose to specify precisely what that philosophical or religious understanding is, that may not be either necessary or even possible. It might turn out that different people would formulate the precise underlying concept somewhat differently but still be able to agree at the level of the standard of death that is to be specified in the law. They might be able to agree that death should be pronounced when the functions of the circulatory and respiratory system are irreversibly lost. Or they might agree that it is the functions of the entire brain that count. They might reach this agreement even though they could not agree what it was about the circulatory system or respiratory system or brain that was so important.

The selection of these basic standards of death is now generally agreed to be a task for the broader public. The only real question is the method that will be used to express public policy. Traditionally, there was such an overwhelming consensus on an apparent concept and standard of death that there was no need for explicit public policy formulation. We relied on the common law and saw very little dispute, except perhaps in questions of inheritance in cases of almost simultaneous death. An example would be an inheritance following the death of spouses in an automobile accident, where a different pattern of inheritance would result if either spouse survived the other.

There is in principle no scientific basis for choosing one set of standards or underlying concepts over another, although once a particular concept or standard is chosen there may be good scientific reasons for selecting a set of criteria or tests or measures that correspond to the standard or concept chosen. This does not necessarily mean, however, that the choice is entirely an arbitrary one. It is possible, in fact it is widely held, that such choices have foundations in objective reality. In deciding to make slavery or murder illegal, for example, there is no scientific proof that either of these activities is wrong. It is not even clear what a scientific proof of such a position would look like. Nevertheless, the society can feel sufficiently sure that slavery and murder are wrong that it can choose to make them illegal without any suggestion that such a decision is arbitrary or capricious. Thus, Henry Beecher, the Harvard physician and chair of the Harvard ad hoc committee, was not speaking precisely when he said that the choice of a definition of death is arbitrary. He probably meant that there is no basis in the natural sciences for making such a choice, although he would, I believe, have conceded that some choices are better than others and some might be so persuasive that it is meaningful to call them the correct choices.

If this is true, then selecting a point when it is appropriate to treat people as dead must be a matter for public policy. In an earlier time the public judgment reflected such a wide consensus that common law was sufficient for expressing that policy judgment. Now, however, when many possible, plausible end points of life have been identified, the public policy question may have to be resolved more explicitly. For this reason many hold that the policy question should be resolved legislatively.[27] Others see it as more appropriately derived from case law—that is, in the courts. The disadvantage of using the courts is that judges deciding many cases will potentially formulate the policy differently.

Still others appear to believe that the policy question can be resolved without any formal expression of policy.[28] Some kind of resolution to the policy question must be reached, however. Deciding what changes in bodily structure or function justify treating an individual as dead is logically before and independent of the question of what tests, measures, or criteria should be used for determining whether those changes have taken place.

There is no need to resolve all of the philosophical problems pertaining to the definition of death to reach a public policy resolution of the question of when people are to be treated as dead. General agreements on the standards may be reached as a matter of public policy, although the philosophical disagreement remains at the most abstract conceptual level.

THE REASON FOR SELECTING A STANDARD FOR DEATH

Some have suggested that a new standard for pronouncing death should be selected because new organs could be available for transplantation and other worthwhile purposes.[29] On reflection, however, others have questioned whether this constitutes an adequate reason for adopting a particular reformulation of the notion of death.[30] Hans Jonas[31] doubts that the interests of others in body parts can be a legitimate basis for deciding when someone has died. Paul Ramsey has expressed similar concern over using the usefulness of organs as a reason for choosing a new definition of death, arguing, "If no person's death should for this purpose be hastened, then the definition of death should not for this purpose be updated. . . ."[32]

Still others have countered, arguing that although it would be wrong to choose a new concept of death for this reason, the new-found potential usefulness to others of being clear on what we mean by being dead might justify the effort at clarification.[33]

The Issues of the Debate Proper

We can now turn to the critical issues in the debate over the definition of death. The first controversy is whether the loss must be irreversible. Next we have to decide whether the critical loss is one of function or one of structure. Then we need to consider whether the loss is at the cellular or the supercellular level.

The Problem of Irreversibility

There are several questions that any public policy over the definition of death must resolve if that public policy is to be clear and complete. One is whether irreversibility is a requirement. The problem is whether we want to speak of people who have temporarily lost some critical body structure or function as dead, even though such functions or structures can be restored and thus the individual would be alive at some point in the future. In the past it has been common in folk discussion of death to talk about someone having died on the operating table or in some other setting, only to be resuscitated and returned to life. This may simply be imprecise use of language, however.[34] Many would hold that irreversibility is inherent in the notion of what it means to be dead.[35] At least for public policy purposes, people who have temporarily lost a critical function like heart function really cannot be thought of as dead. Those mentioned in such an individual's will do not inherit his or her possessions. The president of the United States would not have been removed from office because of such a temporary stoppage. The provisions of the Uniform Anatomical Gift Act giving next of kin authority over the use of organs would not take effect. Irreversibility is an essential requirement for public policies related to treating people as dead.[36] If that is the case, then it is incorrect to talk about people dying temporarily and then coming back to life. Rather, in such cases we can say that the individual continues to live but would have died had not certain critical functions been restored.

Function or Structure

Some recent commentators have argued that the loss that is critical for treating people as dead is not necessarily a functional loss. It may be anatomical. That is, an individual may continue to live until certain anatomical structures are destroyed.[37]

There is no decisive argument for or against such a view. Should a society want to hold that the shape or form of the body is what is critical, rather than its activity, such a policy could be adopted. However, most continue to maintain that the critical loss is a functional one. It may be that those who talk as if the loss is anatomical rather than functional are really just seeking greater certainty of the irreversibility of the functional loss. Such individuals might take the position that what is essential is irreversible functional loss, yet the only empirically certain way to demonstrate irreversible functional loss is by showing anatomical destruction. If so, the anatomical destruction is merely a test or measure or a criterion of irreversible functional loss and probably should not be incorporated into a formally articulated public policy. However, it is possible that some people actually believe that the critical loss is structural, in which case that notion should be made a matter of the public policy formulation.

Cellular versus Higher Levels of Function

The human organism operates at many levels, including cellular and supercellular levels of organization. It is possible to insist that each cell, or at least each cell of a critical organ, be destroyed. After all, as long as one cell remains alive it is possible to say that there is life in the particular tissue or organ. However, many would take the position that mere cellular-level activity is of no significance when it comes to determining when people should be treated as dead. If, for example, one is concerned about the irreversible loss of brain function, one may not really mean the firing of an isolated neuron within the brain but only the organ-level integrated functioning at the supercellular level.

This has potential importance because certain tests or measures may actually indicate the presence of cellular life even though organ-level functioning has irreversibly been lost. For instance, the technical literature pertaining to the use of the electroencephalogram for the measure of the loss of brain function makes clear that what is normally referred to as a flat EEG in fact will still show some activity. It may retain very low microvolt levels of activity. To the uninitiated, it seems certain that if electrical activity is coming from the brain it is not totally dead. If, however, neurologists are able to determine with certainty that particular low levels of activity are really only signs of cellular activity and not consistent with continued capacity for organ-level functioning, it is quite appropriate to exclude such activity if one has adopted a policy of pronouncing death on the basis of the irreversible loss of total brain function at the supercellular level.[38] This appears to be what the legislators in Wyoming had in mind when they passed a statute based on the Uniform Brain Death Act but added the sentence, "Total brain function shall mean purposeful activities of the brain as distinguished from random activity." This still raises the question of what counts as purposeful activity but at least excludes random cellular-level activity. Others make a similar distinction by talking of "integrated"[39] or "clinical"[40] functioning. Recently neurologists have conceded that groups or "nests" of cells may continue to function in brains that are considered "dead."[41] These brains, of course, are not literally dead, but in the opinion of some individuals the remaining functions, even if they are above the cellular level, may be insignificant.[42] The real problem with this position, as we shall see later in the chapter, is that if individuals use their own idiosyncratic judgments to decide what is "insignificant," we can expect countless disputes and personal variations in opinion. We will have abandoned the commitment to the position that literally the whole brain and all its functions must be lost for an individual to be dead.[43]

Which Functions Are Critical?

We are still left with the most fundamental and important public policy question of which functions or structures should be identified as critical for deciding that the individual as a whole should be treated as dead. Several stages have taken place in the debate.

THE LATE 1960s PERIOD

The first stage of the debate began in the late 1960s, especially with the preparation of the Harvard Medical School's ad hoc committee report.[44] At this point, virtually everyone formulated the question in terms of a struggle between two alternatives. One group believed that the critical activity that should be measured is the capacity of the heart and lungs.[45] This seems to be included in the early common law definition of death that says that an individual shall be considered dead when there is "a total stoppage . . . of all animal and vital functions."[46]

Precisely what it was about heart and lung activity that was considered critical is not clear. It seems certain that it was not the functioning of the heart and lungs per se but rather the activities they cause in the body that was thought to be critical. This is made apparent by the recognition that an individual whose lungs have been destroyed but whose blood is oxygenated by a machine is obviously still alive. Likewise, an individual whose heart has been destroyed but whose blood is pumped by a machine would also be considered alive. In fact, an individual who might be maintained indefinitely on a heart–lung machine or artificial heart would obviously be alive according to this formulation. Thus it seems probable that people taking this position hold a concept of death that emphasizes the importance of the flowing of vital bodily fluids—that is, the blood and breath. According to this notion, then, an individual should be considered dead when there is the irreversible loss of the capacity for the flowing of these vital fluids.

This is a rather vitalistic notion of the nature of the human being, one that sees the human as merely physico-chemical forces. It totally excludes any concern for integrated functioning or for mental processes. Yet many have apparently held that anyone who has the capacity for the flowing of these fluids ought to be treated as alive.

During this period the alternative position was that the critical loss that signaled the point at which people ought to be treated as dead was the loss of the capacities of the brain.[47] Defenders of this position were frequently not very precise about exactly what it was in the brain that was considered critical. The empirical measures that were performed implied that the critical functions were quite diverse and inclusive. They included a large number of integrating activities, including reflex pathways in the lower brain as well as the centers that control respiration. Thus it has been suggested that holders of this view might have been taking the position at the conceptual level that people should be treated as dead when they have irreversibly lost the neurological capacity to integrate bodily activities. At this point, according to this view, the individual no longer functions as a whole and can therefore legitimately be treated as dead.

Some people have continued to favor the use of heart- and lung-oriented standards for pronouncing death. Some even explicitly affirm such standards when they are given the alternative of pronouncing death based on the concepts underlying the use of brain-oriented standards.[48] Nevertheless, the defenders of standards related to heart and lung function seem to have decreased substantially.

THE EARLY 1970s PERIOD

In the early 1970s, however, a new and more complicated question emerged—that is, which brain functions (or structures) are so critical that their loss ought to be considered the death of the individual as a whole. Two major camps emerged in this debate. One held fast to the position that all brain function (at least at the supercellular level) must be lost.[49] The second group took the view that some functions, even at the supercellular level, might remain intact, while it would still be appropriate to treat an individual as dead.[50] The choice was presented dramatically in two case reports by Brierley et al. in *The Lancet*.[51]

The first case was that of a 58-year-old man who had suffered cardiac arrest related to bronchospasm. He was resuscitated with cardiac massage and placed on a respirator. The electroencephalogram was flat from day 3 on. He maintained reflexes after day 1 and respired without the aid of the respirator from day 20 on. He died (based on cardiac criteria) after five months.

The second case involved a 48-year-old man who suffered a massive allergic reaction. He was resuscitated with cardiac massage and mouth-to-mouth breathing. He also had reflexes after the first day, but had a flat electroencephalogram from day 2 onward. He also died after five months (based on cardiac criteria). In both cases on examination after death it was found that tissues in the higher brain (neocortex) were dead while lower-brain centers were intact, showing slight to moderate neuronal loss. The patients at no time met the Harvard criteria purported to measure irreversible coma, yet clearly seemed to be irreversibly comatose.[52]

Once these cases are presented, they reveal that there are at least two quite different positions, each reflecting a different concept of death. Those insisting on the destruction of total supercellular brain function would consider these patients alive during the period when they possessed brain reflexes and unaided respiration. They breathed spontaneously. Defenders of this view probably hold fast to a concept that death is something like the irreversible loss of the capacity for bodily integration. They specifically recognize that integrated activities mediated through the lower brain, such as respiratory control mechanisms or the cough reflex, represent a level of bodily integration that would be taken as sufficient to justify treating the individual as still alive.

Others, however, have considered these patients dead. They have abandoned the whole-brain view, making it clear that a very different concept of death is operating. They focus on the activities of the higher-brain centers, including such capacities as remembering, reasoning, feeling, thinking, and the like. One underlying concept of the human's nature that might be implied is that the human is essentially a combination of mental and physical activity, both of which must be present for the individual to be alive. According to this view, a capacity for consciousness would be necessary to treat the individual as alive.

Closely related to this view is a notion having both Greek and Judeo–Christian roots, the notion that the human is essentially a social animal. According to this view, it is appropriate to treat individuals as dead whenever they have irreversibly lost the capacity for social interaction. It is important not to talk about an individual being dead merely because an individual is not interacting socially at a particular time. That would make being dead or alive dependent on the willingness of one's fellow human beings to interact. Rather, what is operating is a concern for a capacity for such interaction.

A standard might be chosen that focuses on higher-brain function rather than total brain function. This standard is often articulated as the irreversible loss of total cerebral or neocortical function. The exact specification would depend on exactly what functional loss was considered crucial and where that function was localized in the brain. There is substantial debate over whether there can be any exact identification between mental functions and brain functions.[53] Possibly we shall never be able to identify precisely which tissues are responsible for the functions often identified, such as consciousness or thinking or feeling and interacting with one's fellow humans. There is general agreement, however, that without cerebral tissue, these functions are all impossible. To the extent that is true empirically, then the standard for death according to a holder of this position would be the irreversible loss of cerebral function. Some, however, are purposely avoiding speaking of cerebral or neocortical definitions of death because they realize that some cerebral or neocortical functions may survive even if the critical functions are completely lost. They are now speaking in purposely vague language of the higher-brain definition of death.[54] For holders of this view, in contrast with the whole-brain standard, quite clearly a different set of empirical measures or tests would be appropriate for confirming death, ones that single out these higher, presumably cerebral functions.

The emergence of the higher-brain-oriented definition of death since the 1970s has been one of the most important theoretical developments in this entire discussion. Although no nation in the world has adopted the higher-brain formulation and it therefore has little practical importance in the clinic for transplantation or any other clinical purposes, it has reshaped our theoretical understanding of what it means to be dead. The development of the higher-brain definition of death will be the subject of Chapter 5.

SINCE THE LATE 1970S

This reformulation of the question so as to ask which brain functions are critical has begun to raise additional questions. For instance, once one has moved to a concept of death based on higher-brain function rather than total brain function, one might appropriately ask whether an individual could be considered dead even though certain higher-brain functions remain intact. If, for example, one retains motor capacities in certain brain centers but has no capacity to feel or think, should such an individual be considered alive? There is no particular reason why this progressive narrowing of the criteria need stop at this point. For instance, one might ask whether an individual could be considered dead solely on the basis of deterioration of mental function even though many higher-brain centers remain intact. It is apparent that one of the dangers of the move from total brain function to higher-brain function is that there may be no obvious and clear point to stop the progression to narrower and narrower formulations. Thus there is the potential that gradually more and more people will literally be defined out of the category of human existence. Some critics of the move to higher-brain function have opposed it not exclusively on the grounds that lower-brain activity is an essential component of life but more on the grounds that once one moves beyond total brain activity it will be impossible to find a point for a public policy at which to stop the regression. They claim that the defenders of the higher-brain positions are on a slippery slope and will not be able to avoid sliding into morally untenable positions that would treat mentally impaired but conscious humans as dead.[55]

Defenders of the move to higher-brain-function notions of death reject this slippery slope or wedge argument.[56] They maintain that it is possible to hold firmly to the notion that an individual should be considered dead when there is loss of consciousness but insist that no compromise be made beyond that point. In fact, I and others who defend the higher-brain formulation have recently begun to turn the slippery slope argument against those who are apparently defending the whole-brain formulations. We argue that there is no principled reason why a line can be drawn between the top of the spinal cord and the base of the brain stem. This means that the defenders of the whole-brain formulations must either acknowledge that activity of the spinal cord should be taken as a sign of life (because it provides integrated nervous system activity not distinguishable from that of the brain stem) or they must concede that some "insignificant" brain functions, even supercellular functions, should be discounted, thus abandoning the true whole-brain position that insists that all functions of the entire brain must be gone for a person to be dead. As we have seen, Bernat and others apparently defending the whole-brain position have done precisely this in conceding that certain functioning of "nests of cells" is "insignificant."[57] They abandon the literal whole-brain definition without providing any principled way of telling which nests of cells are significant. The defenders of the higher-brain position at least offer a basis for distinguishing by insisting that functions are significant that provide integration of mental with organic function.

Still others, including those on the president's commission,[58] may accept the idea in principle that death can be related to the irreversible loss of higher-brain function but believe empirically that there are no solid grounds for measuring such loss. Logically, as a matter of public policy, such people should be willing to adopt a policy that people should be treated as dead when higher-brain function has irreversibly ceased, leaving to those with competent skills in the neurological sciences to determine whether there is any empirical way to measure the mere loss of a higher-brain function. It might turn out empirically that the only reliable test would be one that measures the loss of total brain function. That would seem to be conceptually the correct way to articulate public policy. However, policymakers may be made sufficiently uncomfortable by the possibility of some practitioners prematurely attempting to measure the loss of merely higher-brain function that they would feel it necessary to specify in law that death should be pronounced only when total brain function is lost, even though in principle they would be willing to accept death pronouncement even when certain lower-brain functions remain intact in cases in which all higher function has irreversibly ceased.

The concern about whether irreversible loss of mental function or consciousness can be measured may, in fact, be resolved. At least two major groups have now concluded that, at least in some cases, some irreversible loss of consciousness can be diagnosed with great accuracy.[59]

These practical and theoretical concerns with the attempt to move to a higher-brain-oriented formulation have characterized the debate since the later part of the 1970s. Advocates of higher-brain standards have differed among themselves over exactly which tissues and functions are critical. Other concerns have also emerged, some of which have been mentioned previously. The difference between cellular-level function and more complex function has become increasingly apparent. The tension between those who formulate a concept of death functionally and those who formulate it anatomically has also become recognized. The net effect has been that we have increasingly become aware that there are many different formulations that are plausible and seen as acceptable to different people. It is no longer a debate between two clearly contrasting camps as it was between the heart and the brain seen in the earliest days of the discussion or between the whole brain and higher brain as it was in the early part of the 1970s. It is impossible to reach any consensus on the underlying theological and philosophical issues.

It is probably even impossible to specify clearly what it is about the human that counts as a change so significant that we ought to begin treating that human as if he or she were dead. At best we must come to some common understanding of some general area of bodily structure or function that is so significant that its destruction justifies treating the individual as dead.[60] We may be able to agree that an individual is dead when, say, all brain function is lost even if we cannot agree on exactly what the critical function is.

The question is one that really cannot be taken any further. We must determine what bodily conditions make treating an individual as dead acceptable. It will probably be sufficient to express public policy in terms of general standards for death. Even though those standards have some concept implicit in them, it is clear that greater consensus can be reached on the standards than on the concepts themselves. The three primary candidates are those we have identified: the irreversible cessation of spontaneous respiratory and circulatory functions, the irreversible loss of all spontaneous brain functions, and the irreversible loss of all spontaneous cerebral or higher-brain functions.

The dispute among those holding these positions and the countless variants of the positions has led some of us to conclude that no single whole-brain-oriented concept of death will be able to sustain universal support. Given the countless variations on the three main types of death definitions, there may well be a collapse of the dominant consensus in favor of the whole-brain view. That collapse will be the subject of Chapter 6.

Some Remaining Issues

It is clear that there is and will remain controversy over which of the several plausible concepts or standards for pronouncing death ought to be adopted for public policy. Some standard or combination of standards must be chosen at least for public policy purposes.

Should Safer-Course Arguments Prevail?

This raises the question of whether, as a matter of public policy, we ought not to play it safe and choose the policy that will satisfy the most people that an individual is dead without taking a chance of calling someone dead who really should still be considered alive. Some have argued that when we are in doubt about which of several public policies to adopt, we should take the safer course, especially in matters that are literally life and death. The safer-course argument is presumably the one that will avoid treating people as dead who ought to be considered alive.[61]

This safer-course argument might justify abandoning efforts to incorporate concepts or standards of death related exclusively to higher-brain function because many people hold that an individual can be alive even though higher-brain function is lost. There is real doubt in American society over the use of such a standard for death pronouncement. Under a safer-course argument we would move to the more conservative, now older, definition of death that requires that the whole brain be destroyed.

The problem with this safer-course argument is that we would be even safer and more inclusive were we to insist that not only the whole brain but also the heart and lung activity be irreversibly destroyed. In fact, we would be safer still if we were to insist that not only these functions be destroyed but the anatomical structures as well. If we adopted a position that all heart, lung, and brain function and structure must be destroyed, we would satisfy virtually everyone that an individual is indeed dead before being treated as such.

There are difficulties that now become apparent with the safer-course arguments. If there were no practical or theoretical problems with treating people as alive who are in fact dead, we could safely continue a policy of erring on the side of treating people as alive, but it is clear there are good reasons not to do so. There are bad consequences from treating a dead individual as alive. Some of these consequences are very practical. There are financial costs in medical care as well as human agony. There are organs and tissues that would be lost. None of these concerns about consequences would justify treating someone as dead who was really alive, but they do, at least, justify striving for precision in our social understanding of what it means to be dead. And they give us sufficient reason to avoid the extreme applications of the safer-course arguments. At the very least, this means that we can set some conservative limit on when people ought to be treated as dead. The majority of the population now seems prepared to move at least as far as the whole-brain-oriented formulations—that is, treating people as dead when there has been total destruction of supercellular-level brain function.

Can There Be Variation in the Public Definition of Death?

Because there is such disagreement among members of our society over a definition of death, many have speculated over the difficulties in reaching a policy consensus. In many cases in a pluralistic society, the resolution of this apparent problem is found in pluralism by permitting individual variation based on individual or group preferences. However, the idea of permitting such a variation in the definition of death raises serious problems, each of which should be explored. Three kinds of variation have been considered.

VARIATION BY EXPECTED USE OF THE BODY

First, variation might be based on the expected use of the body. Society could endorse varying definitions of death, depending, in part, on whether the body will be used for transplant, research, therapy, or other important purposes. In fact, the original law passed in the state of Kansas[62] appears to do just that. The Kansas statute includes two alternative definitions of death, one based on respiratory and cardiac function and the other based on brain function. The same alternative definitions appear in the Uniform Determination of Death Act,[63] although that law does not specifically state when a particular definition should be used. The implication, however, is that the latter should be used when transplantation is anticipated and the brain is destroyed and the heart continues to beat (because of mechanical support). Likewise, the new definition of death law in Japan permits the use of a brain-oriented definition of death only when organs are to be procured.

Critics of such a variation argue that it seems that whether one is treated as dead or alive should not be contingent on the anticipated use of the corpse. In fact, one could envision bizarre circumstances were alternative standards permitted. A transplant might be anticipated and death pronounced on that basis. But in the interim before the organ is removed from the newly deceased, the planned recipient dies suddenly, so transplant may no longer be anticipated. Or surgeons may discover that the potential donor had cancer or some other risk that excluded organ procurement. If so, there would be confusion over whether the individual continued to be dead according to the originally relevant definition or should suddenly have the other alternative definition applied for the new circumstance.

VARIATION DEPENDING ON THE PHYSICIAN'S PREFERENCE

Second, there is variation by physicians. The policy question is whether physicians should be required or only permitted to use brain-oriented standards when pronouncing death. Should the physician have the choice of whether to use a brain-oriented definition? As a practical matter, this reduces to the question of whether laws should say that a physician shall pronounce death or that a physician may pronounce death when all functions of the brain are irreversibly lost. A model bill by the American Medical Association (AMA), dated January 1979, says, for example, "A physician, in the exercise of his professional judgment, may declare an individual dead in accordance with accepted medical standards. ..." The immediate bizarre implication is that a physician need not declare an individual dead in accordance with accepted medical standards. He or she might use discretion and choose some other standard. At the very least, this leads to policy confusion. Different physicians seeing the same patient could use different standards for pronouncing death. Thus a physician who sees a patient one afternoon might decide not to use brain-oriented standards, whereas another physician, seeing the patient that evening in exactly the same condition, deciding to use them, could exercise his or her option and pronounce death. In December 1979 at its Interim Meeting the AMA amended its model bill removing the term "may."

In an effort to overcome the ambiguity generated by having several different proposed statutes, the president's commission worked with the AMA, the American Bar Association, and the National Conference of Commissioners on uniform state laws to develop what is referred to as the Uniform Determination of Death Act, which all of these groups have endorsed in place of their previous proposals. It states that:

An individual who has sustained either (1) irreversible cessation of circulatory and respiratory functions, or (2) irreversible cessation of all functions of
the entire brain, including the brain stem, is dead. A determination of
death must be made in accordance with accepted medical standards.[64]

As long as this proposal is interpreted as requiring that death must be
pronounced if either of these conditions is met, there is no problem of variation
from physician to physician. This formulation relies on "accepted medical standards," which, as we have seen, could create a problem if the consensus of the
profession about the relative importance of different types of errors is significantly
different from the consensus of nonprofessionals.

The potential for difficulty is great if variation by physician is permitted.
For example, if standards based on loss of total supercellular brain function are
adopted, but then physicians are given discretion, as in the original AMA model
bill, physicians could presumably opt either for more conservative or more liberal
interpretations. Thus a physician, at his or her discretion, could use traditional
heart and lung standards, higher-brain standards, or even more permissive criteria.
It seems strange that citizens should be considered dead or alive depending on
the preferences of their physician. Many have concluded that such discretion is
not acceptable, that physicians should not be permitted to refrain from pronouncing death in a jurisdiction specifying a whole-brain definition. By the same token
it is an even more serious offense if physicians in the jurisdictions that have not
adopted brain-oriented definition take it on themselves to pronounce death based
on loss of brain function. There is some empirical evidence that physicians have,
in fact, taken it on themselves to use their own standards, pronouncing death
based on brain criteria when states had not authorized such pronouncement.[65]
That was the case with Bruce Tucker, the patient discussed in Chapter 3, who was
apparently pronounced dead based on the individual preference of his physician for
a brain-oriented definition.

In fact individuals with dead brains in the few jurisdictions that have no
legal authorization for death pronouncement based on brain criteria should be
treated as still living. If a patient then really dies (based on heart and lung
function appropriate in that jurisdiction) because treatment stopped because
of erroneous death pronouncement based on brain criteria, a physician might
appropriately be prosecuted for homicide.

VARIATION BASED ON THE PATIENT'S PREFERENCES
Third is the variation based on the views of individual patients or their agents.
There is overwhelming evidence that citizens differ over precisely what standards

should be used for pronouncing death. These differences are rooted in underlying conceptual philosophical and theological differences over the definition of death, having nothing to do with matters requiring knowledge of neurological science. It now seems clear that if any single policy is adopted, some citizens will have their personal convictions about something as basic as the meaning of life and death violated. This suggests that some limited discretion be given to individuals to exercise conscientious objection to a state's chosen definition.

In 1968 M. Martin Halley and William F. Harvey[66] proposed a very early version of a redefinition of death. It contained a provision for pronouncing death apparently using other than cardiac and respiratory standards in "special circumstances" provided that "valid consent" has been given by the appropriate relative or legal guardian. They were criticized for the consent requirement on the grounds that they had apparently made the state of being dead contingent on consent when critics thought they must have intended to make only the withholding of treatment from a dying person dependent on consent.[67]

It does appear that Halley and Harvey had confused two quite different questions. Certainly it is more obvious that decisions to withhold treatment might be contingent on patient or guardian consent. Yet a case can be made that even the choice of a standard for pronouncing death could incorporate discretion of the individual or his or her legal agent. What is at stake is not whether a person's heart or brain has lost function. That presumably is a fact independent of the views of the individual or others. The question is when the person should be treated as dead—that is, when death behaviors become appropriate. Some limited discretion could be given to the individual or others in answering that question. Whether it should be given is, of course, another question.

It seems bizarre that the definition of death should be left to such individual discretion. We have always considered death to be an objective fact. For policy purposes, however, we are not interested in biological, or even in philosophical or theological, formulations, but rather the much more practical question of when people ought to be treated as dead.[68] That clearly is an evaluative question where traditionally individual discretion has been tolerated within limits. The mechanics of tolerating such limited objections or basic philosophical concerns may make the option of permitting variations seem unfeasible to some,[69] yet the alternative of insisting that all operate under the same uniform definition of death regardless of their most deeply held religious and philosophical beliefs is also alien to the American tradition. Although the president's commission recommended adopting the Uniform Determination of Death Act in all jurisdictions in the United States and specifically rejected a "conscience clause" permitting an individual (or family member where the individual is incompetent) to specify the standard to be used for determining death, it also urged ". . . those acting under the statute to apply it with sensitivity to the emotional and religious needs of those for whom the new standards mark a departure from traditional practice," implying possible physician variation in selecting standards.[70] A proposal for a conscience clause permitting limited choice of alternative definitions of death will be the subject of Chapter 7.

Conclusion

The public policy issues raised by the definition of death are more complex than they appear. There is a growing consensus that some form of brain-oriented definition fits the religious and philosophical convictions of the majority of the population, at least of Western societies. But there is growing doubt about the present whole-brain-oriented definition that requires that literally all functions of the entire brain must be lost before death is pronounced. A minority holds religious convictions that support the traditional heart-oriented definition, whereas others favor some form of a newer higher-brain-oriented definition. The choice among the alternative definitions is fundamentally a religious or philosophical one based on personally held beliefs and values. It is for that reason that the dispute is likely to continue.

ENDNOTES

1. David Sell, "Flyers Goalie Lindbergh Is Declared Brain Dead," *Washington Post*, Nov. 11, 1985, pp. D1, D13.

2. Lawrence C. Becker, "Human Being: The Boundaries of the Concept," *Philosophy and Public Affairs* 4 (1975): 334–59; David J. Cole, "The Reversibility of Death," *Journal of Medical Ethics* 18 (1992): 26–30; Michael B. Green and Daniel Wikler, "Brain Death and Personal Identity," *Philosophy and Public Affairs* 9 (2, 1980): 105–33; David Lamb, "Diagnosing Death," *Philosophy and Public Affairs* 7 (1980): 144–53; David Mayo and Daniel I. Wikler, "Euthanasia and the Transition from Life to Death," in *Medical Responsibility: Paternalism, Informed Consent, and Euthanasia*, ed. Wade Robinson and Michael S. Pritchard (Clifton, NJ: Humane Press, 1979); Robert M. Veatch, *Death, Dying, and the Biological Revolution*, rev ed. (New Haven, CT: Yale University Press, 1989); Veatch, "The Definition of Death: Unresolved Controversies," in *Pediatric Brain Death and Organ/Tissue Retrieval*, ed. Howard H. Kaufman (New York: Plenum, 1989), pp. 207–18.; Daniel Wikler and Alan J. Weisbard, "Appropriate Confusion over 'Brain Death,' " *Journal of the American Medical Association* 261 (15, April 21, 1989): 2246; Stuart J. Youngner, C. Seth Landefeld, Claudia J. Coulton, Barbara W. Juknialis, and Mark Leary, " 'Brain Death' and Organ Retrieval," *Journal of the American Medical Association* 261 (15, April 21, 1989): 2205–10.

3. David J. Bleich, "Neurological Criteria of Death and Time of Death Status," in *Jewish Bioethics*, ed. J. David Bleich and Fred Rosner (New York: Sanhedrin Press, 1979), pp. 303–16; Bleich, "Of Cerebral, Respiratory, and Cardiac Death," *Tradition: A Journal of Orthodox Jewish Thought* 24 (3, 1989): 44–66; John Fletcher, "Our Shameful Waste of Human Tissue," in *Updating Life and Death*, ed. Donald R. Cutler (Boston: Beacon Press, 1969), pp. 1–27; Bernard Haring, *Medical Ethics* (Notre Dame, IN: Fides Press, 1973); Stanley Hauerwas, "Religious Concepts of Brain Death and Associated Problems," in *Brain Death: Interrelated Medical and Social Issues*, ed. Julius Korein (New York: New York Academy of Sciences, 1978), pp. 329–38; Pope Pius XII, "The Prolongation of Life: An Address of Pope Pius XII to An International Congress of Anesthesiologists," *The Pope Speaks* 4 (1958): 393–98; Paul Ramsey, *The Patient as Person* (New Haven, CT: Yale University Press, 1970), pp. 59–164.

4. Michael B. Green and Daniel Wikler, "Brain Death and Personal Identity"; cf. Karen Grandstand Gervais, *Redefining Death* (New Haven, CT: Yale University Press, 1986).

5. Stephen Ashwal and Sanford Schneider, "Brain Death in Children, I, II," *Pediatric Neurology* 3 (1987): 5–10, 69–78; P. M. Black, "Brain Death," *New England Journal of Medicine* 299 (1978): 338–44, 393–401; Collaborative Study, "An Appraisal of the Criteria of Cerebral Death—A Summary Statement," *Journal of the American Medical Association* 237 (1977): 982–86; R. Cranford, "Uniform Brain Death Act," *Neurology* 29 (1979): 417–18; Harvard Medical School, "A Definition of Irreversible Coma: Report of the Ad Hoc Committee of the Harvard Medical School to Examine the Definition of Brain Death," *Journal of the American Medical Association* 205 (1968): 337–40; M. D. O'Brien, "Criteria for Diagnosing Brain Stem Death," *British Medical Journal* 301 (July 14, 1990): 108–09; Report of the Medical Consultants on the Diagnosis of Death to the President's Commission for the Study of Ethical Problems in Medicine and Biomedical and Behavioral Research, *Defining Death: Medical, Legal and Ethical Issues in the Definition of Death* (Washington, DC: U.S. Government Printing Office, 1981); D. Alan Shewmon, "Commentary on Guidelines for the Determination of Brain Death in Children," *Annals of Neurology* 24 (1988): 789–91; Task Force for the Determination of Brain Death in Children, "Guidelines for the Determination of Brain Death in Children," *Neurology* 37 (1987): 1077–78.

6. Bernard Haring, *Medical Ethics*; Paul Ramsey, *The Patient as Person*, pp. 59–164.

7. Robert Fulton and Julius Fulton, "Anticipatory Grief: A Psychosocial Aspect of Terminal Care," in *Psychosocial Aspects of Terminal Care*, ed. Bernard Schoenberg, Arthur C. Carr, David Peretz, and Austin H. Kutscher (New York: Columbia University Press, 1972), pp. 227–42.

8. C. H. Fellner, "Selection of Living Kidney Donors and the Problem of Informed Consent," *Seminars in Psychiatry* 3 (1971): 70–85; John Mahoney, "Ethical Aspects of Donor Consent in Transplantation," *Journal of Medical Ethics* 1 (1975): 67–70; John A. Robertson, "Organ Donations by Incompetents and the Substituted Judgment Doctrine," *Columbia Law Review* 3 (1976): 48 ff.; Roberta G. Simmons and Julius Fulton, "Ethical Issues in Kidney Transplantation," *Omega* 2 (1971): 179–90.

9. William F. May, "Attitudes toward the Newly Dead," *Hastings Center Studies* 1 (1, 1973): 3–13.

10. In 1979 efforts surfaced in Britain to circumvent the requirement that next of kin give permission for removal of organs by means of the device of claiming that the health authorities are normally in possession of a dead body until such time as it is claimed by the person with the right to possession of it. This would, in principle, open the door for "donation" by health authorities. The British law requires that such a person must have no reason to believe that the spouse or any surviving relative objects, having made "reasonable enquiry as may be practicable." A British Working Party has implied that this may not be a serious restraint since they emphasize that, "The designated person's duty is only to make such reasonable enquiry as may be practicable." They point out that, "if a donor's relatives are found to be inaccessible it would be impracticable to ask them." The American discussion has not progressed to this point in looking for ways of excluding the next of kin and other family members from the decision to donate. Should the British recommendation be incorporated into law, Britain would have moved some distance away from the donation of organs in the direction of a policy based on salvaging. See *Removal of Cadaveric Organs for Transplantation: A Code of Practice*. Report of a Working Party set up by the United Kingdom Health Department under chairmanship of Lord Smith of Marlow, 1979; Robert M. Veatch, *Death, Dying, and the Biological Revolution* (New Haven, CT: Yale University Press, 1976); and Paul Ramsey, *The Patient as Person* (New Haven, CT: Yale University Press, 1970).

11. Amir Halevy and Baruch Brody, "Brain Death: Reconciling Definitions, Criteria, and Tests," *Annals of Internal Medicine* 119 (6, 1993): 519–25; Robert D. Truog, "Is It Time to Abandon Brain Death?" *Hastings Center Report* 27 (1, 1997 Jan.–Feb.): 29–37.

12. Robert Morison, "Death—Process of Event?" *Science* 173 (1971): 694–98.

13. Leon Kass, "Death As An Event: A Commentary on Robert Morison," *Science* 173 (1971): 698–702.

14. M. B. Green and Daniel Wikler, "Brain Death and Personal Identity"; Michael Tooley, "Decisions to Terminate Life and the Concept of Person," in *Ethical Issues*

Relating to Life and Death, ed. John Ladd (New York: Oxford University Press, 1979), pp. 62–93.

15. Ibid.

16. Harvard Medical School, "A Definition of Irreversible Coma, Report of the Ad Hoc Committee of the Harvard Medical School to Examine the Definition of Brain Death," *Journal of the American Medical Association* 205 (1968): 337–40.

17. Ibid., p. 337.

18. Joseph F. Sullivan, "Lawyer Outlines Arguments He'll Use in Coma Case," *New York Times*, October 3, 1975, p. 39.

19. S. Saperstein, "Maryland Law on Brain Death Was Unclear to Jurors," *Washington Post*, March 22, 1979, pp. C1, C13.

20. James L. Bernat, "The Boundaries of the Persistent Vegetative State," *Journal of Clinical Ethics* 3 (Fall 1992): 176–80; Council on Scientific Affairs and Council on Ethical and Judicial Affairs, "Persistent Vegetative State and the Decision to Withdraw or Withhold Life Support," *Journal of the American Medical Association* 263 (1990): 426–30; R. Donald Cranford and Harmon L. Smith, "Some Critical Distinctions between Brain Death and the Persistent Vegetative State," *Ethics in Science and Medicine* 6 (4, 1979): 199–209; Bryan Jennett and F. Plum, "Persistent Vegetative State after Brain Damage," *Lancet* 1 (1972): 734–37; D. E. Levy, R. P. Knill-Jones, and F. Plum, "The Vegetative State and Its Prognosis Following Non-traumatic Coma," in *Brain Death: Interrelated Medical and Social Issues*, ed. Julius Korein (New York: New York Academy of Sciences, 1978), pp. 293–304.

21. *In re Quinlan*, 70 N.J. 10, 355 A.2d 647 (1976); Julius Korein, "Terminology, Definitions, and Usage," in *Brain Death: Interrelated Medical and Social Issues* (New York: New York Academy of Sciences, 1978), 6–10; Korein, "Editor's Comment," *Brain Death: Interrelated Medical and Social Issues*, pp. 320–21.

22. Gunner Biorck, "On the Definition of Death," *World Medical Journal* 14 (1967): 137–39.

23. Alexander M. Capron and Leon Kass, "A Statutory Definition of the Standards for Determining Human Death: An Appraisal and a Proposal," *University of Pennsylvania Law Review* 121 (1972): 87–118; President's Commission for the Study of Ethical Problems in Medicine and Biomedical and Behavioral Research, *Defining Death: Medical, Legal and Ethical Issues in the Definition of Death* (Washington, DC: U.S. Government Printing Office, 1981); Robert M. Veatch, *Death, Dying and the Biological Revolution*.

24. Harvard Medical School, "A Definition of Irreversible Coma."

25. A. Mohandas and Shelley N. Chou, "Brain Death: A Clinical and Pathological Study," *Journal of Neurosurgery* 35 (Aug. 1971): 211–18.

26. Robert M. Veatch, *Death, Dying, and the Biological Revolution*, pp. 43–44.

27. Don Harper Mills, "The Kansas Death Statute: Bold and Innovative," *New England Journal of Medicine* 285 (1971): 968–69; D. R. Richardson, "A Matter of Life and Death: A Definition of Death: Judicial Resolution of a Medical Responsibility," *Harvard Law Journal* 19 (1976): 138–48; P. D. G. Skegg, "Case for a Statutory 'Definition of Death,'" *Journal of Medical Ethics* 2 (1976): 190–92.

28. David A. Frenkel, "Establishing the Cessation of Life," *Legal Medical Quarterly* 2 (3, 1978): 162–68; C. Anthony Friloux, "Death? When Does It Occur?" *Baylor Law Review* 27 (1975): 10–21; Ian M. Kennedy, "The Kansas State Statute on Death—An Appraisal," *New England Journal of Medicine* 285 (17, 1971): 946–49; Kennedy, "A Legal Perspective on Determining Death," *The Month* 8 (1975): 46–51; Kennedy, "The Definition of Death," *Journal of Medical Ethics* 3 (1977): 5–6; John F. Mackert, "Should the Law Define Brain Death?" *Hospital Progress* 60 (3, 1979): 6 ff.; Ralph B. Potter, "The Paradoxical Preservation of a Principle," *Villanova Law Review* 13 (Summer 1968): 784–92.

29. John Fletcher, "Our Shameful Waste of Human Tissue," pp. 1–27.

30. A. C. Forrester, "Brain Death and the Donation of Cadaver Kidneys," *Health Bulletin* 34 (1976): 199–204.

31. Hans Jonas, "Against the Stream: Comments on the Definition and Redefinition of Death," in his *Philosophical Essays: From Ancient Creed to Technological Man* (Englewood Cliffs, NJ: Prentice-Hall, 1974), pp. 132–40.

32. Paul Ramsey, *The Patient as Person*, p. 103

33. Robert M. Veatch, *Death, Dying and the Biological Revolution*, pp. 33–34.

34. See David J. Cole, "The Reversibility of Death," for a philosophical argument to the contrary.

35. David Lamb, "Reversibility and Death: A Reply to David Cole," *Journal of Medical Ethics* 18 (March 1992): 31–33.

36. John Ladd, "The Definition of Death and the Right to Die," in *Ethical Issues Relating to Life and Death*, ed. John Ladd (New York: Oxford University Press, 1979), pp. 118–45.

37. Lawrence C. Becker, "Human Being: The Boundaries of the Concept"; S. O'Reilly and P. M. Quay, "Brain Death: An Opposing Viewpoint," *Journal of the American Medical Association* 242 (1979): 1985–90.

38. Collaborative Study, "An Appraisal of the Criteria of Cerebral Death—A Summary Statement."

39. Ake Grenvik, D. J. Pawner, James V. Snyder, M. S. Jastremski, R. A. Babcock, and M. G. Loughhead, "Cessation of Therapy in Terminal Illness and Brain Death," *Critical Care Medicine 1978*, 6 (1978): 284–91.

40. Ibid.

41. James L. Bernat, "How Much of the Brain Must Die on Brain Death?" *Journal of Clinical Ethics* 3 (1, Spring 1992): 21–26.

42. Ibid.

43. Robert M. Veatch, "Brain Death and Slippery Slopes," *Journal of Clinical Ethics* 3 (3, Fall 1992): 181–87.

44. Harvard Medical School, "A Definition of Irreversible Coma. Report of the Ad Hoc Committee of the Harvard Medical School to Examine the Definition of Brain Death."

45. Hans Jonas, "Philosophical Reflections on Experimenting with Human Subjects," *Daedalus* 98 (Spring 1969): 243–45; R. B. Potter, "The Paradoxical Preservation of a Principle," *Villanova Law Review* 13 (Summer 1968): 784–92.

46. *Black's Law Dictionary*, 4th ed., rev. (St. Paul, MN: West, 1968), p. 488.

47. Henry K. Beecher, "The New Definition of Death, Some Opposing Views," paper presented at the meeting of the American Association for the Advancement of Science, Chicago, IL, 1970; Vincent Collins, "Considerations in Defining Death," *Linacre Quarterly* (May 1971): 94–101; John Fletcher, "Our Shameful Waste of Human Tissue"; Task Force on Death and Dying, Institute of Society, Ethics and the Life Sciences, "Refinements in Criteria for the Determination of Death: An Appraisal" *Journal of the American Medical Association* 221 (1972): 48–53; James F. Toole, "The Neurologist and the Concept of Brain Death," *Perspectives in Biology and Medicine* 14 (1971): 599–607; Carl E. Wasmuth, "The Concept of Death," *Ohio State Law Journal* 30 (1969): 32–60.

48. Robert M. Arnold and Stuart J. Youngner, "Ethical, Psychological, and Public Policy Implications of Procuring Organs from Non-Heart-Beating Cadavers," *Kennedy Institute of Ethics Journal* (Special Issue 3, 1993): 103–278; William C. Charron, "Death: A Philosophical Perspective on the Legal Definitions," *Washington University Law Quarterly* 4 (1975): 979–1008.

49. Peter M. Black, "Three Definitions of Death," *The Monist* 60 (1, 1977): 136–46; Dennis J. Horan, "Euthanasia and Brain Death: Ethical and Legal Considerations," *Linacre Quarterly* 45 (3, 1978): 284–96; "Diagnosis of Death," *Lancet* 1 (1, 8110): 261–62; D. L. Stickel, "The Brain Death Criterion of Human Death," *Ethics in Science and Medicine* 6 (Winter 1979): 177–97.

50. Bernard Haring, *Medical Ethics* (Notre Dame, IN: Fides Press, 1973), pp. 131–36; Robert M. Veatch, "The Whole-Brain-Oriented Concept of Death: An Outmoded Philosophical Formulation," *Journal of Thanatology* 3 (1975): 13–30; S. D. Olinger, "Medical Death," *Baylor Law Review* 27 (Winter 1975): 22–26; William H. Sweet, "Brain Death," *New England Journal of Medicine* 299 (1978): 410–11.

51. J. B. Brierley, J. A. H. Adam, D. I. Graham, and J. A. Simpson, "Neocortical Death After Cardiac Arrest," *Lancet* (Sept. 11, 1971): 560–65.

52. Van Till d'Aulnis de Bourouill, Adrienne. "How Dead Can You Be?" *Medical Science Law* 15 (1975): 133–47.

53. John C. Burnham, "The Mind-Body Problem in the Early Twentieth Century," *Perspectives in Biology and Medicine* 20 (2, 1977): 271–84; H. Feigl, *The "Mental" and the "Physical"* (Minneapolis: University of Minnesota Press, 1967); G. G. Globus, "Consciousness and Brain I: The Identity Thesis," *Archives of General Psychiatry* 29 (1973): 153 ff.; David L. Wilson, "On the Nature of Consciousness and of Physical Reality," *Perspectives in Biology and Medicine* 19 (1976): 569 ff.

54. Robert M. Veatch, "Whole-Brain, Neocortical, and Higher Brain Related Concepts" in *Death: Beyond Whole-Brain Criteria*, ed. Richard M. Zaner (Dordrecht, Holland: D. Reidel, 1988), pp. 171–86.

55. James L. Bernat, "How Much of the Brain Must Die on Brain Death?"

56. Robert M. Veatch, "Brain Death and Slippery Slopes."

57. James L. Bernat, "How Much of the Brain Must Die on Brain Death?"

58. "Report of the Medical Consultants on the Diagnosis of Death to the President's Commission for the Study of Ethical Problems in Medicine and Biomedical and Behavioral Research," President's Commission for the Study of Ethical Problems in Medicine and Biomedical and Behavioral Research. *Defining Death: Medical, Legal and Ethical Issues in the Definition of Death* (Washington, DC: U.S. Government Printing Office, 1981), pp. 159–66.

59. Ibid; Council on Scientific Affairs and Council on Ethical and Judicial Affairs. "Persistent Vegetative State and the Decision to Withdraw or Withhold Life Support," *Journal of the American Medical Association* 263 (1990): 426–30.

60. Robert M. Veatch, "The Definition of Death: Ethical, Philosophical, and Policy Confusion," in *Brain Death: Interrelated Medical and Social Issues*, ed. Julius Korein (New York: New York Academy of Sciences, 1978), pp. 307–21.

61. B. Currie, "The Redefinition of Death," in *Organism, Medicine and Metaphysics*, ed. S. F. Spicker (Boston: D. Reidel, 1978), pp. 177–97; Hans Jonas, "Philosophical Reflections on Experimenting with Human Subjects," *Daedalus* 98 (Spring 1969): 244.

62. Kansas State Ann. 77-202 (Supp. 1974).

63. President's Commission for the Study of Ethical Problems in Medicine and Biomedical and Behavioral Research. *Defining Death: Medical, Legal and Ethical Issues in the Definition of Death* (Washington, DC: U.S. Government Printing Office, 1981), p. 2.

64. Ibid.

65. Peter M. Black and Nicholas T. Zervas, "Declaration of Brain Death in Neurosurgical and Neurosurgical Practice," *Neurosurgery* 15 (Aug. 1984): 170–74.

66. M. Martin Halley and William F. Harvey, "Medical and Legal Definitions of Death," *Journal of the American Medical Association* 204 (1968): 423–25.

67. Alexander M. Capron and Leon Kass, "A Statutory Definition of the Standards for Determining Human Death: An Appraisal and a Proposal," *University of Pennsylvania Law Review* 121 (1972): 87–118.

68. John Ladd, "The Definition of Death and the Right to Die," In *Ethical Issues Relating to Life and Death*, ed. John Ladd (New York: Oxford University Press, 1979), pp. 118–45.

69. Paul Ramsey, *Ethics at the Edges of Life* (New Haven, CT: Yale University Press, 1978).

70. S. D. Olinger, "Medical Death"; President's Commission for the Study of Ethical Problems in Medicine and Biomedical and Behavioral Research. *Defining Death: Medical, Legal and Ethical Issues in the Definition of Death* (Washington, DC: U.S. Government Printing Office, 1981), p. 43.

FIVE

THE WHOLE-BRAIN-ORIENTED CONCEPT OF DEATH: AN OUTMODED PHILOSOPHICAL FORMULATION

DEBATE OVER THE past 25 years between holders of concepts of death that focus on the brain and those with the more traditional focus on the heart and lungs has created a situation wherein defenders of the neurological concepts of death have not been forced to be particularly precise in specifying the meaning of terms. The seemingly endless prolongation of cellular and organ functioning (in what can be appropriately called *human corpses)* has been brought about by new death-assaulting technologies giving rise to a new and inhuman form of existence. Although the potential for use of human organs for therapeutic transplantation should never justify adopting a new understanding of what is essentially significant to human life and death, it may require a philosophically responsible clarification of imprecise use of these terms adequate only in a time when little that was morally critical was at stake. These developments have led to an infatuation with the neurologically oriented concepts, which have made the more traditional heart-and-lung definition of death appear totally inadequate and outmoded. The thesis of this chapter, however, is that the time has come when crude formulations of the so-called "brain definition of death" can no longer be tolerated.

Holders of the brain-oriented concept of death would probably grant that the only practical problem with the more traditional concept, which focuses on the heart and lungs, is that it will in special occasions produce false-positive tests for human life. In these rare cases, individuals who should be considered dead are labeled alive because heart and lung functions continue even though brain function may have permanently and irreversibly ceased. Traditional moralists, however, or at least those who tend to hold a more rigorous, life-preserving position regarding moral obligation to an individual human being, have followed the principle of erring in the direction of following the morally safer course. Thus

Hans Jonas[1] has argued that unless one can be certain of philosophical foundations (technical uncertainty is not being considered here) of the more limited brain-oriented concept, one should opt for the false-positive judgment of continuing life rather than running the moral risk of a false-positive pronouncement of death.

The holders of the brain-oriented concept, however, have apparently satisfied themselves that there is no significant risk of making the philosophical mistake of considering an individual dead because his or her brain function has ceased when, in fact, the correct moral judgment would be that the individual is still alive, although brain function has irreversibly ceased.

This chapter attempts to turn the tables on the holders of the concept of death that focuses on the function of the whole brain and asks them precisely the same question that they have put to holders of the more traditional heart-and-lung-oriented concepts. Because they have opted for a system that would eliminate the rare false-positive pronouncement of life, I consider it fair to ask whether the whole-brain concept of death might also lead to conditions in which there would be a false-positive judgment that life continues. Is it then possible that there could be a condition wherein portions of the brain retain their normal functioning and yet for all practical purposes the individual should, according to our philosophical understanding of the nature of the human, be pronounced dead? In this chapter I argue that this indeed is the case, that our concept or standard of death must be further refined, and our technical criteria for death must be modified accordingly so that our concept and criteria most accurately reflect our understanding of what is essentially significant to the nature of humans.

Preliminary Philosophical Assumptions

Before turning to an assessment of the brain-based definition of death itself, I need to make clear that my main focus is on the concept of death (not the criteria) and that any discussion will be in the context of a formal definition of death that can be stated in very general terms.

The Concept of Death as a Philosophical Rather Than a Technical–Medical Issue

To make the argument of this chapter, it will be necessary to assume a great deal of the debate about the definition of death that has taken place over the past 25 years. The first major document in this debate was the report of the Ad Hoc Committee of the Harvard Medical School to Examine the Definition of Brain Death.[2] It is crucial for philosophical understanding of this debate to realize that this committee did not in any sense offer a new definition of death or even a new definition of brain death. It merely offered, as the title of the report states, criteria for irreversible coma. In no place in the committee's report did the formulators argue that irreversible coma measured by the criteria it presented is to be equated with brain death and, in turn, that brain death is to be equated with death of the whole human being. In 1968 the distinction between the technical measures of the irreversible loss of a body function and the much more philosophical or moral judgment about the nature of life and death was not clear. This distinction has been made increasingly clear over the years that followed. I have argued previously[3] that the criteria for loss of a body function must be kept radically separate from the philosophical argumentation. This distinction is also emphasized in a report of the Task Force on Death and Dying of the Institute of Society, Ethics and the Life Sciences, which reviewed the Harvard criteria for death[4] (1972). In this chapter, as in the previous one, I shall keep this distinction clear by using the term *concept* or *standard* when referring to a philosophical understanding of that which is essentially significant to a human's nature and by using the term *criteria* in reference to technical measures of the capacity of a body organ or organ system to function. It should be clear that the validity of a "concept" is to be tested philosophically, whereas "criteria" are to be verified by the empirical methods of biomedical science.

Death Formally Defined as Irreversible Loss of That Which Is Considered to Be Essentially Significant to the Nature of Humans

The distinction between the technical measures of criteria for loss of a body function and the philosophical argumentation needed for a concept of death can be seen if one begins with a completely formal definition of death. I propose such a formal definition:

> Death is the irreversible loss of that which is essentially significant to the nature of humans.

Death, as the term is used in the present debate, is not in any sense a biological statement of cessation of cellular respiration or functioning, as the term might be used in referring to the death of a plant or nonhuman animal. When we say that an amoeba has died, we mean that cellular respiration has ceased or mobility of the cellular protoplasm has ceased—and nothing more. When we speak of human death, however, we mean something radically different. We are making a practical statement with policy implications. We are saying that it is now appropriate to behave toward the individual in a different way, what in the previous chapters we called "death behaviors." Human death is a social and moral concept quite beyond the biological. It may still be appropriate to talk about the death of an individual's cells or even an organ in the more narrow biological sense, but the only reason the definition of death receives any attention at all in the realm of public policy is that the term summarizes and legitimates these "death behaviors," a radically different set of social relationships and actions.

The formal definition of death given here reveals that that formal definition can be given substantive content only by further philosophical analysis. It is necessary to reach some understanding about what is essentially significant to the nature of the human. This can never be determined by biological investigation but only by philosophical or theological reflection.

The Difficult Case for a Brain-Oriented Concept of Death

Before offering criticism of the whole-brain-oriented concept of death and a proposal for refinements that I feel are necessary, I shall first explore some preliminary arguments pertaining to adopting any concept of death that is brain oriented. It is apparent that it is only with difficulty and only by very careful statement of our precise meaning that we are able to justify adoption of any brain-oriented concept. First, I shall deal with the problem of moral doubt, second with the distinction between the death of the whole human being and the death of the brain, and third, I shall examine candidates for a concept of death that would give substantive content to the formal definition I have offered.

The Problem of Moral Doubt

The reason why a brain-oriented concept of death is replacing the more traditional heart-and-lung-oriented concept is that focus on the heart and lungs produces what must be called false-positive diagnosis of the presence of human life. Advocates of the brain-oriented concept, however, must deal with the traditional principles for resolving moral doubt. If there is uncertainty about whether a course of action is acceptable, there are several principles for resolving this doubt. One view (sometimes termed *tutiorism*) holds that it is never right to perform an action for which there is some reason to think it may perhaps be wrong. A less rigorous position for resolving doubt (called *probabiliorism*) holds that an action may be performed only if arguments in favor of its being legitimate are more probable than the arguments against.

In regard to moral doubt about whether a human with heart and lung but no brain function may morally be treated as dead, many people would plausibly argue that there is sufficient doubt to require taking the safer course and treating the human as if he or she were living. Certainly, this would be the position of the tutiorist and, conceivably, of the probabilist. Even for the probabilist (i.e., for one who considers a probable moral opinion as justifying an action even though another course of action is as probable or more probable), there are special cases of exclusion for which the safer course is required. One of these cases is that in which a life may be saved when the safer course is taken. Thus even for the probabilist, in the case of deciding whether to treat a being with heart and lung but no brain function as if he or she were dead, there is a strong moral tradition that would support opting for the safer course.

The problem with this method of handling moral doubt is that it tends to assume that only one of two courses of action will lead to morally wrong behavior. In the case of determining whether or not human life exists, however, it appears that immoral behavior results when either of the two concepts of death is incorrectly chosen. If the patient is really alive in the absence of brain activity and is pronounced dead, the more obvious moral infringement occurs: A human life might be terminated improperly. However, we must also consider that there will be moral infringement if a patient who should be considered dead is considered living. There are two problems with the false-positive diagnosis of human living. The first must be the more significant—it is simply an immoral assault on human dignity to treat a corpse as if it were living. It is a moral infringement to fail to distinguish between a living individual and a formerly living individual, who should now be appropriately treated as a corpse. To fail to recognize that the essential qualities of humanness have left an individual is a serious assault on the dignity of humans. To treat an individual who has lost that which is essential to human life as if he or she still had it is to say about that individual and about humanity in general that we fail to perceive the essential dignity and humanness of life.

There is another consideration as well. This is clearly of secondary moral significance, but nevertheless must be introduced. This is the harm done to others by treating a human corpse as if it were still a living human being. The introduction of social, economic, and political considerations into decisions about the treatment of the individual patient is a dangerous act and violates the traditional Hippocratic maxim that the medical obligation is to seek only the benefit of the patient. To compromise patient care for social, economic, or political purposes is a basic violation. If the body before us, however, is a corpse and we continue to treat it as if it were a living being, we are compromising the welfare of others with no benefit to the patient whatsoever. Equipment and space are wasted; resources are squandered. This is true independent of the introduction of the dramatic and over-publicized consideration of the possible use of body parts for transplantation. To change our concept of death for the benefit of the family or to provide organs for transplant is clearly a moral outrage. To fail to clarify our concept of death simply through philosophical laziness is equally outrageous, however, if the result is harm to the dignity of the patient or harm to the welfare of others. To fail to provide help to others when the individual patient has absolutely nothing further to gain is simply irresponsible.

The implication of these arguments is that if there is moral doubt about the concept of death, it is a case in which the conscience is truly perplexed.

There are good reasons to anticipate that there will be moral wrong in either case, whether the action be treating living individuals as if they were corpses or treating corpses as if they were living beings. For some, this will be seen as sufficient reason for abandoning the now no-longer "safer course" of treating the patient with heart and lung function but no brain function as if he or she were living. However, for those persuaded of the necessity of excluding life-risking actions from the general principles for handling cases of doubt, even these arguments based on the probability of wrong from treating the corpse as if it were human may not be persuasive. Thus the movement to a brain-oriented concept of death from the more conservative concept is a difficult case at best. Those who make such a choice do not do so without moral risk.

The Death of the Whole Being and the Death of the Brain

It is also difficult to make the case for "brain death" for another reason. The term *brain death* suggests that only the brain dies, not the whole organism. Yet it should be clear that it is the entire human being who dies. The behavior of others changes vis-à-vis the entire human and not just the brain, although the brain may be the criterion by which the moral status of the entire individual is assessed. Although this might seem to be only a technical distinction, the point is philosophically important in rejecting arguments about death being arbitrary or a continual process.[5] It avoids the notion that there are many different human deaths—of cells and organs and organ systems. In the early days of the definition of death debate the case was argued forcefully by High.[6]

We no longer can accept imprecise uses, especially when these imprecise uses give rise to the compartmentalizing of the human into a number of isolated organ systems and functions. It is the human as a whole who dies, and our language must reflect this, especially at times when we are trying to be precise. Thus we may speak of a "brain-oriented" concept of death, but if this indicates only the death of a whole individual by loss of bodily function that (according to our current empirical understanding of the body) has an anatomical locus in the brain, we should not use the term *brain death*. That term implies it is simply the brain that is dying, not the individual as a whole.

Candidates for a Concept of Death

We saw in the previous chapter that several definitions might specify what is essentially significant to the nature of the human such that its loss should appropriately be called death. Traditional religious thought in the Western world characterized death as the departure of the soul. This traditional religious notion of death was gradually replaced by the modern concept of death, which was oriented to the irreversible loss of the ability of the body to maintain the flowing of vital body fluids—in other words, the blood and breath.

Against these more traditional understandings of death, contemporary intellectual thinkers posed a concept of death that focuses on humans and has a neurological locus. Whether it is stated explicitly or not, this recent understanding of what is essential to the nature of humans was something closely related to the individual's capacity to integrate bodily functioning through the neurological system. Starting with the Harvard report of 1968 and the state laws beginning in 1970 the human was considered to be living so long as minimal capacity for integration of the functions remained. Our scientific understanding of anatomy and physiology led us to believe that this function, considered to be philosophically significant, has its locus in the human brain.

Thus the difficult case for a brain-oriented concept of death rests on the plausibility of the philosophical argument for this integrating capacity, or some similar function, as that which is essential to the human's nature. Only if one adequately handles the problem of moral doubt, the distinction between death of the human and death of the brain, and the argument for the plausibility of the neurological concept over the other concepts can one make any move in the direction of a brain-oriented concept.

Given these difficulties, there appear to be strong reasons against moving to a brain-oriented concept. The remainder of the chapter, however, assumes that these difficulties can be overcome by the arguments I have presented, provided the case is stated carefully enough. I shall now turn to the problems involved in focusing on the whole brain as the locus for the functions that are thought to be essential to the human's nature. Previously I argued that in one sense the brain is much too narrow a focus for determining what dies. Now I shall argue that in another sense, it is much too gross and crude a locus.

The Essentially Significant to the Nature of the Human

The Harvard committee had as its objective, if we are to believe its title, the examination of the definition of brain death. Yet the title of its report clearly indicates that what the committee did was attempt to provide criteria for irreversible coma. Whether the "death" of the brain can be equated without remainder to the state of irreversible coma is in large part a scientific, empirical question. In the perspective of the years since the Harvard report was written, however, it seems on the surface that there may well be a great difference between the death of the entire brain and the state of irreversible coma. Some people who are irreversibly comatose may nevertheless retain some brain-stem functions.

This forces us to be much more precise about exactly what in the functioning of the brain is of critical importance. First, we must gain a clearer understanding of what is so essentially significant to the nature of the human that its loss is called *death* and appropriately initiates death behavior.

Capacity to Integrate Bodily Function

So far, I have argued that one candidate is the capacity of the body to function as an integrated whole. If we are speaking of the death of the organism as a whole, and not simply the death of isolated cells, organs, or organ systems, it at first seems plausible to consider the complex integrating capacity of an organism as that which is essential to it. If this is the case, then the loss of that integrating capacity could appropriately be equated to the organism's death. From what we know of the integrating capacity of the human body, the brain is far and away the dominant locus of this capacity. To be sure, the spinal cord and peripheral nerves are also important, but these do not really provide integration. The spinal reflex at most provides a primitive and pale imitation of integrating function. The mysterious integrating capacity of the nervous system, which has fascinated humans and been conceptualized so influentially by Claude Bernard is, by comparison, so much more grand as to make the difference between a simple animal and the human organism.

It seems reasonable from what we think we know about the brain to relate this concept of integrating capacity to the whole brain. If this is what is seen as essentially significant to the human, then the examination of the whole brain for signs of functioning may be a plausible test for death of the individual.

Yet the simple equation of brain death to "irreversible coma" by the Harvard committee should give us pause. Was it really this integrating capacity the committee members had in mind? If so, why did they substitute the term *irreversible coma*? Henry Beecher, the committee's chair, writing elsewhere, makes clear which functions he deemed essential, and he does not seem to include all of the brain's functions. He states that a human is dead when there is irreversible loss of

> personality, his conscious life, his uniqueness, his capacity for remembering, judging, reasoning, acting, enjoying, worrying, and so on.

Beecher goes on to argue

> We have proof that these and other functions reside in the brain. . . . It
> seems clear that when the brain no longer functions, when it is destroyed,
> so also is the individual destroyed; he no longer exists as a person; he is
> dead.[7]

Certainly this conclusion follows from what we know about the brain, but there is a fundamental error in the argument. We have suggested that the practical problem with the more conservative heart-and-lung-oriented concepts is that they occasionally produce false-positive tests for life. If the argument is to be made for brain-oriented criteria at all (and we have already argued that this is a difficult but possible case to make), then certainly that argument must be subject to the same criticism. The functions mentioned by Beecher and summarized by the term *irreversible coma* certainly are in the brain but clearly do not exhaust the brain's functions. Focusing on the destruction of the whole brain may include additional nonessential functions, just as focusing on the heart and lungs did.

Capacity for Rationality
Beecher's list of characteristics includes the human's ability to reason. The Latin name for our species (*Homo sapiens*) clearly implies that reasoning capacity is somehow an essential characteristic. Could it be that it is reasoning capacity, rather than integrating capacity, that is essential? I believe not. Our considered moral judgments about those members of the species who do not have any capacity for reasoning is that they are still to be considered living in a very real way. They are still to have human rights, protected by both moral and positive law. Babies lacking a language, a culture, and a capacity to reason certainly are living in a human sense in spite of the fact that they have never executed the reasoning function. One might, of course, argue that babies have the potential for reasoning—the capacity for future reasoning. In this sense, they might be included among the category of living humans using this definition. But what of those afflicted with senile dementia, mentally retarded individuals, persons who have apparently permanent psychosis? They also lack a capacity for rationality and in some cases will never regain that capacity. Yet it is clear that they are still living in a meaningful sense of the term. In fact, one of the great dangers of moving to any brain-oriented concept of death is that it might place us on an evolutionary course, a "slippery slope" leading to the eventual exclusion of individuals who lack a certain minimal quality of life from the category of the human. Unless this tendency can be avoided, the dangers of movement to brain-oriented concepts may well exceed the moral right-making tendencies. Whatever may be our propensity to see rationality as the pinnacle of human functioning, it must

not be the characteristic that is essential to consider humans living. We must look elsewhere.

Capacity to Experience

Most of the other functions mentioned in lists of essentially human characteristics—consciousness, capacity for remembering, enjoying, worrying, acting voluntarily—characterize the human as an experiential animal. *Experience* is here taken in the broadest sense. Humans experience cognitively and emotionally. They cathect, comprehend, experience through sense organs and through much more complex experiential modes. It seems clear that a human who has some vestige of consciousness, some capacity to experience in this broadest sense could never be considered dead. To be sure, this human life may not be on the highest plane. It may be limited to blurred vision of reality and stunted emotional experience, but it is nevertheless life of a form that must be protected. Death behavior for such an individual is inappropriate.

Capacity for Social Interaction

Although humans may be experiential, they are also social creatures. At least in the Western tradition, the human's capacity to relate to fellow humans is fundamental. Is it meaningful to speak of a living human who lacks the capacity for social interaction? We must make clear that we are not at all saying that actual social interaction must take place for a creature to be alive. We are not even saying that such interaction has ever taken place. To say this would place the human's existence at the mercy of fellow humans. The cruel treatment of a baby who has been abandoned in a room with no human interaction should not define that baby out of existence. Presumably the capacity for social interaction nevertheless remains.

What is the relationship between the capacity for experience and the capacity for social interaction? It appears that they may be synonymous. It is conceivable that a condition could exist that would differentiate the two capacities. But to be able to experience in general but not experience others in particular would certainly be a bizarre form of existence. In practical terms, it would appear to be impossible. If it is the case that capacity to experience and capacity to experience others are coterminus, then we need pursue the matter no further. For practical purposes this seems to be sufficient. We conclude, then, that if we abandon the more traditional concepts of death (those focusing on the departure of the soul or the irreversible cessation of fluid flow) we may well find it more plausible to opt for a concept focusing on the irreversible loss of the capacity for experience or social interaction rather than the irreversible loss of integrating capacity of the body. If this is the case, the implications for the whole-brain-oriented criteria for death are great.

Before exploring those criteria, there must be one final comment about that which is essential to the nature of the human. Is it simply capacity for experience and social interaction per se or must there also be some embodiment of the capacity? Consider the bizarre and purely hypothetical case in which all of the information of the human brain were transferred to a computer hard drive together with sufficient sensory inputs and outputs to permit some form of rudimentary experiential and social function. Would the deleting of this information be murder? The thought is so novel that perhaps we cannot even conceive clearly of the philosophical significance of the question. It seems quite possible that our concept of the essential must include some embodiment. The human is, after all, something more than a sophisticated computer. At least in the Judeo–Christian tradition the body is an essential element, not something from which humans escape in liberation. If this is the case, then the essential element is embodied capacity for experience and social interaction.

Problems with the Whole-Brain-Oriented Criteria of Death

Our methodology at this point will be to begin by reviewing the criteria for brain death as outlined by the Harvard report and defined and endorsed by the Task Force on Death and Dying of the Institute of Society, Ethics and the Life Sciences[8]. I shall attempt to determine the functions implied as being morally significant that are being tested by the various criteria of the Harvard report. I shall then extend the analysis by examining other brain foci, the functions of which might constitute the essentially significant in the nature of the human.[9]

The Harvard committee, in proposing the criteria, and the institute's task force, in endorsing the criteria, simply failed to deal with the apparent gap between criteria for irreversible coma on the one hand and criteria for complete cessation of brain function on the other. Although empirically the two sets of criteria may be the same, they certainly represent different ranges of function. And there is no theoretical reason why the criteria should be identical, nor is there any clarification given in the reports as to which set of functions is of concern.

Brain-Mediated Reflexes

The first criterion for irreversible coma I shall examine will be the absence of brain-mediated reflexes. The Harvard criteria for irreversible coma indicate that there should be no central nervous system reflexes present that are routed through the brain. The contraction of the pupil in response to light is given as the typical case. In later writings, Beecher,[10] the chair of that committee, makes clear that one must exclude spinal cord reflexes in applying this test. The presence of a spinal reflex arc in a decapitated corpse, according to this view, should not be considered a test for the presence of life. The problem that the committee members did not face, however, is whether a brain reflex, such as the pupillary reflex, should not similarly be excluded. The difference between these reflexes and spinal reflexes is simply that they are mediated through the lower brain stem rather than the spinal cord.

I shall assume for purposes of this discussion that these brain reflexes are used directly as criteria for irreversible cessation of brain function. That is to say, it is the functioning of the brain stem and the ability to dilate and contract the pupil that are considered significant, and the reflex arc is not considered to be some indirect measure of some other brain function. If we can make this assumption, it seems very doubtful that the ability to contract and dilate the pupil and to execute any other reflex arc that happens to pass through the brain stem is in any way a significant sign of human living. If we can exclude a spinally mediated withdrawal reflex, which might be elicited by pricking an extremity with a pin, as being insignificant in the diagnosis of living, it seems that the same argument must apply to brain-stem reflexes. The ability to maintain nerve circuitry to carry out one of these reflexes does not really add significantly to the human's integrating capacity. Certainly it does not directly measure capacity to experience or inter-act socially.

Spontaneous Respiration or Breathing

Another criterion in the Harvard report is the observation of the presence of spontaneous respiration or breathing. The technique used is to turn off any artificial respiratory device for a period of three minutes and make observations. The moral question that is raised by this criterion is somewhat more difficult than the presence of brain-mediated reflexes. We traditionally had a societally dictated belief that a respiring individual is living. The holder of whole-brain-oriented criteria, however, has made the moral decision that artificial respiration is not a sufficient indicator of human life. Now the same question must be asked with regard to spontaneous respiration. Is the presence of the ability to respire spontaneously essentially significant to humanness? The question is not merely a philosophical one. Early in the brain death discussion, Brierley et al.[11] reported two cases in which comatose individuals respired spontaneously for long periods of time, four months in one case and five months in the other. The individuals apparently had no higher-brain function, as indicated by repeated isoelectric electroencephalogram. There was generalized necrosis within the neocortex when examined macroscopically and microscopically after cessation of spontaneous respiration.

Those individuals with spontaneous respiration are capable of a continued existence closely related to biological life as seen in plants and other animal species (the ability to respire, together with ability to carry out some rudimentary circulatory and excretory function, is the minimal essential characteristic of nonhuman biological life). The view that humans are closely related to the animal species is a very modern one, growing in part out of Darwinian evolutionary theory. Nevertheless, there are serious problems with this approach. To view humans as essentially respiratory creatures is to ignore most of the faculties that philosophers and anthropologists have considered essential to the species. It ignores humans' rational capacity, their ability to experience emotion and to reflect on that feeling systematically. It ignores their capacity for consciousness and memory, which gives rise to the systematic organization of experience and, in turn, gives rise to purposes, actions, and the eventual building of language and culture.

It should be clear that no philosophical or scientific argument can be definitive beyond the appeal to that which is reasonable or "obvious on reflection." The claim I make, however, is that one who would see the experiential and social function of the human as essential to its nature would not find spontaneous respiration a sufficient indicator of human life.

It may be that the criterion of spontaneous respiration incorporated into the Harvard criteria is an indirect measure of one of these functions (the experiential or social). The committee may have taken the position, for instance, that consciousness is the essential characteristic of the nature of the human, but the absence of spontaneous respiration is the only criterion that ensures the loss of the future capacity for consciousness. The Harvard committee, however, was established to determine criteria for brain death, not for the irreversible loss of consciousness. It appears that in the absence of any arguments in the report to the contrary, its authors incorporated the criterion of spontaneous respiration as a direct measure of a function of a part of the brain (i.e., the lower-brain center, which is responsible for spontaneous respiratory function). If that was their intention, they have indeed given a measure of functioning of a part of the whole brain. But they have not necessarily given a criterion for diagnosing the presence of a living individual any more significant than spontaneous beating of a heart supported by artificial oxygenation, which are now widely taken to be irrelevant for deciding if death has occurred.

Unreceptivity and Unresponsivity

The third criterion of irreversible coma, according to the Harvard report, is the presence of unreceptivity and unresponsivity: "There is a total unawareness to externally applied stimuli and inner need and complete unresponsiveness." It is incontrovertible that were either receptivity or responsiveness present, the individual would be alive, whether the concept of death being used is the irreversible loss of integrating function or the irreversible loss of experiential and social interaction capacity. What is confusing, however, is that the report's authors state explicitly that this characteristic of total unawareness is their definition of irreversible coma. In effect, they are saying that one of the four criteria for diagnosing irreversible coma is the presence of irreversible coma. The criterion would be more plausible had they claimed that complete unreceptivity and unresponsiveness were their definition of "coma"; however, they make the confusing claim that it is their definition of irreversible coma. One wonders whether that can be maintained empirically with any normal understanding of the meaning of the words.

In any case, we are left with unreceptivity and unresponsiveness (i.e., coma, but surely not necessarily irreversible coma) as a criterion of irreversible coma. We are left wondering, however, whether the committee is really interested in criteria for complete loss of the capacity for consciousness and experiential and social functioning or criteria for complete loss of all brain function. In the preceding paragraph of the report the authors claim that the criteria for irreversible coma are "characteristics of a permanently nonfunctioning brain," implying that they are seeking the latter in spite of their avowed purpose. The question remains whether parts of the brain may retain the capacity for function in the presence of unreceptivity and unresponsiveness and even apparently permanent unreceptivity and unresponsiveness. The answer cannot come from these gross behavioral observations alone. The condition of the patient–corpse described by Brierley et al.,[12] however, implies that some parts of the brain may indeed retain that capacity.

Thus far, we have seen that the criteria of the Harvard report are not particularly helpful in resolving the underlying philosophical debate about which concept of death is justifiable. In principle, they could not be, for the concept of death is independent of the verification of criteria. The fourth criterion, however, suggests the existence of scientific techniques for confirming the absence of experiential and social function in spite of ongoing lower brain activity that continues to carry out complex integrating functions.

Flat Electroencephalogram

The flat electroencephalogram is proposed by the Harvard report as being of "great confirmatory value" for the diagnosis of irreversible coma. Although the justification of this claim rests both on the definition of irreversible coma and empirical tests, I suggest, based on my understanding of the available data, that this claim must be questioned. On the one hand, the claim may be a simple one—that an EEG with some activity is incontrovertible evidence that there is some brain function. The flat EEG helps confirm the existence of a permanently nonfunctioning brain.

The problem, however, is one we have faced before. Is the EEG measuring whole-brain function or something more limited? From the scientific evidence, the EEG apparently measures simply the presence of neocortical electrical activity. If this is true, it is quite possible that some brain activity could remain in the presence of a flat electroencephalogram. There are two implications. If one is interested in a concept of death such as integrating capacity, which is oriented to the whole brain, it is quite possible (as Brierley et al. reported)[13] that a flat EEG would be present with brain activity remaining. Thus although EEG activity refutes the cessation of the functioning of the whole brain, the absence of EEG reading does not necessarily mean the absence of brain function.

More significant for our purposes, if the EEG measures only neocortex activity and one chose a concept of death that is oriented more to functions centered in that portion of the brain, the EEG may not be a confirmatory test but the central one. The use of tests centered on lower brain function may well be irrelevant (or at least not direct) ones for the irreversible loss of consciousness and experiential and social functions. Thus the EEG may be the most important test. Whether this is true will depend on empirical tests.

One argument against sole reliance on the EEG would be doubt of its empirical validity. The early evidence seemed very convincing, however. Silverman et al.[14] report 2,642 comatose patients with isoelectric EEGs, none of whom recovered (except three influenced by central nervous system [CNS] depressants and thus excluded from the data). The institute's report authors, who endorsed the Harvard criteria, were aware of this but chose not to pursue its implications because they wanted to avoid the critical question of which of the alternative concepts of death was being tested for by the proposed criteria. The implication is clear. If an integrating function or related concept oriented to the whole brain is maintained, the EEG alone is not sufficient for a diagnosis of death and is of only limited confirmatory value. If, however, an experiential and social interaction concept of death is held, or a related one oriented to more narrow brain functions apparently localized in the neocortex, then the EEG does not confirm at all: It is the definitive test. The 2,642 cases are quite persuasive. Perhaps they are so convincing that reasonable doubt of their validity for diagnosing irreversible loss of experiential capacity is removed. If this is the case, the adoption of this criterion for death will still depend on the adoption of the related concept, but a test would be available for measuring this higher-brain-based notion of death.

The Significant Portions of the Cortex

There is one final step in clarifying the concepts of death related to brain function that go beyond the older, more simplistic whole-brain-oriented concepts. If the EEC measures neocortical function, it presumably may measure any neocortical activity. Yet we have concluded that experiential and social integrating function is the essential element in the nature of the human, the loss of which is to be called death. Once again the danger of false-positive diagnosis of living must be raised. The neocortical cells and nerve circuits responsible for experiential and social integrating function are certainly complex. They would have to include some sensory portions of the cortex, as well as the limbic system and other areas responsible for emotion.

Yet is it not theoretically possible that some cortical cells could retain viability and yet the person would be dead in the sense we have discussed? What, for instance, if only motor cortex cells continued to survive through some freak preservation of blood supply to a small area of the cortex or some theoretical artificial perfusion? Whether or not the EEG would be present and whether the existence of only this kind of cortical activity could be distinguished are empirical questions. At the philosophical level, however, for one who sees the essence of the human to be an embodied experiential and social capacity, the presence of viable motor cells would be of no more significance than the presence of the spinal or cranial reflex arc. Thus the concept of death being dealt with cannot be reduced without remainder to the criterion of a flat EEG. The irreversible loss of these essential functions may be compatible with the presence of some form of EEG reading. Whether empirical tests can be made to make such a distinction and whether such solely motor-cell capacity could ever exist are beyond this discussion.

The problem of doubt returns once again—this time with doubt between the older, broader whole-brain-oriented integrating function and the more limited experiential function. This newer concept of death I have called the *higher-brain-oriented concept of death*. Exactly which functions should be singled out as "higher" will take further philosophical debate. What is critical is that we now have identified a new, significantly different concept of death that must be distinguished from the older, now-outdated *whole-brain-oriented concept*. As for me, the case for the concept of the human that sees experiential and social functioning as central is persuasive. The debate about the competing philosophical concepts is complex, much more complex than the original proponents of the older and more naive concept of brain death ever realized. They seemed satisfied to orient attention to brain function, failing to perceive that irreversible coma and the death of the whole brain were not exactly the same. Moreover, they failed to perceive that neither of these might be exactly the same as the irreversible loss of experiential functions that the Harvard committee's chair indicated were crucial to being alive.

Conclusion

Although I personally favor the more limited experiential concept and am now convinced of the empirical validity of the related EEG criterion, I am not convinced that a philosophical issue so complex requires universal conformity. I would thus favor a law that recognizes the complexity of the debate and permits the patient or the patient's agent to choose among the plausible death concepts—a position I will defend in Chapter 7. My objective in this discussion has been to push beyond the older, simpler whole-brain-oriented concept of death, which is now often used in the literature without careful definition, to obtain more precise usage of terms. Whether a person dies when he or she loses functions that have a primary locus in the whole brain, in a part of the brain, or in some other organs, it is the person who dies. The choice of the concept of death will require a more precise philosophical choice among these alternatives, and the use of criteria for death will, in turn, depend on those philosophical choices.

ENDNOTES

1. Hans Jonas, "Philosophical Reflections on Human Experimentation," *Daedalus* 98 (2, 1969): 219–47.
2. Ad Hoc Committee of the Harvard Medical School to Examine the Definition of Brain Death, "A Definition of Irreversible Coma," *Journal of the American Medical Association* 205 (1968): 337–40.
3. See Chapter 3, this volume.
4. Task Force on Death and Dying, Institute of Society, Ethics, and the Life Sciences, "Refinements in Criteria for the Determination of Death: An Appraisal," *Journal of the American Medical Association* 221 (1972): 48–53.
5. Leon Kass, "Death as an Event: A Commentary on Robert Morison," *Science* 173 (1971): 698–702; Robert Morison, "Death: Process or Event?" *Science* 173 (1971): 694–98.
6. Dallas High, "Death: Its Conceptual Elusiveness," *Soundings* 55 (1972): 438–58; Institute of Society, Ethics, and the Life Sciences, Task Force on Death and Dying, "Refinements in Criteria for the Determination of Death," *Journal of the American Medical Association* 221 (1972): 48–53.
7. Henry Beecher, the committee's chair, writing elsewhere: Beecher, "The New Definition of Death: Some Opposing Views," paper presented at the American Association for the Advancement of Science, Annual Meeting, Symposium on Meaning of Death, Chicago, IL, Dec. 27–29, 1970, p. 4.

8. Op. cit. Task Force.

9. It is important to distinguish between criteria that are apparently closely and directly linked to functions considered essentially significant to living and criteria that are more remote and less direct. The most crucial example is the criterion of spontaneous respiration. The observation of spontaneous movement of respiratory muscles might be a direct criterion for the observation of spontaneous respiratory function. On the other hand, it might be an indirect criterion for the irreversible loss of consciousness. It is crucial to distinguish between these two types of criteria. We do not want to rule out a criterion apparently linked to a function that we might decide to be nonessential to human living, when, in fact, that criterion is really an indirect empirical measure of some functions that we indeed can consider to be significant.

10. Henry K. Beecher, "The New Definition of Death: Some Opposing Views."

11. J. B. Brierley et al., "Neocortical Death After Cardiac Arrest," *Lancet* (Sept. 1971): 560–65.

12. Ibid.

13. Ibid.

14. D. Silverman et al., "Irreversible Coma Associated with Electrocerebral Silence," *Neurology* 20 (1970): 525–33.

Six

THE IMPENDING COLLAPSE
OF THE WHOLE-BRAIN
DEFINITION OF DEATH

As WE HAVE SEEN in the previous chapter, for many years there has been lingering doubt, at least among theorists, that the currently fashionable "whole-brain-oriented" definition of death has things exactly right.* The presently accepted standard definition, the Uniform Determination of Death Act, specifies that an individual is dead who has sustained "irreversible cessation of all functions of the entire brain, including the brain stem."[1] It also provides an alternative definition, specifying that an individual is also dead who has sustained "irreversible cessation of circulatory and respiratory functions." The President's Commission for the Study of Ethical Problems in Medicine and Biomedical and Behavioral Research made clear, however, that circulatory and respiratory function loss are important only as indirect indicators that the brain has been permanently destroyed.[2]

---

*I have long resisted the term "brain death" and use it only in quotation marks to indicate the still common, if ambiguous, usage. As we have seen, the term is ambiguous because it fails to distinguish between the biological claim that the brain is dead and the social/legal/moral claim that the individual as a whole is dead because the brain is dead. An even greater problem with the term arises from the lingering doubt that individuals with dead brains are really dead. Hence, even physicians are sometimes heard to say that the patient "suffered brain death" one day and "died" the following day. It is better to say that the patient "died" on the first day, the day the brain was determined to be dead, and that the cadaver's other bodily functions ceased the following day. For these reasons I insist on speaking of persons with dead brains as individuals who are dead, not merely persons who are "brain dead." I will therefore use the term "brain-oriented definition of death" to indicate that I am speaking of the definition of the death of the individual based on measurement of brain function. I will use the term "whole-brain-oriented definition of death" to refer to a concept of the death of the individual based on the irreversible loss of all functions of the entire brain.

Doubts about the Whole-Brain-Oriented Definition

It is increasingly apparent, however, that this consensus is coming apart. Chapter 5 revealed that as long ago as the early 1970s some of us doubted that literally the entire brain had to be dead for the individual as a whole to be dead.[3]

Must All Cellular Functions Be Destroyed?

From the early years, it was known, at least among neurologists and theorists who read the literature, that individual, isolated brain cells could be perfused and continue to live even though integrated supercellular brain function had been destroyed. When the uniform definition of death said all functions of the entire brain must be dead, there was understanding that cellular-level functions did not count. The commission recognized this, positing that "cellular activity alone is irrelevant."[4] This willingness to write off cellular-level functions is more controversial than it may appear. After all, the law does not grant a dispensation to ignore cellular-level functions, no matter how plausible that may be. Keep in mind that those who were to oppose the soon-to-be-developed higher-brain definitions of death would need to emphasize that the model statute called for loss of all functions.

Must All Electrical Functions Be Destroyed?

By 1977 an analogous problem arose regarding electrical activity. The report of a multicenter study funded by the National Institutes of Neurological Diseases and Stroke found that all of the functions it considered important could be lost irreversibly while very small (2 microvolt) electron potentials could still be obtained on EEG. These were not artifact but real electrical activity from brain cells. Nevertheless, the committee concluded that there could be "electrocerebral silence," and therefore the brain could be considered "dead" even though these small electrical charges could be recorded.[5]

It is possible that the members of the committee believed that these were the result of nothing more than cellular-level functions, so that the same reasoning that permitted the president's commission to write off little functions as unimportant would apply. However, no evidence was presented that these electron potentials were exclusively arising from cellular-level functions. It could well be that the reasoning in this report expanded the existing view that cellular functions did not count to the view that some minor supercellular functions could be ignored as long as they were small.

Must All Supercellular Functions Be Destroyed?

More recently neurologist James Bernat, a defender of the whole-brain-oriented definition of death, has acknowledged that it is possible that:

the bedside clinical examination is not sufficiently sensitive to exclude the possibility that small nests of brain cells may have survived . . . and that their continued functioning, although not contributing significantly to the functioning of the organism as a whole, can be measured by laboratory techniques. Because these isolated nests of neurons no longer contribute to the functioning of the organism as a whole, their continued functioning is now irrelevant to the dead organism.[6]

The idea that functions of "isolated nests of neurons" can remain when an individual is declared dead based on whole-brain-oriented criteria certainly stretches the plain words of the law that requires, without qualification, that all functions of the entire brain must be gone. That exceptions can be granted by individual private citizens based on their personal judgments about which functions are "contributing significantly" certainly challenges the integrity of the idea that the whole brain must be dead for the individual as a whole to be dead.

Must All Brain Structure Be Destroyed?

There is still another problem for those who favor what can now be called the "whole-brain definition of death." It is not altogether clear that the "death of the brain" is to be equated with the "irreversible loss of function." At least one paper appears to hold out not only for loss of function but also destruction of anatomical structure.[7] Thus we are left with a severely nuanced and qualified whole-brain-oriented definition of death. For it to hold as applied at the turn of the twenty-first century, one must assume that for the whole brain to be dead it must be function rather than structure that is irreversibly destroyed and that not only can certain cellular-level functions and microvolt-level electrical functions be ignored as "insignificant" but also certain "nests of cells" and associated super-cellular-level functions can as well.

By the time the whole-brain-oriented definition of death is so qualified, it can hardly be referring to the death of the whole brain any longer. What is particularly troublesome is that private citizens—neurologists, philosophers, theologians, and public commentators—seem to be determining just which brain functions are insignificant.

The Higher-Brain-Oriented Alternative

The problem is exacerbated when one reviews the early "brain death" literature. Writers trying to make the case for a brain-based definition of death over a heart-based one invariably pointed out that certain functions were irreversibly lost when the brain was gone. Then, implicitly or explicitly, they made the moral/philosophical/religious claim that individuals who have irreversibly lost these key functions should be treated as dead.

Although this function-based defense of a brain-oriented definition of death served the day well, some of us realized that the critical functions cited were not randomly distributed throughout the brain. We saw, for instance, in the previous chapter that Henry Beecher, the chair of the Harvard Ad Hoc Committee, identified the following functions as critical: "the individual's personality, his conscious life, his uniqueness, his capacity for remembering, judging, reasoning, acting, enjoying, worrying, and so on."[8]

Of course, all these functions are known to require the cerebrum. If these are the important functions, the obvious question is why would any lower-brain functions signal the presence of a living individual?

This gave rise to what is now best called the higher-brain-oriented definition of death—in other words, that one is dead when there is irreversible loss of all "higher" brain functions.[9] At first, this was referred to as a cerebral or a cortical definition of death, but it seems clear that just as some brain-stem functions may be deemed insignificant, likewise some functions in the cerebrum may be deemed so as well.* Moreover, it is not clear that the functions of the kind Beecher listed are always necessarily localized in the cerebrum or the cerebral cortex. At least in theory someday we may be able to build an artificial neurological organ that could replace some functions of the cerebrum. Someone who was thinking, feeling, reasoning, and carrying on a conversation through the use of an artificial brain would surely be recognized as alive even if the cerebrum that it had replaced was long since completely dead. I have preferred the purposely ambiguous term "higher-brain function" as a way to make clear that the key philosophical issue is which of the many brain functions are really important.

Although that way of putting the question may offend the defenders of the more traditional whole-brain definition of death, once they have made the move of excluding the cellular, electrical, and supercellular functions they consider "insignificant," they are hardly in a position to complain about the project of sorting functions into important and unimportant ones.

---

*With the suggestion that the critical functions for diagnosing that an individual is alive are localized in the cerebrum, a serious problem arises with an older, inaccurate usage. Some early commentators, including the authors of the National Institute of Neurological Diseases and Stroke report previously mentioned, use the term "cerebral death" to refer to the death of the entire brain. It is odd that trained neurologists would do so because they clearly know that the cerebrum is only one part of the brain. Once the important distinction is made between the death of the whole brain and the death of the cerebrum, using the adjective "cerebral" to refer to the whole brain is a serious and confusing error.

Criticisms of the Higher-Brain Formulations

Several criticisms have been offered of the higher-brain-oriented formulation in defense of the whole-brain-oriented one.

Reluctance to Change the Concept of Death

Several defenders of the whole-brain-oriented concept have claimed that defining death in terms of loss of certain significant brain functions involves a change in the concept of death. This, however, rests on the implausible claim of Alex Capron, the executive director of the president's commission, that the move from a heart-oriented to a whole-brain-oriented definition of death is not a change in concept at all but merely the recognition of new diagnostic measures for the traditional concept of death.[10] It is very doubtful, however, that the move to a whole-brain-oriented concept of death is any less of a fundamental change in concept than movement to a higher-brain-oriented one. From the beginning of the debate many people with beating hearts and dead brains would have been alive under the traditional concept of death focusing on fluid flow but are clearly dead based on a then-newer whole-brain-oriented concept. Most understood this as a significant change in concept. In any case, even if there is a greater change in moving to a definition of death that identifies certain functions of the brain as significant, the mere fact that it is a conceptual change should not count against it. Surely, the critical question is which concept is right, not which concept squares with traditional views.

Difficulty in Measuring Higher-Brain Functions

A second major charge against the higher-brain-oriented formulations has been that neurophysiologists are unable to measure precisely the irreversible loss of these higher functions based on current techniques.[11] By contrast it has been assumed that the irreversible loss of all functions of the entire brain is measurable based on current techniques.

Although lay people generally do not realize it, the measurement of death based on any concept can never be 100 percent accurate. The greatest error rates have certainly been with the heart-oriented concepts of death. Many patients have been falsely determined to have irreversibly lost heart functions. In earlier days we simply did not have the capacity to measure precisely. Even today there may be no reason to determine precisely whether the heart could be restarted in the case of a terminally ill, elderly patient who is ready to die.

There is even newly found ambiguity in the notion of irreversibility.[12] We are moving rapidly toward the day when organs for transplant will be obtained from non–heart-beating cadavers who have been determined to be dead based on heart function loss (see Chapter 13, where this possibility is discussed). It will be important for death to be pronounced as quickly as possible after the heart function has been found irreversibly lost. It is not clear, however, whether death should be pronounced when the heart has permanently stopped (say following a decision based on an advance directive to withdraw a ventilator) but could be started again. In the minutes when it could be started but will not be because the patient has refused resuscitation, can we say that the stoppage is "irreversible" and that therefore the individual is dead?

Likewise, it is increasingly clear that we must acknowledge some, admittedly very small, risk of error in measuring the irreversible loss of all functions of the entire brain. Alan Shewmon has argued that the determination of the death of the entire brain cannot be made with as great a certainty as some neurologists would claim.[13] Some neurologists have persisted in claiming that brains are dead (or have irreversibly lost all function) even though electrical function still remains.[14] Clearly, brains with electrical function must have some living tissues; claims these brains are dead must rest on the assumption that the functions that remain are insignificant.

None of this should imply that the death of the brain cannot be measured with great accuracy. But it is wrong to assume that similar or greater levels of accuracy cannot be obtained in measuring the irreversible loss of key higher functions, including consciousness. The literature on the persistent vegetative state repeatedly claims that we can know with great accuracy that consciousness is irreversibly lost.[15] The AMA's Councils on Scientific Affairs and Ethical and Judicial Affairs have concluded that the diagnosis can be made with an error rate of less than 1 in 1,000.[16] In fact the president's commission itself said that "the Commission was assured that physicians with experience in this area can reliably determine that some patients' loss of consciousness is permanent."[17]

Even if we could not presently measure accurately the loss of key higher functions such as consciousness, that would have bearing only on the clinical implementation of the higher-brain-oriented definition, not the validity of the concept itself. Defenders of the higher-brain formulation might continue to use the now old-fashioned measures of loss of all brain function, but only because of the assurance that if all functions are lost, the higher functions *certainly* are. Such a conservative policy would leave open the question of whether we could some day measure the loss of higher functions accurately enough to use the measures clinically.

The Higher-Brain Formulation's Link to Personhood
Still another criticism of the higher-brain formulations is the claim that any higher-brain formation would rely on a concept of personhood or personal identity that is philosophically controversial.[18] Personhood theories are notoriously contro-

versial. It is simply wrong, however, to claim that any higher-brain-oriented concept of death is based on either personhood or personal identity theories. I, for one, have acknowledged the possibility that there are living human beings who do not satisfy the various concepts of personhood. As long as the law is only discussing whether someone is a living individual, the debate over personhood is irrelevant.

The Slippery Slope Problem

Perhaps the most serious charge against the higher-brain-oriented formulations is that they are susceptible to the so-called slippery slope argument.[19] Once one yields on the insistence that all functions of the entire brain must be irreversibly gone before an individual is considered dead, there seems to be no stopping the slide of eliminating functions considered insignificant. The argument posits that once totally and permanently unconscious individuals who have some other brain functions (such as brain-stem reflexes) remaining are considered dead, someone will propose that those with only marginal consciousness similarly lack significant function, and soon all manner of functionally compromised humans will be defined as dead. Because being labeled dead is normally an indicator that certain moral and legal rights cease, such a slide toward considering increasing numbers of marginally functional humans as dead would be morally horrific.

But is the slippery slope argument plausible? In fact, there is a good case to be made that it is more plausible as an argument against the now more traditional whole-brain-oriented concept of death.

A slippery slope argument, in its most significant form, involves a claim that the same principle underlying one, apparently tolerable, judgment also entails other, clearly unacceptable judgments. For example, imagine we were trying to determine whether elderly individuals could be excluded from access to certain health care services based on the utilitarian principle of choosing the course that produced the maximum aggregate good for society. The slippery slope argument might be used to show that the same principle entails implications presumed clearly unacceptable, such as the exclusion of health care from socially unproductive individuals. To the extent that one is certain that the empirical assumptions are correct (for example, that the utilitarian principle does entail excluding care from unproductive individuals) and one is confident that such an outcome would be morally unacceptable, then one might attempt to challenge the withholding of health care from the elderly population on slippery slope grounds. The same principle used to support one policy also entails other policies that are clearly unacceptable.

The slippery slope argument is valid insofar as it shows that the principle used to support one policy under consideration entails clearly unacceptable implications when applied to different situations. In principle, there is no difference between the small, potentially tolerable move and the more dramatic, unacceptable move. However, as applied to the definition of death debate, the slippery slope argument can actually be used to show that the whole-brain-oriented definition of death is less defensible than the higher-brain-oriented one.

As we have seen, the whole-brain-oriented definition of death rests on the claim that irreversible loss of all functions of the entire brain is necessary and sufficient for an individual to be dead. That, in effect, means drawing a sharp line between the top of the spinal cord and the base of the brain (i.e., the bottom of the brain stem). But is there any principled reason why one would draw a line at that point?

In the early years of the definition of death debate, the claim was made that an individual was dead when the central nervous system no longer retained the capacity for integration. It was soon discovered, however, that that could be taken to imply that one was "alive" as long as some spinal cord function remained. That was counterintuitive (and also made it more difficult to obtain organs for transplant). Hence very early on it was agreed that simple reflexes of the spinal cord did not count as an indicator of life. Presumably the principle was that reflex arcs that do not integrate significant bodily functions are to be ignored.

But why, then, do brain-stem reflexes mediated through the base of the brain stem count? By the same principle, if spinal reflexes can be ignored, it would seem that some brain-stem reflexes might be as well. An effort to show that brain-stem reflexes are more integrative of bodily function is doomed to fail. At most there are gradual, imperceptible gradations in complexity between the reflexes of the first cervical vertebra and those of the base of the brain stem. Some spinal reflexes that trigger extension of the foot while the contralateral arm is withdrawn certainly cover larger distances.

Whatever principle could be used to exclude the spinal reflexes surely can exclude some brain-stem reflexes as well. We have seen that the defenders of the whole-brain-oriented position admit as much when they exclude cellular-level functions and electrical functions. Certainly, those who exclude "nests of cells" in the brain as insignificant have abandoned the whole-brain position and are already sliding along the slippery slope.

By contrast the defenders of the higher-brain-oriented definition of death can articulate a principle that avoids such slipperiness. Suppose, for example, they rely on classical Judeo–Christian notions that the human is essentially the integration of the mind and body and that the existence of one without the other is not sufficient to constitute a living human being. Such a principle provides a bright line that would clearly distinguish the total and irreversible loss of consciousness from serious but not total mental impairments. Likewise, it provides a firm basis for telling which functions of nests of brain cells count as significant. It avoids the hopeless task of trying to show why brain-stem reflexes count more than spinal ones or trying to show exactly how many cells must be in a nest before it is significant. There is no subjective assessment of different bodily functions; no quibbles about how much integration there must be for the organism to function as a whole. The principle is simple. It relies on qualitative considerations: When, and only when, there is the capacity for organic (bodily) and mental function present together in a single entity is there a living human being. That, I would suggest, is the philosophical basis for the higher-brain-oriented definition of death. Rather than placing one on a slippery slope, it avoids the slippery slope on which the defenders of the whole-brain-oriented position have found themselves. It, and only it, provides a principled reason for avoiding the slippery slope.

Conscience Clauses

There is one final development that signals the demise of the whole-brain-oriented definition of death as the single basis for declaring death. It should be clear by now that the definition of death debate is actually a debate over the moral status of human beings. It is a debate over when humans should be treated as having moral standing as full members of the human community. When humans are living, full moral and legal human rights accrue. Saying people are *alive* is simply shorthand for saying that they are bearers of such rights. That is why the definition of death debate is so important. It is also why, in principle, there is no scientific way in which the debate can be resolved. The choice of who is alive—who has full moral standing as a member of the human community—is fundamentally a moral, philosophical, or religious choice, not a scientific one.

In a pluralistic society, we are not likely to reach agreement on such moral questions, which is why no one definition of death has carried the day thus far. When one realizes that there are many variants on each of the three major definitions of death, each of which has some group of adherents, it seems unlikely that any one position is likely to gain anything close to a majority any time soon. For example, my defense of the higher-brain-oriented position stands or falls on the claim that the essence of the human being is the integration of a mind and a body, a position reflecting religious and philosophical assumptions that are not beyond dispute. Other defenders of the higher-brain position are more Manichaean, holding that only the mind is important; they apparently are committed to a view that a human memory transferred to a computer with a capacity to continue mental function would still have all the essential ingredients of humanness, and we would continue to have the same living human being on the computer hard drive. These are disputes not likely to be resolved soon.

As a society we have a method for dealing with fundamental disputes in religion and philosophy. We tolerate diversity and affirm the right of conscience to hold minority beliefs as long as actions based on those beliefs do not cause insurmountable problems for the rest of society. That is precisely what I initially proposed doing in 1976.[20] I proposed a definition of death with a conscience clause that would permit individuals to choose their own definition of death based on their religious and philosophical convictions. I did not say at the time, but should have, that the choices would have to be restricted to those who avoid violating the rights of others and avoid creating insurmountable social problems for the rest of society. The possibility of permitting individuals to pick their own definition of death is the issue of the next chapter.

ENDNOTES

1. President's Commission for the Study of Ethical Problems in Medicine and Biomedical and Behavioral Research, *Defining Death: Medical, Legal, and Ethical Issues in the Definition of Death* (Washington, DC: U.S. Government Printing Office, 1981), p. 2.

2. Ibid., p. 74.

3. Robert M. Veatch, "The Whole-Brain-Oriented Concept of Death: An Outmoded Philosophical Formulation," *Journal of Thanatology* 3 (1975): 13–30.

4. President's Commission for the Study of Ethical Problems in Medicine and Biomedical and Behavioral Research, *Defining Death: Medical, Legal, and Ethical Issues in the Definition of Death.*

5. A. Earl Walker, "An Appraisal of the Criteria of Cerebral Death—A Summary Statement," *Journal of the American Medical Association* 237 (1977): 983.

6. James L. Bernat, "How Much of the Brain Must Die on Brain Death?" *The Journal of Clinical Ethics* 3 (1, Spring 1992): 25.

7. Paul A. Byrne, Sean O'Reilly, and Paul M. Quay, "Brain Death—An Opposing Viewpoint," *Journal of the American Medical Association* 242 (1979): 1985–90.

8. Cited in Robert M. Veatch, *Death, Dying, and the Biological Revolution* (New Haven, CT: Yale University Press, 1976), p. 38.

9. Robert M. Veatch, "Whole-Brain, Neocortical, and Higher Brain Related Concepts," in *Death: Beyond Whole-Brain Criteria*, ed. Richard M. Zaner. (Dordrecht, Holland: D. Reidel, 1988), pp. 171–86.

10. President's Commission for the Study of Ethical Problems in Medicine and Biomedical and Behavioral Research, *Defining Death: Medical, Legal, and Ethical Issues in the Definition of Death*, p. 41.

11. Ibid., p. 40.

12. David J. Cole, "The Reversibility of Death," *Journal of Medical Ethics* 18 (1992): 26–30.

13. Alan D. Shewmon, "Caution in the Definition and Diagnosis of Infant Brain Death," in *Medical Ethics: A Guide for Health Professionals*, ed. John F. Monagle and David C. Thomasma (Rockville, MD: Aspen, 1988), pp. 38–57.

14. Stephen Ashwal and Sanford Schneider, "Failure of Electroencephalography to Diagnose Brain Death in Comatose Patients," *Annals of Neurology* 6 (1979): 512–17.

15. Ronald B. Cranford and Harmon L. Smith, "Some Critical Distinctions between Brain Death and the Persistent Vegetative State," *Ethics in Science and Medicine* 6 (Winter 1979): 199–209; Phiroze L. Hansotia, "Persistent Vegetative State," *Archives of Neurology* 42 (1985): 1048–52.

16. Council on Scientific Affairs and Council on Ethical and Judicial Affairs, "Persistent Vegetative State and the Decision to Withdraw or Withhold Life Support," *Journal of the American Medical Association* 263 (1990): 428.

17. President's Commission for the Study of Ethical Problems in Medicine and Biomedical and Behavioral Research, *Deciding to Forego Life-Sustaining Treatment: Ethical, Medical, and Legal Issues in Treatment Decisions* (Washington, DC: U.S. Government Printing Office, 1983), p. 177.

18. President's Commission for the Study of Ethical Problems in Medicine and Biomedical and Behavioral Research, *Defining Death: Medical, Legal, and Ethical Issues in the Definition of Death*, pp. 38–39.

19. James L. Bernat, "How Much of the Brain Must Die on Brain Death?"

20. Robert M. Veatch, *Death, Dying, and the Biological Revolution*.

SEVEN

THE CONSCIENCE CLAUSE: HOW MUCH INDIVIDUAL CHOICE CAN SOCIETY TOLERATE IN DEFINING DEATH?

ON THE MORNING of March 1, 1994, a blue 1978 Chevrolet Impala pulled next to a van as it began to cross the Brooklyn Bridge. The van was carrying 15 students from the Lubavitch Hasidic Jewish sect returning from a prayer vigil in Manhattan. As the car neared the van, a lone gunman shouted "Kill the Jews" in Arabic and fired at least five rounds of bullets from two separate semiautomatic weapons into the side of the van. Four students were injured, two critically. One, 15-year-old Aaron Halberstam, was "declared brain dead, but he remained on life support."[1]

New York has adopted a brain-oriented definition of death through administrative regulation of the State Hospital and Planning Council and with the endorsement of the state health commissioner, which reads, "Both the individual standard of heart and lung activity and the standard of total and irreversible cessation of brain function should be recognized as the legal definition of death in New York."[2] That would seem to imply that Halberstam was dead once the diagnosis of the death of the brain was confirmed. However, the parents, following widely held Jewish beliefs, insisted that the individual does not die when the brain dies. They would accept only a criterion based on respiratory function. The rabbis for the Halberstam family were reported to have said that Halberstam should be kept on support systems as long as his heart could beat on its own.[3] The physician, honoring the parents' wishes, refused to pronounce the death. Depending on the interpretation, this may have been legal in New York. A sentence in the regulation permits (but does not require) physicians to accommodate family views on the definition of death.

One can hardly imagine what the result would have been had the family placed their ventilator-dependent, brain-dead, but not legally pronounced dead son in an ambulance and driven him through the Holland Tunnel to New Jersey. In New Jersey, they would be in a jurisdiction with an even more complex legal situation. New Jersey has a whole-brain-oriented criterion of death, but the law explicitly permits religious objectors to reject the use of that criterion in their own cases, thus making the patient alive until cardiac function ceases irreversibly.[4] Had Halberstam been known to hold such views, he would clearly be alive in New Jersey, assuming the law applies to minors. The present law, however, does not explicitly permit family members to choose a cardiac criterion of death based on their own religious beliefs. Thus, unless his own views were known or the law were extended to permit surrogate decision making, he could not have been treated as alive.

The New York case is not the only one that has raised these complex issues surrounding religious and other dissent from the legal definition of death. In California and Florida two additional cases at about the same time pressed the issue. In California on March 27, 1994, two students, whose parents live in Japan and who had been shot in a senseless act of violence, were declared "brain dead." According to the report, they were diagnosed as brain dead, taken off respirators, and then pronounced dead even though the family was from a culture that still does not recognize brain criteria for death pronouncement.[5] The families were not given discretion to opt for a criterion of death that was preferred in their culture.

At about the same time, in Florida, 13-year-old Teresa Hamilton, a severe diabetic who had been left in a coma, had been diagnosed as "brain dead." Although Florida, like California, has a law stating that people with dead brains are dead people, the parents insisted that she was still alive and demanded that she kept on what was called "life support."[6] Although the hospital insisted that the patient was dead and its personnel wanted to stop ventilatory support on the body, they yielded to the family wishes that her body be treated as if it were alive. They pressed for a plan to send the girl home on the ventilator without pronouncing her dead. Here the family got its wishes in spite of the Florida law.

The Present State of the Law

The New Jersey law, until recently, was unique in the world. Japan has recently adopted an even more complex law that permits brain criteria to be used to pronounce death, but only if the individual while alive has explicitly consented to both the brain-based death pronouncement and organ procurement and then only if the family also consents.[7] A few countries (primarily in Asia) have not yet adopted a whole-brain concept of death.[8] They continue to use the traditional cardiac definition. All other jurisdictions have adopted a whole-brain-oriented definition without any provision for individuals to conscientiously object for religious or other reasons. The New York regulation appears to introduce some discretion, based on family objections to a brain-oriented definition, but actually gives the discretion to the physician who is contemplating death pronouncement based on a brain-oriented concept of death. A family could express dissent to one physician who is willing to accommodate, whereas if they happen to be dealing with another physician, that physician could refuse the request to refrain from pronouncing death.

The law in most American jurisdictions specifies that if the criteria for measuring the irreversible loss of all functions of the entire brain are met, "death shall be pronounced." In other jurisdictions, the law actually reads "death may be pronounced." This seems to imply that the physician has the discretion, much as in New York, except that the discretion is actually broader. The physician could refuse to pronounce based on his or her own personal values, economic considerations, or other factors in addition to family wishes. Clearly, these laws seem defective if they give the physician the opportunity legally to choose whether to pronounce death based on the physician's values. The problem under consideration in this chapter is whether such discretion could be tolerated by the society if the dissent comes from the patient or the patient's next of kin.

The common wisdom has been that such discretion makes no sense. After all, being dead seems to be an objective matter to be determined by good science (or perhaps good metaphysics) rather than by individual conscientious choice. Concern is often expressed that such discretion not only makes no sense but would produce public chaos leading to situations in which some patients are dead while medically identical patients are alive. I will make the case for the legitimacy of a conscientious objection to a uniform definition of death, which will permit patients to choose while competent an alternative definition of death provided it is within reason and does not pose serious public health or other societal concerns. In cases in which the patient has not spoken while competent (in cases of infants, children, and adults who simply have not expressed themselves), I will argue that the next of kin should have this discretion within certain limits.

Concepts, Criteria, and the Role of Value Pluralism

As we have seen, early in the definition of death debate commentators insisted that a basic distinction be made between two elements of the discussion. What at first appeared to be one question turned out to include at least two separate issues.

The Early Fact–Value Distinction

The first question seems primarily scientific: How can we measure that the brain has been irreversibly destroyed (that it has "died")? That seems like the kind of question that those skilled in neurology could answer. The neurological community, sometimes aided by others, has offered many sets of criteria with associated tests and measures for determining that the brain will never again be able to conduct any of its functions.[9] We have come to understand this as primarily a question for competent medical scientists.[10]

The second question is quite different in character. It asks whether we as a society or as individuals ought to treat an individual with a dead brain as a dead person. This question is clearly not something about which the neurological community can claim expertise. No amount of neurological study could possibly determine whether people with dead brains should be considered dead people. This is a religious, philosophical, ethical, or public policy question, not one of neurological science. When society determines someone is dead, many social behavioral changes occur. These are not neurological issues; they are social, normative issues about which all citizens may reasonably voice a position relying on their personal religious, philosophical, and ethical view of the world.

Democratic Pluralism and Value Variation

In a democratic, pluralistic culture we have great insight into how to deal with religious, philosophical, and ethical controversies about which there are strongly held views and unresolvable controversy. At the level of morality, we agree to tolerate diverse opinion, and we even let a person act on those opinions, at least until the impact on the lives of others becomes intolerable. This is the position we take regarding religious dissent.

RELIGIOUS AND OTHER POSITIONS

To the extent that the disagreement is a religious or quasi-religious disagreement, toleration of pluralism seems the appropriate course. It permits people with differences to live together in harmony. And at least one major source of division over the definition of death is surely theological. The case with which this chapter opened appears not only to have been *caused* by Jewish/Arab tensions; the moral disagreement about whether to declare Halberstam dead also has religious roots. Judaism has long been known to include persons who oppose brain criteria for death pronouncement. Not all Jews oppose it. Rabbi Moses Tendler, a well-known moral commentator, has supported it.[11] But many Orthodox rabbinical scholars strongly oppose using brain criteria to pronounce death, maintaining that where there is breath there is life.[12] Some Japanese individuals, influenced by Buddhist and Shinto belief systems, see the presence of life in the whole body, not just in the brain.[13] Some Native Americans also hold religious beliefs that oppose a brain-oriented definition of death.[14] Fundamentalist Christians, sometimes associated with the right-to-life movement, and some Catholics focusing on prolife issues, press for a consistent prolife position by opposing death pronouncement of brain dead individuals.[15]

On the other hand, many Christians, both Protestant[16] and Catholic,[17] support a brain-oriented definition, claiming that being prolife does not foreclose being clear on when life ends. As we have seen in the previous chapter, one Christian theological argument supporting brain-oriented definitions starts with the ancient Christian theological anthropology that sees the human as the integration of body and mind or spirit. When the two are irreversibly separated, then the human is gone. This view, as we have seen, places some Christian theologians in the higher-brain camp. In doing so these theologians sometimes differentiate themselves from secular defenders of higher-brain concepts. The latter group, under the influence of philosophers such as Derek Parfit,[18] stresses mentalist conceptions of the person that sometimes lead to support of a higher-brain conception that focuses exclusively on the irreversible loss of mental function without concern about the separation of mind from body.[19] By contrast those working within Christian theology are more likely to insist on the importance of both mind and body.[20]

There are, of course, also many secular persons who support a cardiac definition of death. One survey, now dated, found that about a third of those questioned continued to support a cardiac definition.[21] The only plausible conclusion is that the definition of death is heavily influenced by theological and metaphysical beliefs along with theories of value. We have learned that in a pluralistic society it is unrealistic to expect unanimity on such questions. Hence a tolerance of pluralism may be the only way to resolve the public policy debate.

This conclusion seems even more inevitable when one realizes—as I argued in the previous chapter—that there are not just two or three plausible definitions (cardiac, whole-brain, and higher-brain definitions); there are literally hundreds of possible variants. Some insist on irreversible loss of anatomical brain structure at the cellular level; others only on irreversible loss of function. Some insist on loss of cellular-level functions, and others insist only on irreversible loss of supercellular functions of integration of bodily function. Some might insist on loss of all central nervous system functions including spinal cord function (an early position of Henry Beecher, the chair of the Harvard ad hoc committee), and others draw a line between spinal cord and brain. Among higher-brain defenders, there are innumerable variations on what counts as "higher": everything above the brain stem, the cerebrum, the cerebral cortex, the neocortex, the sensory cortex, and so on. As we have seen, some who insist on loss of all brain functions ignore electrical functions, limiting their attention to clinical functions.[22] Some are even willing to ignore functions of "nests of cells," claiming they may be "insignificant."[23] When all the possible variants are combined, there will be a large number of positions; no group is likely to gain the support of more than a small minority of the population. The only way to have a single definition of death is for those with power to coerce others to use their preferred definition. If that single definition were the current "whole-brain" one with a requirement that literally all functions of the brain must be gone before death is pronounced, the result could be disastrous. No one really believes that every last function of the entire brain must be irreversibly lost for a brain to be dead. That would include all electrical functions, all neurohumoral functions, and cellular functions. Because clinicians would necessarily have to exercise discretion in deciding which functions are to be ignored, patients would be at the mercy of the discretion of the clinician who happens to be present when the question of pronouncing death arises. Even if we were willing to let some ride roughshod over others, it is very unlikely that any one position could gain majority support; in fact, it is unlikely that any single position could come close to a majority. There may be no alternative but to tolerate multiple views.

CONSTITUTIONAL ISSUES

Once the choice of a definition of death is cast in terms of theological or philosophical issues, the necessity of conscientious choice among the definitions seems more plausible. The constitutional issue of separation of church and state presses us in the direction of accepting definitions with religious groundings. Of course, the constitutional provision prohibiting the establishment of religion does not give absolute freedom of religious action. Many religious beliefs, if acted on, could cause significant harm to others. The "harm to others" principle (or perhaps some more complex social ethical principle such as the principle of justice) necessitates the state's right to limit action based on many belief systems. Snake-handling cults, religious groups that support extremes of corporal punishment for children, religious groups using hallucinogenic drugs, and sects that would practice human and animal sacrifice have all been constrained for the safety and welfare of others.

Nevertheless, the burden on the state to justify interference with religious practice is great. Defenders of compulsory imposition of a single definition of death on a large group of religious conscientious objectors to that definition would have to be supported by significant social harms to other parties. I shall argue later in the chapter that such harms cannot be demonstrated. Thus the New Jersey law authorizes religious objection to the state's default definition of death when there is a religious basis for objecting to the whole-brain definition.

Problems Limiting Conscientious Objection to Religious Objectors

A state limiting conscientious objection to religious objectors as New Jersey has done is likely to face potentially difficult constitutional challenges. We learned from laws permitting religious conscientious objection to service in the military that restricting objection to certain types may be legally indefensible. During the Vietnam War era, some objectors had views that were clearly moral or philosophical, but they had a hard time accepting or demonstrating to others that they were religious. Especially if *religious* is defined as involving belief in a Supreme Being, many individuals whose objections seemed very similar to religious objections could not qualify. Even members of certain groups often classified as *religions* could not meet the belief in a Supreme Being test: Buddhists, Confucians, and Native American belief systems all look much like religions, but fail the Supreme Being test. Gradually the restriction of conscientious objection to religious objection was challenged and found to be discriminatory. The concept of religious objection was gradually broadened to include many belief systems that may not, at first, appear to be overtly religious.

Some scholars who have studied the New Jersey criterion of death law (including some most closely involved with the drafting of the law) believe that restricting the beliefs supporting objection to the brain-oriented definition of death to those that were narrowly religious would be interpreted to include more broadly moral objections as well. That at least is the opinion of Robert Olick (personal communication, Oct. 23, 1996), an attorney and bioethicist who served as the executive director of the commission that developed the New Jersey law.[24] The only reason that the New Jersey Commission on Legal and Ethical Problems in the Delivery of Health Care and the New Jersey legislature limited its provision to religious objection was political. Even during the debates before passage, some commentators said that objections that were not religious (if religion is narrowly construed) would be sustained in a legal challenge.

There are also enormous practical problems as well as moral problems with narrowly construed attempts to limit the law to religion. At a practical level, enforcement officials would have to establish mechanisms for verifying whether an objection was truly religious. A nonpracticing Jew who had a nonreligious objection to a brain-oriented definition of death could cite his or her religious background, and it would be almost impossible for the state to establish whether the objection was religious. Morally, the principle of equal respect would seem to require that if religious objections were permitted, equally sincere, and equally deeply held, nonreligious philosophical objections would be equally acceptable. If little is at stake in terms of public interest, little is lost by accepting both on equal terms.

Explicit Patient Choice, Substituted Judgment, and Best Interest

Assuming that the case is made that individuals should be able to exercise religiously or nonreligiously based conscientious choice of an alternative definition of death, should that discretion be extended to surrogate decision makers in the manner that terminal illness treatment refusal decisions are? I see no reason to limit the choice to competent and formerly competent persons who have executed advance directives.

Consider a formerly competent adult or adolescent who has never formally written a document choosing an alternative definition of death but who has left an oral record or a lifestyle pattern that appears to the surrogate to favor an alternative. Halberstam was returning from an Orthodox Jewish prayer service when he was shot. Assuming he had not written an instruction stating a preference for a cardiac-oriented definition of death, should parents (or other next of kin) be permitted formally to choose it for him (as, in fact, Halberstam's did through the informal decisions in New York)? It appears that Halberstam had continued to live the religious life of his parents, and I see no reason to doubt that he would choose as they did. Just as the next of kin can presently exercise substituted judgment in forgoing of treatment decisions, his parents likewise should be permitted to choose on his behalf based on the values he is most likely to have held.

Some might claim that this subordinates the interests of the patient or society to the whim of the idiosyncratic beliefs of the next of kin. Later I shall argue that there is little at stake for the society. As for Halberstam's interests, as an unconscious individual he seems to have no explicit contemporaneous interest. If it can be said that he has any residual interests, it surely must be to have his prospective autonomy preserved. Insofar as the parents can deduce what he would have autonomously chosen had he been able to exercise such judgment, surely they must be permitted, indeed required, to exercise that choice on his behalf.

But suppose we had no idea what Halberstam's wishes were about which definition of death should be used in his case. Or suppose he suffered his injury when he was 1 rather than 15 or 21. Clearly in this case respecting autonomy is out of the question. The only moral alternative is to use what is considered the best concept of death. But should it be the concept of death considered best by the society—perhaps some version of a whole-brain oriented death assuming that is the law of the state—or should it be the concept considered best by his next of kin? In the context of forgoing treatment decisions I have long argued that in such cases the discretion should go to the next of kin under the doctrine of what I have called *limited familial autonomy*.[25] Just as the individual has an autonomy right to choose a definition of death (or a treatment plan), so families have a right to a range of discretion in deciding what is best for their wards.

They select the schooling and religious education that so dramatically shapes the system of values and beliefs of the child. They are expected to socialize the child into some value system. In a liberal pluralistic society, we do not insist that familial surrogates choose the best possible value system for their wards; we expect them to exercise discretion drawing on their own beliefs and values. As long as the ward's interests are not jeopardized too substantially and the interests of the society are not threatened, parents should not only be permitted but actually expected to make a choice of a definition of death for their wards.

Limits on the Range of Discretion

In my early writing on the subject of individual choice of a definition of death I assumed without stating it that the range of choice would be limited among a range of tolerable alternatives. If the risks to the society became too great, surely a limit would have to be placed. Hence, probably, no one should be able to decide that he or she should be treated as alive if cardiac, respiratory, and brain function have all completely and irreversibly ceased. At least such choice should be foreclosed if it would pose public health problems or be grossly unfair to spouse and beneficiaries. Likewise, I believe no one should be able to choose to be considered dead when he or she retains all of these functions. Also, for pragmatic reasons, a state should choose a default definition leaving it up to individuals to exercise conscientious objection if they disagree with the default. What I now make explicit is that the choice must be within a range of reasonable or tolerable alternatives.

WHOLE-BRAIN VERSUS CARDIAC CONCEPTIONS OF DEATH

The New Jersey law gives the narrowest of options: between the default whole-brain-oriented definition and the single alternative of a cardiac definition. That would be a clearly acceptable choice assuming there are no significant societal or third-party consequences. The New Jersey plan would seem to offer a minimal range of choice.

INCLUDING HIGHER-BRAIN CONCEPTS OF DEATH

For many years I and many other people have argued that it is no longer plausible to hold to a literal whole-brain definition in which every last function of the entire brain must be dead before death can be pronounced.[26] A case can be made that some versions of higher-brain formulations of a definition of death should be among the choices permitted. Under such an arrangement, a whole-brain definition might be viewed as the centrist view that would serve as the default definition, permitting those with more conservative views to opt for cardiac-oriented definitions and those with more liberal views to opt for certain higher-brain formulations. Of course, this would permit people with brain-stem function including spontaneous respiration to be treated as dead. Organs could be procured that otherwise would not be available (assuming the dead donor rule is retained), bodies could be used for research (assuming proper consent is obtained), and life insurance would pay off.

Some might be concerned that this would give surrogates the authority to make their wards treated as dead while some brain and cardiac functions remain. They see this as posing risks for unacceptable choices, for ending a lingering state of disability, for example. Assuming that the only cases that could be classified as dead by surrogates would be those who have lost all capacity for consciousness— that is, who have lost all higher-brain functions—the risks to the individual classified as deceased would be minimal. We must keep in mind that surrogates are already presumed to have the authority to terminate all life support on these people. Often this would mean that they would soon be dead by the most traditional definitions of death. This would occur within minutes in many cases. The effect on inheritance and insurance would be trivial if they were simply called dead before stopping medical support rather than stopping before pronouncing death. Even for those vegetative or comatose patients who had sufficient lower-brain function to breathe on their own, a suspension of all medical treatment would lead to death fairly soon. Adding a higher-brain option to the range of discretion would have only minimal effect on practical matters and would be a sign that we can show the same respect to the religious and philosophical convictions of those favoring the higher-brain position as we do now in New Jersey for the holders of the cardiac position. If there are actually scores of potential definitions of death within the range from higher-brain to cardiac positions, then only a relatively small minority is likely to be in agreement with the default position, whatever it may be. The wise thing to do seems to be to pick some intermediary position and permit people to deviate both to somewhat more liberal and somewhat more conservative positions. The choices would probably have to be limited to this range. Both public health and moral problems become severe if the scope of choice is expanded much further.

The Problem of Order: Objections to a Conscience Clause

All of this, of course, depends on my as-yet-undefended claim that there are no significant societal or third-party harms from permitting conscientious objection to a default definition within the range I have specified. The President's Commission for the Study of Ethical Problems in Medicine and Biomedical and Behavioral Research prepared an important report in 1981 reviewing the definition of death debate.[27] In that report the commission examined the cardiac, whole-brain, and higher-brain options. In spite of the fact that I and Dan Wikler, their two philosophical consultants on the issue, endorsed versions of a higher-brain formu-lation, the commission endorsed the whole-brain position. They gave serious consideration to the higher-brain position before rejecting it for a number of reasons, most of which can be summarized under the heading of the problems that would be created for social order.

Death as a Biological Fact

One preliminary objection that was not dwelled on by the commission but that arises in many discussions of the issue is the claim that death is not a matter of religious or philosophical or policy choice but rather a matter of biological fact.[28] It is now generally recognized that the choice of a concept of death (as opposed to formulation of criteria and tests) is really normative[29] or ontological.[30] We are debating when, as a matter of social policy, we ought to treat someone as dead. No amount of biological research can answer that question at the conceptual level. Of course many people could still hold that although the definition of death is a normative or ontological question, there is still only one single correct formulation. That seems to me to be a very plausible position, but we are not discussing the issue of whether there can only be one true definition of death; we are discussing whether society can function for public policy purposes while tolerating differences in beliefs about what the true definition of death is. Tolerat-ing a Jew's or Native American's belief in a definition that is perceived by the rest of society as wrong is no different from having a society tolerate more than one belief about whether abortion or forgoing life support in the living is morally correct. We are asking whether society can treat people as dead based on their own beliefs rather than whether people are really dead—that is, really conform to some metaphysically correct conception of what it means to be dead in such circumstances. It is possible to hold that there is one and only one metaphysically correct concept of death but that, out of respect for minority views, society can treat some people who conform to this meaning of death as if they were alive.

Policy Chaos

One of the consistent themes in the criticism of higher-brain definitions, especially with the conscience clause I am defending, is that its adoption would lead to policy chaos. Presumably critics have in mind stress of health professionals, insurers, family members, and public policy processes such as succession of the presidency. But a very similar substituted-judgment and best-interest discretion is already granted surrogates regarding decisions to forgo life support on still-living patients. One would think that the potential for abuse and for chaos would be much greater granting this discretion. It remains to be seen what chaos would be created from conscientious objection to a default definition of death. If each of the envisioned policy problems can be addressed successfully, then we are left with a religious/philosophical/policy choice for which we should be tolerant of variation if possible and if there existed no good social reasons to reject individual discretion.

Potential Problems with a Conscience Clause That Includes Higher-Brain Formulations

Some of the rebuttal against the charge of policy chaos has already been suggested. Some additional arguments need to be addressed.

PROBLEMS WITH STOPPAGE OF TREATMENT

One concern is that life-sustaining medical treatment would be stopped on different people with medically identical conditions at different times if conscientious choice among definitions of death is permitted. That assumes, however, that decisions to stop treatment are always linked to pronouncement of death. We now know that normally it is appropriate to consider suspension of treatments in a manner that is decoupled from the question of whether the patient is dead.[31] A large percentage of in-hospital deaths now occur as a result of a decision to stop treatment and let the patient die. Presumably any valid surrogate who was contemplating opting for a higher-brain definition of death would, if told that option were not available, immediately contemplate choosing to forgo treatment, letting the patient die. In either case the patient will be dead within a short period of time.

The decoupling of the decision to forgo treatment from that of the pronouncement of death has led some to further decouple what I have called *death behaviors*, leaving agreed on points for various behaviors such as initiating grief, procuring organs, and terminating insurance coverage.[32] I considered such decoupling in the 1970s before rejecting it for two reasons.

First, even if we further decouple death behaviors, different people with different cultural beliefs and values will still consider different times appropriate for each of these behaviors. Some will consider widowhood to begin with loss of higher-brain function, others only with the death of the whole brain or the cessation of circulatory and respiratory function. We would still need a conscience clause, but now we would need one for the societally defined point for each of the list of death behaviors.

Second, even though some death behaviors surely must be decoupled (such as deciding to forgo treatment), we should not underestimate the importance of having something resembling a moment of death. Socially and psychologically, we need a moment, no matter how arbitrary, that loved ones can identify as a symbolic transition point at least for a large cluster of these death behaviors.

Relatives cannot send flowers one at a time as each moment arrives during a drawn out process of death involving many different death-related behaviors. Kass won the 1970 argument about whether death was a process or an event.[33] Although dying might be a process, death is not. There must be one defining moment of transition to which at least many of the death-related behaviors may attach.

ABUSE OF TERMINALLY ILL INDIVIDUALS

For the same reasons the risk of abuse of the terminally ill should not be a problem. There could be more concern about a family member dependent on the terminally ill person's pension, opting for a cardiac definition of death. That, however, seems remote. The same risk currently exists when family members make decisions to forgo life support. Moreover, there is no record of that having occurred in New Jersey where the option for a cardiac definition is available. If the problem did arise, the procedures currently available for review of suspected patient abuse would be available so that the next of kin could be removed from the surrogate role just as they would be now if a surrogate refused life support in a situation in which the motive appeared to be the financial gain of the surrogate.

HEALTH INSURANCE

I have already mentioned the potential impact on health insurance if someone chooses a definition of death that would have the effect of making someone live longer, if, for instance, a cardiac definition were chosen. (If some version of a higher-brain definition were chosen, the effect would more likely be a savings in health insurance.) There is good reason to believe that the effect on health insurance would be minimal. A relatively small number of people would actively make a protreatment choice based on their preference for a cardiac definition or any alternative that would require longer treatment. The small costs would probably be justified in the name of preserving respect for individual freedom on religious or philosophical matters. If the problem became significant, a health insurance policy could easily address the problem. Any health insurance policy must have some limits on coverage. Cosmetic surgery is usually not covered; there are often limits on the number of days of inpatient care for psychiatric services. Many marginal procedures including longer days of stay in the hospital are rejected. If an insurer were worried about unfair impact on the subscriber pool if its funds were used to provide care for patients without brain function who had selected a cardiac definition of death, they could simply exclude care for living patients with dead brains.

LIFE INSURANCE

The concern of life insurance companies is exactly the opposite. Insisting on a cardiac definition would simply delay payment, which would be in the insurer's interest; however, selecting a higher-brain definition would make the individual dead sooner, potentially quite a bit sooner. However, most living persons with dead brains die fairly soon either because such patients are hard to maintain or because an advance directive or surrogate opts for termination of treatment.

INHERITANCE

As in the case of pensions and life insurance, some surrogate might be inclined to manipulate the timing of death to gain an inheritance more quickly. This could lead to choosing a higher-brain definition. However, the same surrogate already has the power to decline medical treatment, which would theoretically expose the patient to similar risks, and such cases are exceedingly rare. If a surrogate is suspected of abusing a patient by choosing an inappropriate concept of death, such a surrogate can always be challenged and removed. If one compares the risk of abuse from surrogate discretion in deciding to forgo treatment with that from deciding on a variant definition of death, surely the discretion in forgoing treatment is more controversial and more subject to abuse. Yet that has not proved to be a significant problem.

SPOUSAL/MARITAL STATUS

Another social practice that can be affected directly by the timing of a death is the marital status of the spouse. Spouses may want to retain their status as spouses rather than become widows/widowers for various psychological and financial reasons. Or they may want to become widows/widowers so that they can get on with their lives. Conceivably some may be ready to remarry. For example, a spouse who had been caring for a persistent vegetative state (PVS) patient for years may have already separated psychologically from his or her mate even though she or he was not actually dead. This person could be ready to remarry, which could be done legally once the spouse were deceased. This problem seems quite farfetched, but it could happen. Such spouses would probably already have contemplated refusing life support and could be removed as inappropriate surrogates if it is clear they are motivated for nonpatient-centered reasons.

ORGAN TRANSPLANT

One significant impact of the definition of death is the availability of organs for transplant. If someone insists on a cardiac-based definition of death, that person would not be able to donate organs when heart function remains even though brain function has ceased. However, any who selected cardiac definition of death would be unlikely to be a donor of organs if he or she were forced to be pronounced dead based on brain criteria in any case. On the other hand, a person who chose to be considered dead even though lower-brain function remained would be a potential organ source. Someone who wanted to have organs procured when his or her higher brain functions were irreversibly lost potentially could have his or her organs procured earlier by selecting a higher-brain definition. As long as this were limited to cases in which an active choice were made in favor of the higher-brain formulation, it is hard to see why there would be strong objection. With the evolution of the non–heart-beating cadaver protocols (which I will discuss in Chapter 13), such persons could accomplish something similar by refusing life support to the point of death followed by organ procurement. The outcome would be similar except that the donor would be forced to participate in the use of a concept of death that he or she rejected, and the quality of the organs might be jeopardized. As long as the cases are limited to those in which there was a valid choice for a higher-brain definition, I cannot see why moral or societal concern should be raised.

Many people have pressed for a law authorizing organ procurement from living anencephalic infants (a proposal I will consider in Chapter 14).[34] Recently the AMA's Council on Ethical and Judicial Affairs temporarily endorsed such a view.[35] It seems they must be muddled. If we mean by *death* nothing more than being in a condition in which it is appropriate for others to engage in death-associated behaviors and we include procuring organs in the list of such behaviors, then anyone who is an appropriate candidate for procuring so-called life-prolonging organs is dead.[36] By this logic if members of the AMA council really believed it was acceptable to procure organs from an anencephalic infant with remaining brain-stem function, then to be consistent they should have claimed that such anencephalic infants are already dead (or, more accurately, have never been alive). In effect, they have adopted a version of a higher-brain-oriented definition of death and, if they wanted to be consistent, should really have claimed that it is acceptable to procure organs from anencephalic infants because they are dead (or have never been living, in the social policy sense of the term). In fact, the AMA reversed its endorsement of anencephalic organ procurement, making their position once again consistent with a whole-brain view of the definition of death.

SUCCESSION TO THE PRESIDENCY

Another potential implication of choosing an alternative definition of death is that succession to the presidency or to other roles could be affected. In the United

States, the vice president automatically is elevated to the presidency on the death of the president. Similar policies affect monarchies in which the successor is automatically made king. A president who chose a cardiac definition of death could thereby end his term of office at a different time than one who chose a whole-brain or higher-brain definition. Because one in certain circumstances can retain cardiac function for years, the succession of the vice president could be delayed.

Obviously, this reflects a flaw in the succession law. Under present law a permanently vegetative president is not dead and there would be no automatic succession. But as soon as permanent vegetative state is diagnosed, there should be immediate succession regardless of whether the president is dead. One could imagine a next of kin being pressured to choose a definition with an eye toward timing the succession. That could happen now in an effort to delay succession of the governorship in New Jersey. It could happen elsewhere if discretion were permitted, although the possibility of this seems extremely remote. A constitutional amendment provides a mechanism for temporary assumption of the office, but once a president is known to be permanently incapacitated, he or she clearly should be replaced.

THE EFFECT ON HEALTH PROFESSIONALS

A final potential problem with authorizing conscientious choice is the possible effect on health professionals providing care for the patient. Nurses will be required to suffer potential emotional stress at having to continue care or cease care at a time they believe inappropriate. Physicians will face similar problems. But this is hardly a problem unique to a choice of a definition of death. Some living patients or their surrogates refuse life-supporting therapy before the nurse or physician believes appropriate. They are simply obliged to stop according to laws about informed consent and the right to refuse treatment. More recently, health professionals have been disturbed about requests for care the clinicians deem "futile." Patients who insisted on not being pronounced dead until their heart stopped potentially could insist on hospital-based treatment even though their brains were dead. That is potentially the situation in New Jersey now. But the responsibility of the health professional to deliver care deemed futile against his or her will is already a matter of considerable controversy. It remains to be determined whether other states will adopt the New Jersey conscience clause. Most patients demanding such care are clearly not dead by any definition. The resolution could be the same for patients with dead brains as it is for terminally ill or vegetative patients, or it could be different. The law could determine, for instance, that conscious patients would have a right of access to normatively futile care (perhaps with the proviso that they have independent funding), but that permanently unconscious patients or those with dead brains would have no right of access. In any case, the impact on caregivers is not a problem unique to patients who might exercise an option for an alternative definition of death.

Implementing a Conscience Clause

The procedural implementation of a conscience clause would require some additional planning, but the problems would not be novel. Most are addressed in the existing Patient Self-Determination Act and required request laws (see Chapter 9). The former requires that someone inquire about the existence of an advance directive on admission to a hospital and provide assistance in executing an advance directive if the patient desires. The latter requires that the next of kin be notified of the opportunity to donate organs in suitable cases. The most plausible way to record a choice of something other than a default concept of death would be in one's advance directive. That is the kind of document that ought to be on the minds of those caring for a patient who is near death. An addition specifying a choice of an alternative concept of death would be easy; it would be crucial in the case of those who are writing an advance directive demanding that life support continue even though the brain is dead. It would be a simple clarification in the case of one asking that support be forgone when the patient is permanently unconscious. A sentence choosing a higher-brain concept of death (and perhaps donating organs at that point) would be a modest addition.

Whether the new definition of death laws authorizing a conscience clause should also impose a duty on health professionals to notify patients or their surrogates of alternative concepts of death is a pragmatic question that would have to be addressed. I do not think that would be necessary. Just as Orthodox Jews presently carry the burden of notifying others of their requirements for a kosher diet and Jehovah's Witnesses carry the burden of notifying about refusal of blood transfusions, so those with alternative concepts of death would plausibly carry that burden. Something akin to the subjective standard for informed consent would apply. According to that standard, health professionals, when they negotiate a consent, are required to inform the patient of what the patient would reasonably want to know, but they are not expected to surmise all unusual views and interests of the patient. According to this approach, they would be expected to initiate discussions on alternative definitions of death only when they knew or had reason to know that the patient plausibly would have an interest in such a discussion. A clinician who knew his or her patient was an Orthodox Jew and knew that many Orthodox Jews prefer a more traditional concept of death would have such an obligation, but if he or she had no reason to believe the patient might be inclined toward an alternative concept there would not be such an obligation.

Some might claim that adding a conscience clause is unnecessary because only a small group of people would favor an alternative. In fact, a not insignificant number seem to prefer a more traditional cardiac or respiratory concept of death (Jews, Native Americans, Japanese, and others who are still committed to the importance of the heart or lungs). If a higher-brain-oriented concept of death were among the options, a much larger minority would have an interest in exercising the conscience clause. In fact, there have been a number of court cases and anecdotal reports of families objecting to the use of whole-brain-based concepts. It seems reasonable to assume that these represent only a fraction of the total number of cases in which patients or families would prefer either a more traditional or a more innovative concept of death.

Even if it could be shown that few people would care enough about the concept and criteria of death used to pronounce them or their loved ones dead, this is still an important issue to clarify. It is important if only the rights of a small minority are violated. It is also important as a matter of conceptual clarity and of principle. The knee-jerk revulsion with a conscience clause for alternative concepts of death probably reflects lingering belief that deciding when someone is dead is a matter of biological fact (for which individual conscience seems irrelevant). But insisting that the choice of a concept of death be treated as a matter of philosophical and theological dispute seems to follow naturally once one realizes the true nature of the issues involved. Getting people to think why a conscience clause is appropriate for this issue has an important teaching function as well as serving to respect the rights of minorities on deeply held religious and philosophical convictions.

Conclusion

Once one grasps that the choice of a definition of death at the conceptual level is a religious/philosophical/policy choice rather than a question of medical science, the case for granting discretion within limits in a liberal pluralistic society is a very powerful one. There seems to be no basis for imposing a unilateral normative judgment on the entire population when the members of the society are clearly divided. When one realizes that there are many variants and that no one is likely to receive the support of a majority, pluralism appears the only answer. Having a state choose a default definition and then granting individuals a limited range of discretion within the limits of reason seems to be the only defensible option. There is no reason to limit this discretion to religiously based reasons and no reason why familial surrogates should not be empowered to use substituted judgment or best-interest standards for making such choices just as they presently do for forgoing treatment decisions that determine even more dramatically the timing of death. A default with an authorization for conscientious objection seems the humane, respectful, fair, and pragmatic solution.

ENDNOTES

1. "Man Charged in Shooting of Jewish Students," *New York Times*, March 3, 1994, pp. A1, A6.

2. "Failure of Brain Is Legal 'Death,'" New York Says," *New York Times*, June 19, 1987, pp. A1, B4.

3. "In Hospital Hallways, Family and Friends Pray for Victims," *New York Times*, March 3, 1994, p. B4.

4. The New Jersey Declaration of Death Act, signed April 8, 1991. *New Jersey Statutes Annotated*. Title 26, 6A-1 to 6A-8. It reads, in part:

   The death of an individual shall not be declared upon the basis of neurological criteria . . . of this act when the licensed physician authorized to declare death, has reason to believe, on the basis of information in the individual's available medical records, or information provided by a member of the individual's family or any other person knowledgeable about the individual's personal religious beliefs that such a declaration would violate the personal religious beliefs of the individual. In these cases death shall be declared, and the time of death fixed, solely upon the basis of cardio-respiratory criteria. . . .

5. "Slaying Suspects Share a Past Marred by Crime," *New York Times*, April 1, 1994, p. A24.

6. "Florida Hospital Seeks to End Life Support of Comatose Girl," *New York Times*, Feb. 13, 1994, p. A24; "Brain-Dead Florida Girl Will Be Sent Home on Life Support," *New York Times*, Feb. 19, 1994, p. 9.

7. "The Law Concerning Human Organ Transplants" (Law No. 104 in 1997).

8. Rihito Kimura, "Japan's Dilemma with the Definition of Death," *Kennedy Institute of Ethics Journal* 1 (1991): 123–31.

9. Harvard Medical School, "A Definition of Irreversible Coma. Report of the Ad Hoc Committee of the Harvard Medical School to Examine the Definition of Brain Death," *Journal of the American Medical Association* 205 (1968): 337–40; Task Force on Death and Dying, Institute of Society, Ethics, and the Life Sciences, "Refinements in Criteria for the Determination of Death: An Appraisal," *Journal of the American Medical Association* 221 (1972): 48–53; President's Commission for the Study of Ethical Problems in Medicine and Biomedical and Behavioral Research, "Report of the Medical Consultants on the Diagnosis of Death to

the President's Commission for the Study of Ethical Problems in Medicine and Biomedical and Behavioral Research," *Defining Death: Medical, Legal, and Ethical Issues in the Definition of Death* (Washington, DC: U.S. Government Printing Office, 1981), pp. 159–66; Ronald E. Cranford, "Minnesota Medical Association Criteria: Brain Death—Concept and Criteria. Part I," *Minnesota Medicine* 61 (1978): 561–63; Law Reform Commission of Canada, *Criteria for the Determination of Death* (Ottawa: Minister of Supply and Services, 1981); Earl A. Walker et al. "An Appraisal of the Criteria of Cerebral Death—A Summary Statement," *Journal of the American Medical Association* 237 (1977): 982–86.

10. More recent analysis has challenged the blatant fact–value dichotomy implied in this separation of the criteria question as one for medical science and the concept question as one of religious, philosophical, or public policy. See Robert M. Veatch, *Death, Dying, and the Biological Revolution*, rev. ed. (New Haven, CT: Yale University Press, 1989), pp. 43–44.

11. M. D. Tendler, "Cessation of Brain Function: Ethical Implications in Terminal Care and Organ Transplant," in *Brain Death: Interrelated Medical and Social Issues*, ed. Julius Korein (New York: New York Academy of Sciences, 1978), pp. 394–97; Frank J. Veith, Jack M. Fein, Moses S. Tendler, Robert M. Veatch, Marc A. Kleiman, and George Kalkinis, "Brain Death: I. A Status Report of Medical and Ethical Considerations," *Journal of the American Medical Association* 238 (1977): 1651–55.

12. J. David Bleich, "Establishing Criteria of Death," *Tradition* 13 (1973): 90–113; Bleich, "Neurological Criteria of Death and Time of Death Statutes," in *Jewish Bioethics*, eds. Fred Rosner and J. David Bleich (New York: Sanhedrin Press, 1979), pp. 303–16; Fred Rosner, "The Definition of Death in Jewish Law," *Tradition* 10 (4, 1969): 33–39.

13. Rihito Kimura, "Japan's Dilemma with the Definition of Death."

14. President's Commission for the Study of Ethical Problems in Medicine and Biomedical and Behavioral Research, *Defining Death: Medical, Legal, and Ethical Issues in the Definition of Death*, p. 41.

15. Paul A. Byrne, Sean O'Reilly, and Paul M. Quay, "Brain Death—An Opposing Viewpoint," *Journal of the American Medical Association* 242 (1979): 1985–90.

16. Stanley Hauerwas, "Religious Concepts of Brain Death and Associated Problems," in *Brain Death: Interrelated Medical and Social Issues*, ed. Julius Korein (New York: New York Academy of Sciences, 1978), pp. 329–38; Ralph B. Potter, "The Paradoxical Preservation of a Principle," *Villanova Law Review* 13 (Summer 1968): 784–92; Paul Ramsey, "On Updating Death," in *Updating Life and Death*, ed. Donald R. Cutler (Boston: Beacon Press, 1969), pp. 31–53.

17. Bernard Haring, *Medical Ethics* (Note Dame, IN: Fides, 1973), pp. 131–36.

18. Derek Parfit, *Reasons and Persons* (Oxford: Clarendon Press, 1984).

19. Michael B. Green and Daniel Walker, "Brain Death and Personal Identity," *Philosophy and Public Affairs* 9 (2, Winter 1980): 105–33.

20. Paul Ramsey, *The Patient as Person* (New Haven, CT: Yale University Press, 1970), p. xiii; Robert M. Veatch, *Death, Dying, and the Biological Revolution*, p. 42.

21. William C. Charron, "Death: A Philosophical Perspective on the Legal Definitions," *Washington University Law Quarterly* 4 (1975): 979–1008.

22. Stephen Ashwal and Sanford Schneider, "Failure of Electroencephalography to Diagnose Brain Death in Comatose Patients," *Annals of Neurology* 6 (1979): 512–17.

23. James L. Bernat, "How Much of the Brain Must Die on Brain Death?" *The Journal of Clinical Ethics* 3 (1, Spring 1992): 21–26.

24. Robert S. Olick, "Brain Death, Religious Freedom, and Public Policy," *Kennedy Institute of Ethics Journal* 1 (Dec. 1991): 275–88. Also see C. K. Goldberg, "Choosing Life after Death: Respecting Religious Beliefs and Moral Convictions in Near Death Decisions," *Syracuse Law Review* 39 (4, 1988): 1197–1260 (see especially p. 1256).

25. Robert M. Veatch, "Limits of Guardian Treatment Refusal: A Reasonableness Standard," *American Journal of Law and Medicine* 9 (4, Winter 1984): 427–68.

26. Robert M. Veatch, "The Whole-Brain-Oriented Concept of Death: An Outmoded Philosophical Formulation," *Journal of Thanatology* 3 (1975): 13–30 (see also Chapter 3 of this volume); H. Tristram Engelhardt, "Defining Death: A Philosophical Problem for Medicine and Law," *American Review of Respiratory Disease* 112 (1975), 587–90; James L. Bernat, "How Much of the Brain Must Die on Brain Death?"; Bernard Haring, *Medical Ethics*.

27. President's Commission for the Study of Ethical Problems in Medicine and Biomedical and Behavioral Research, *Defining Death: Medical, Legal, and Ethical Issues in the Definition of Death*.

28. For a discussion see Karen Grandstand Gervais, *Redefining Death* (New Haven, CT: Yale University Press, 1986), pp. 45–74; David Lamb, "Diagnosing Death," *Philosophy and Public Affairs* 7 (1978): 144–53; and Lawrence C. Becker, "Human Being: The Boundaries of the Concept," *Philosophy and Public Affairs* 4 (1975): 334–59.

29. Robert M. Veatch, *Death, Dying, and the Biological Revolution*.

30. Michael B. Green and Daniel Wikler, "Brain Death and Personal Identity."

31. The general problem of decoupling of behavioral correlates of pronouncing death is the subject of Norman Fost's chapter cited in note 32 and will not be examined in detail in this paper.

32. Baruch Brody, "How Much of the Brain Must Be Dead?" in *The Definition of Death: Contemporary Controversies*, ed. Stuart J. Youngner, Robert M. Arnold, and Renie Schapiro (Baltimore: Johns Hopkins University Press, 1999), pp. 71–

82; Norman Fost, "The Unimportance of Death," *The Definition of Death: Contemporary Controversies*, pp. 161–78.

33. Leon R. Kass, "Death as an Event: A Commentary on Robert Morison," *Science* 173 (1971): 698–702.

34. Michael Harrison, "The Anencephalic Newborn as Organ Donor," *Hastings Center Report* 16 (April 1986): 21–23; John Fletcher, John Robertson, and Michael Harrison, "Primates and Anencephalics as Sources for Pediatric Organ Transplants," *Fetal Therapy* 1 (2–3, 1986): 150–64; James Walters and Stephen Ashwal, "Organ Prolongation in Anencephalic Infants: Ethical & Medical Issues," *Hastings Center Report* 18 (Oct./Nov. 1988): 19–27.

35. American Medical Association, Council on Ethical and Judicial Affairs, "The Use of Anencephalic Neonates as Organ Donors," *Journal of the American Medical Association* 273 (20, May 24–31, 1995): 1614–18.

36. Of course, some organs (single kidneys and liver lobes) can be procured from living people. We do not insist on people being declared dead in these cases. It is considered appropriate behavior even for the living, assuming that proper consents have been obtained.

EIGHT

CRAFTING A NEW DEFINITION OF DEATH LAW

CHANGING CURRENT LAW to conform to the suggestions made in the preceding chapters will be complex and should be done with deliberate speed, but it should be done. Two changes are needed in the current definition of death: (1) incorporating the higher-brain function notion of death and (2) incorporating some form of the conscience clause.

Incorporating the Higher-Brain Notion

Present law makes humans dead when they have lost all functions of the entire brain. It is uniformly agreed that the law should incorporate only this basic concept of death, not the precise criteria or tests needed to determine that the whole brain is dead. That is left up to the consensus of neurological experts.

All that is needed to shift to a higher-brain formulation is a change in the wording of the law to replace "all functions of the entire brain" with some relevant, more limited alternative. There are at least three options: references to higher-brain functions, cerebral functions, or consciousness. Although we could simply change the wording to state that an individual is dead when there is irreversible cessation of all higher-brain functions, that poses a serious problem. We are now suffering from the problems created by the vagueness of referring to "all functions of the entire brain." Even though referring to "all higher-brain functions" would be conceptually correct, it would be even more ambiguous. This could be given substance by referring to irreversible loss of cerebral functions, but I have already suggested two problems with that wording. Just as we now know there are some isolated functions of the whole brain that should be discounted, so there are probably some isolated cerebral functions that most would not want to count either. For example, if, hypothetically, an isolated "nest" of cerebral motor neurons were perfused so that if stimulated the body could twitch, that would be a cerebral function—but not a significant one for determining life any more

136

than a brain-stem reflex is. Second, in theory some really significant functions, such as consciousness, might someday be maintainable even without a cerebrum—if, for example, a computer could function as an artificial center for consciousness. The term "cerebral function" adds specificity, but is not satisfactory.

The language that seems best if integration of mind and body is what is critical is "irreversible cessation of the capacity for consciousness." That is, after all, what the defenders of the higher-brain formulations really have in mind. (If someone were to claim that some other "higher" function is critical, that alternative could simply be plugged in.) In Chapter 5 I actually endorsed a concept of death related not only to consciousness but also to capacity for social interaction, claiming that this was critical in the Judeo–Christian conception of human existence with full moral standing. I went on, however, to suggest that I could envision no cases in which the presence of consciousness would not also permit social interactions—at least inputs. Likewise, I cannot envision one who possesses capacity for social interaction without consciousness. The two, I argued, were coterminous. I am therefore content to propose a higher-brain definition of death based on irreversible loss of capacity for consciousness. As is the case now, we will leave the specifics of the criteria and tests for measuring irreversible loss of capacity for consciousness up to the consensus of neurological expertise.[1] If the community of neurological expertise claims irreversible loss of consciousness cannot be measured, so be it. We will have at least clarified the concept and set the stage for the day when it can be measured with sufficient accuracy. We have noted, however, that neurologists presently claim that they can measure irreversible loss of consciousness accurately, at least when they are diagnosing persistent vegetative state in the context of decisions to forgo life support.

The Conscience Clause

A second significant change in the definition of death would be required to incorporate the conscience clause. It would permit individuals, while competent, to execute documents choosing alternative definitions of death that are, within reason, not threatening to significant interests of others. Although the New Jersey law permits only choosing a heart-oriented definition as an alternative, my proposal, assuming some version of a whole-brain formulation—adjusted to acknowledge that minor, cellular electrical activity and probably also hormonal regulatory functions should be ignored—were the default definition, would permit choosing either heart-oriented or higher-brain-oriented (consciousness-based) definitions as alternatives.

As I have indicated, the New Jersey law presently only permits competent adults to execute such conscience clauses. This, of course, excludes the possibility of parents choosing alternative definitions for their children. I had long ago proposed that, just as legal surrogates have the right to make medical treatment decisions for their wards provided the decisions are within reason, so they should be permitted to choose alternative definitions of death provided the individual had never expressed a preference. Although the New Jersey law tolerates only explicitly religiously based variation, I would favor variation based on any conscientiously formulated position.

As a shortcut the law could state that patients who had opted for the consciousness-based definition who had clearly irreversibly lost consciousness because of the stopping of heart and lung function could continue to be pronounced dead based on criteria measuring heart and lung function. It would have to be made more clear than in the present Uniform Determination of Death Act that this was simply an alternative means for measuring loss of consciousness. I see no reason to continue including the alternative forms of measurement in the legal definition itself. I would simply leave that to the criteria to be articulated by the consensus of experts.

A Proposed New Definition of Death for Public Policy Purposes

This leads to a proposal for a new definition of death that would read as follows:

> An individual who has sustained irreversible loss of all functions of the entire brain (excluding cellular-level and hormonal regulatory functions) is dead. This shall be referred to as the "default" definition of death. A determination of death must be made in accordance with accepted medical standards.
>
> However no individual shall be considered dead based on irreversible loss of these functions if he or she, while competent, has asked to be pronounced dead based on some other acceptable definition of death. These alternative definitions of death could include or exclude other bodily functions, however no individual shall be treated as dead for public policy purposes unless he or she has sustained irreversible cessation of all consciousness, and no individual shall be treated as alive for public policy purposes if he or she has irreversibly lost all circulatory and respiratory functions.
>
> Unless an individual has, while competent, selected a definition of death to be used for his or her own death pronouncement, the legal guardian or next of kin (in that order) may do so relying on substituted judgment insofar as information is available about the patient's own wishes. If no such information is available the decision maker shall rely on a best-interest determination. The definition selected by the individual, legal guardian, or next

of kin shall serve as the definition of death for all legal purposes. If no such alternative is selected, then the default definition shall be used.

There are alternative approaches to this one. If one favored only the shift to consciousness as a definition of death without the conscience clause, only paragraph one would be necessary. "Irreversible loss of consciousness" would be substituted for "irreversible loss of all functions of the entire brain." One could also craft a similar definition using the whole-brain-oriented definition of death as the default definition without permitting conscientious objection. Some have proposed an additional paragraph prohibiting a physician with a conflict of interest (such as an interest in the organs of the deceased) from pronouncing death. I am not convinced that paragraph is needed, however.

Conclusion

It has been puzzling why what at first seemed like a rather minor debate over when a human was dead should have persisted as long as it has. Many thought the definition of death debate was a technical argument that would be resolved in favor of the more fashionable, scientific, and progressive brain-oriented definition as soon as the old romantics attached to the heart died off. It is now clear that something much more complex and more fundamental is at stake. We have been fighting over the question of who has moral standing as a full member of the human moral community, a matter that forces on us some of the most basic questions of human existence: the relation of mind and body, the rights of religious and philosophical minorities, and the meaning of life itself.

I am not certain whether some version of the higher-brain-oriented definition of death will be adopted in any legal jurisdiction anytime soon, but I am convinced that the now old-fashioned whole-brain-oriented definition of death is becoming less and less plausible as we realize that no one really believes that literally all functions of the entire brain must be irreversibly lost for an individual to be dead. Unless there is some public consensus expressed in state or federal law conveying agreement on exactly which brain functions are insignificant, we will all be vulnerable to a slippery slope in which private practitioners choose for themselves exactly where the line should be drawn from the top of the cerebrum to the caudal end of the spinal cord. There is no principled reason to draw it exactly between the base of the brain and the top of the spine. Better that we have a principled reason for drawing it. To me, the principle is that for human life to be present—that is, for the human to be treated as a member in full standing of the human moral community—there must be integrated functioning of mind and body. That means some version of a higher-brain-oriented formulation relying on the presence of capacity for consciousness and social interaction.

Endnote

1. I have argued elsewhere that, in theory, even determining the criteria for measuring irreversible loss of capacity for a brain function such as consciousness involves fundamentally nonscientific value judgments. The community of neurologists, for example, would have to choose a probability level at which the prediction of irreversibility can be made. They would have to add nuanced meaning to the terms critical for the enterprise. They would have to assume certain concepts in their work. None of these are matters about which neurologists have expertise. In theory the lay community could disagree with the consensus of neurological experts, and in such disputes over these matters the lay population would have a legitimate claim to have their preferences and assumptions used in choosing the criteria for measuring irreversible loss of consciousness. For example, if the lay population wanted greater levels of statistical significance than the community of neurological experts, there is no rational reason why the neurologists' choice of a significance level should prevail. See Robert M. Veatch, *Death, Dying, and the Biological Revolution*, rev. ed. (New Haven, CT: Yale University Press, 1989), pp. 41–44; and Veatch, "Consensus of Expertise: The Role of Consensus of Experts in Formulating Public Policy and Estimating Facts," *Journal of Medicine and Philosophy* 16 (1991): 427–45.

PART TWO

PROCURING ORGANS

NINE

GIFT OR SALVAGE: THE TWO MODELS OF ORGAN PROCUREMENT

WE SAW IN Chapter 1 that the major religious and cultural traditions of the world do not have clear-cut, principled objections to life-saving organ transplants. The groundwork is in place for establishing the basic approach of a society to transferring organs from potential organ sources to others who need these organs. The focus of Part Two of this book is the ethics of organ procurement. In this part I examine the general options for a basis for ethical procurement, and then, a number of specific areas of controversy—for example, ways to reward those who donate organs. I will ask whether we can presume consent of those who have not explicitly objected to donation, whether we can require hospitals or other institutions to request donation or require people to respond to such requests, and whether we can procure organs from those who are "non–heart-beating cadavers"—in other words, "people who have died by cardiac arrest either from accidents or intentional termination of life-support. We will also look at the ethics of procuring organs from living people and anencephalic infants, the role of age in procurement, procuring organs from HIV-positive donors and others with potentially contagious medical problems, and the use of organs from nonhuman animals. I begin with the basics: Are organs the society's to salvage and use as it sees fit, or are they the individual's so they must be presented as a gift before another makes use of them?

In about 1970 Western society made a choice. By this time we were beginning to accept human-to-human (homologous) transplant as morally licit. Some pockets of resistance reflecting deep cultural beliefs remained in some cultures: Asians, especially Japanese people, found transplant difficult to accept. In part this was because of serious doubts that the essence of a human being could be localized in the brain. In part it resulted from a 1968 attempt by surgeon Juro Wada to transplant a heart in which there was widespread doubt that the surgeon had waited until the person from whom the organ was taken was really dead when the heart was procured. Native Americans were also skeptical, as were some people who continued to worry about the impact of organ transplant on the abortion debate. But most people in Western culture, both secular and religious, had come to accept the exciting new technology of organ replacement. Most of Christianity—both Catholic and Protestant—was strongly approving. Although Judaism continued to resist a brain-oriented definition of death, some of its Talmudic scholars treated organ transplant as morally required, more than most Christian ethicists were willing to claim.

Two Models for Justifying Organ Procurement

Given the increasing acceptance of organ procurement and the enormous good that can come from these organs, the remaining issue is establishing the basis on which the organs can be removed. As was suggested in Chapter 1, two polar positions surfaced in the early debate. They reflect two major ethical approaches.

Routine Salvaging

The earliest thinking about the basis for procuring organs reflected the common-sense view that the body of the deceased—the "mortal remains"—were no longer of any use to the dead person. It was not even of any use to the surviving family. Thus lawyer Jesse Dukeminier and physician David Sanders proposed a model they called *routine salvaging*.[1] The idea was that no harm—in fact great good—could come from cadaver salvaging, so it was appropriate for the society to routinely take any leftover viable parts without any formal permission.

In moral terms the view was utilitarian. The morally right course was to be determined by estimating the total consequences of alternative courses of actions and choosing the one doing the greatest good. In this case it meant estimating the net good (the good minus any envisioned harms) that could come from simply treating useful body parts of the deceased as state property and then estimating the net good expected from alternative policies, including those that require some sort of permission be obtained to take the organs. Their conclusion was that because no one would be harmed and some organ recipients could be given enormous benefits, the organs could simply be taken. "Salvage" without permission of deceased or next of kin was the recommended policy.

This policy has in more recent times sometimes been called organ procurement with *presumed consent*.[2] This naming, as I shall suggest later, is a mistake. Thus I shall continue to use the original, more graphic, term: routine salvaging. I do so without any implication that this approach is morally unacceptable before a review of the issues involved.

The case for routine salvaging requires careful scrutiny. "Salvaging" is probably an unfortunate term, but it implies exactly what its defenders have in mind:

picking over trash and taking, without permission, what seems to have some residual value. The assumption that the human body can be used by the state without permission suggests the troublesome analogy of Nazi medical research. There, as well, the presumption was made that certain humans could be used for the service of the state without permission.

The Nazi analogy is sometimes overused, however. An important difference in the case of salvaging organs is that the humans who are being used are dead. Nevertheless, there are similarities in the reasoning. In both cases, certain human bodies were considered to be outside the bounds of moral standing. Because of their lower status, they were considered accessible for others to use for their own purposes. In the case of Nazi research we used to believe that the experiments were not even good science, so the "purpose" being pursued was without any defense. More recently some analysts have suggested that some of that research was, in fact, scientifically valid and some of the studies were pursuing important scientific questions (such as how the body responds to extremes of temperature).[3]

Even if those purposes were to turn out to be important and worthwhile, however, critics of the utilitarian approach to the use of one person's body by another consider the moral premise totally inadequate. The most obvious lesson of the Nazi experience is that one cannot use another person's body for the good of society without permission. That is the first and most critical point of the Nuremberg Code:

1. The voluntary consent of the human subject is absolutely essential.

This means that the person involved should have legal capacity to give consent; should be so situated as to be able to exercise free power of choice, without the intervention of any element of fire, fraud, deceit, duress, over-reaching, or other ulterior form of constraint or coercion; and should have sufficient knowledge and comprehension of the elements of the subject matter involved as to enable him to make an understanding and enlightened decision. The latter element requires that before the acceptance of an affirmative decision by the experimental subject there should be made known to him the nature, duration, and purpose of the experiment; the method and means by which it is to be conducted; all inconveniences and hazards reasonably to be expected; and the effects upon his health or person which may possibly come from his participation in the experiment.

The duty and responsibility for ascertaining the quality of the consent rests upon each individual who initiates, directs or engages in the experiment. It is a personal duty and responsibility which may not be delegated to another with impunity.[4]

This notion of consent, which is so central to the Nuremberg approach to research with human subjects, is equally critical for the second approach to organ procurement.

Donation Model

The *donation model* is built on the moral notion that there is a duty to respect the bodily integrity of members of the moral community and that this obligation remains even after death. Just like there is a duty to respect the will of the individual whose assistance is sought in a research project, so likewise must that individual's integrity be respected even after his or her death. We have long acknowledged the right of the individual to control the disposal of his or her assets after death. Just like there is a duty to respect the will of the individual for disposition of assets, so we must respect his or her wishes about what will happen with his or her body.

The Foundation of the Duty to Respect the Wishes of the Deceased

This donation model is not based primarily on concerns about consequences. True, a sophisticated utilitarian might argue that routine salvaging could produce such hostility that fewer organs would be procured using that model, but the primary argument in favor of donation is not that the society (or the individual) will be harmed by the use of the body. Some who believe in reincarnation might, theoretically, have concerns about consequences, but, as we saw in Chapter 1, those who hold traditional Orthodox Christian beliefs about the resurrection of the body need have no fears of organ procurement. The real concern is grounded in the ethical principle of *autonomy*. That principle holds that others have a duty to permit individuals to live out their lives according to their own life plans—regardless of whether they have calculated the consequences so as to maximize their personal well being.

A question is sometimes raised about whether autonomy has any bearing after one dies. If the duty is to permit people to live out a life plan, some would ask how contravening the individual's wishes after that person's death could be a violation of autonomy. The question has generated a philosophical literature.[5] For example, a distinction is sometimes made between "*experiential interests*" and "*critical interests*."[6] Experiential interests are the normal interests we have in having certain experiences. These obviously cannot be fulfilled after death. Critical interests, however, are interests that are not thwarted by death. Our interest in having a particular relative receive a personal treasure, for example, can be fulfilled or blocked even after we die. Likewise, our interest in how our body is treated need not cease with death. Just as a person's objection to cremation or postmortem research binds those who survive, creating obligations that remain after a person's death, so interests in giving or refusing to give organs also can survive one's death and create obligations that remain.

Suffice to say for our purposes, most people accept the idea that their autonomy would be violated if their wishes about the disposal of their assets are not followed after they die. So much the more would they feel their autonomy would be violated if their wishes about the disposal of their body were not followed.

The mere fact that one will no longer be around to be aware one's choice was violated is not really the essential issue. For one thing if there were a general policy of disregarding people's interests, great distress would result. In the case of economic wills, if society believes that the will could be disregarded whenever more good would come if the assets were used in some other way, then all would live with the discomfort of knowing that their wishes about the future uses of their assets are not secure. More critically, we tend to feel a wrong is committed if the individual's will is not honored, even if we believe that individuals cannot know about this when it occurs.

A similar concern is reflected in the donation model for the use of body parts. We owe respect to the individual, limiting what we can do ethically to a person without consent. That duty of respect does not cease with the individual's death. The body is still the *mortal remains* of the individual, and his or her wishes deserve respect. Therefore, we can use the body for research, education, therapy, or transplantation only if that individual grants us permission, only if the body is made a gift to others. The reasoning is what philosophers would call *deontological*. Derived from the Greek word for "duty," the term is used to convey the idea that there are certain duties we owe to others *regardless of the consequences*. The ethical principle of respect for autonomy is one of the most profound and widely affirmed deontological duties in Western culture. It is the foundation of the donation model. That model won the debate in the United States and most of the rest of the world. In the United States there could be no other solution.

Surrogate Permission

There is one important qualification to the application of the principle of respect for autonomy to organ donation. What should happen if there is no reason to expect the individual has objected to donating his or her body but that individual has left no direct evidence that the gift was intended? Can we presume that, because no objection was on record, the individual intended that his or her body be used to benefit others? As we shall see in the next chapter, there is no reason to make such a presumption. We know that a significant portion of the American population does not want their organs used for transplant. In other cultures the percentage who would object may be even higher.

Nevertheless, even though we reject the presumption that a person who was silent about organ procurement would have wanted to donate organs, we have opened the door to donation by a surrogate—either a surrogate named by the individual while alive or, if that has not happened, the next of kin. There are several reasons to support allowing such surrogates to make this choice. For one, the named person or nearest relative might be in the best position to know the deceased's wishes. For another, drawing on the analogy of the economic will, we could view the body as property left at death to the family or other named parties. Just as someone who inherits assets has the right to make a gift of them to another, so it might be argued that, once the "beneficiary" receives the body, he or she then has a certain ownership interest, including the authority to make a gift of it for valid medical purposes. Finally, we may view the surrogate as having some limited range of discretion in choosing how to honor the dead and dispose of the remains. For some combination of these reasons, the surrogate named by the individual or, absent such naming, the family is, therefore, given the authority to choose a mode of burial, the kind of funeral or memorial service, and to make many other choices pertaining to the final rituals for the deceased.

There are, however, severe limits on the discretion of the next of kin or other surrogates. They cannot do literally anything they want with the body. As I discussed in the introduction, they have duties as well as rights—including the duty to dispose of the remains in a respectful manner. They are therefore said to have "quasi-property rights" in the body.[7] It is a right but with certain duties attached that constrain the amount of discretion the surrogate has.

The interesting case is what should happen when the wishes of the deceased conflict with those of the next of kin or other surrogate when one party wants organs to be procured and the other does not. The ethical principle of autonomy is the basis for rights for the individual. Especially in a highly individualistic society such as that of the United States, it should be clear that the deceased's own wishes must prevail. Hence the Uniform Anatomical Gift Act makes clear that an individual's refusal to agree to organ procurement takes precedence over the willingness of relatives to make the gift.

In principle, a valid donation of the bodily remains made while one is alive and competent should also take precedence over the objection of the next of kin. Thus someone with a valid donor card expressing a willingness to have organs taken for transplant should be enough to authorize organ procurement even if the family objects.

This could pose practical problems, however. For one, it is the family that is alive at the end. They are the ones who could sue the organ procurement organization and the surgeons who procured the organs. The law is quite clear that the family would eventually lose such a suit, but it could make life unpleasant for the health professionals involved for a while.

A second reason procurement personnel are reluctant to procure against the wishes of the family is that to procure organs that are useful for transplant, the procuring team needs to obtain a medical and social history to help rule out disease or high-risk lifestyle that could suggest the danger of exposure to HIV or other contagious diseases. If the family objects to organ procurement, there is a good chance it will fail to cooperate in obtaining an adequate history.

There are special cases, however, in which an adequate history can be obtained even though the family objects to the transplant. If the individual dies from the irreversible stoppage of brain function following an accident, it is possible that the person was alive long enough to give an adequate medical and social history to the physicians before death. Perhaps the deceased was living with someone who is emotionally very close, but not the next of kin, who could supply the important history. In those situations, both law and ethics support organ procurement on the basis of the gift of the deceased, regardless of familial objection. In fact, I would argue that if the organs are otherwise suitable and adequate medical and social history are available, the organ procurement organization has a moral duty—not merely the right—to follow the deceased's wishes and procure organs over the objection of the next of kin. Doing so may mean a confrontation with the family, but it is clearly supported by the law. If someone has gone out of his or her way to make a potentially lifesaving donation, that is a noble gift. Those in the transplant community, those who are generally committed to the good that can come from organ transplant, owe it to the memory of the deceased to take on the added burden of confronting the family not only to honor the deceased but also to make the effort to save the lives that hang in the balance— lives the deceased was actively committed to saving. If we accept the model of donation and the moral principles on which it is based, we will show respect for the deceased by honoring his or her wishes, honoring any wish to refuse to participate in organ procurement but also honoring the deceased's wish, whenever possible, to procure organs so that he or she may make a final gift of life to others.

Variants on the Two Models of Organ Procurement

The donation model has carried the day, at least in the United States and other countries that stress the importance of human rights. As we shall see in the next chapter, even in those countries that claim to have taken a more communitarian approach that places the interests of the community of living people over those of the individual who is deceased, the donation model has great power. Countries that authorize procurement of useful organs without individual permission still attempt to dress their more social approach in the language of gift-giving. They still talk about those from whom organs are procured as "donors." They still honor individual objections from those who explicitly refuse to donate. Most tellingly, they still tend not to take organs when family members object. Scholars are beginning to understand the uses and abuses of the "donation model" as the dominant metaphor for organ transplantation. It not only places moral pressure on recipients to "maintain their gift" responsibly, it also puts pressure on potential organ sources to cooperate in the gift-giving system. Laura Siminoff and Kata Chillag have recently provided an insightful analysis of these pressures.[8]

Limits to the Donation Model

There is only one problem with the donation model: It does not work. The policy of taking organs only after donation—from the individual or the surrogate—has not produced enough donations.

As of February 2000, there were in the United States 67,340 people on the waiting list for organs. A total of 4,791 cadaveric organs were recovered in 1998, together with 3,268 from living donors, for a total of 8,059 organs. It is clear that the need is great. The disparity between organs needed and procured is growing rapidly. In 1998, 4,855 Americans died while on the waiting list for an organ.[9]

Determining the number of organs that could be procured if all medically suitable patients donated their organs or had them donated on their behalf is more complicated than it seems. The number will depend on exactly which potential sources of organs are considered medically suitable, whether we include medically suitable candidates that are excluded because the medical examiner objects,[10] how we count organs actually donated that are not recoverable (because the patient "crashes" before procurement or the medical examiner objects postconsent), whether non–heart-beating donors are included, and so forth. The overall result from many different studies, however, leaves the impression that between 40 and 60 percent of the total potential donors actually donate (or have surrogates donate on their behalf) and have their organs used.[11] This suggests that, assuming the usable organs in the medically suitable donors who do not donate are comparable to those in the people who do donate, we could approximately double the number of usable organs procured each year if we had a maximal recovery.

We know that although about half the population would be willing to donate, only about 30 percent have signed an organ donor card.[12] In many cases, people who would be willing to donate simply have not done so for reasons of inertia. They simply do not know how to go about making the donation or have not taken the time and energy to do so. We also know that when family members are asked to donate organs, almost half refuse to do so. In some of these cases, it may simply be because the family is too traumatized at the time of a loved one's death to think about the difficult subject of organ donation. Some may even regret at a later date that they failed to make the donation.

The donation model is probably not the most efficient way of obtaining all the organs that people, under ideal circumstances, would be willing to donate. It certainly is not the most efficient way of obtaining all the lifesaving organs that could be obtained. Routine salvaging, even considering the potential backlash, is probably more efficient.

That the donation model may not be maximally efficient in preserving the lives that could be preserved through transplant is not surprising because it was not supposed to be a model based on maximizing good consequences in the first place. The realization that there are useful organs not being used that could save lives if procured and may be missed simply through inertia is distressing. If some people would, in fact, be willing to donate but simply have never expressed those wishes, it is a tragedy. This has led to a search for a more nuanced system of organ procurement that maintains the moral high ground of donation while providing more efficiency in getting the organs into the transplant system that people would be willing to donate.

More Subtle Options

Although many will die for lack of an organ, many people who are willing to give an organ never make the effort to fill out a donation card. Planning for the disposal of one's body parts is not a pleasant subject. Dying in a manner that would make organ procurement possible is something that is unlikely to happen, and especially not likely to happen soon. Some people may not even know how to go about making a donation. What is needed is a set of more subtle options for facilitating donation.

MARKETS IN ORGANS

One good American way of making the supply of organs match the demand more closely would be to create a market in organs. Several analysts have suggested that the inertia in donation could be overcome by paying people who donate organs.[13] According to free-market principles, the price could be increased until a much greater portion of the potential is donated. In the introductory chapter, we saw that this method is used to increase live kidney supply in India.

Of course, our language would have to change. We would then more properly speak of the *sale* of organs, not the *donation*. It is strange to see advocates of markets to buy and sell organs referring to "donation." The one from whom the organ was obtained would be a *vendor*, not a donor.

The relation of the market to the donation model. Nevertheless, the market model may be more compatible with the donation model than many people realize. As we have seen, the donation model is built on the premise that one's body, in some important sense, belongs to one's self. We have the authority to give away body parts or refuse to make such as gift. There is a way in which we own our bodies. If so, selling body parts when they are no longer of any use to us but very valuable to others is not obviously incompatible with the underlying premises of the donation model. It at least avoids the assumption that the body parts of the deceased belong to the state and can be salvaged without permission.

As mentioned in Chapter 1 a market for kidneys already exists in India. I have met K. C. Reddy, the Indian surgeon who procures such organs and who serves as a kind of broker between those who want to buy and those who must sell. He seems like a decent, respectable professional concerned about benefiting patients. He claims that if he does not facilitate a market in organs, some other, less reputable people will (and he is probably right). He claims he gives the poor their only chance to obtain vitally needed goods.

Many Westerners find this situation repulsive. However, whether markets for organs are justifiable in a culture like that in Bombay is difficult for a Westerner to determine. The cultural and economic conditions are so radically different in Bombay that it is hard to provide a definitive moral assessment. I am convinced that if I had no way to feed my child and could obtain enough income to buy a substantial food supply by selling a kidney, I would be terribly distressed with anyone who had the nerve to tell me I should refrain because of some theoretical principle about the repulsiveness of selling my body parts.

A similar scheme was proposed in the early 1980s for the United States by Virginia physician H. Barry Jacobs. In a statement before the Subcommittee for Investigations and Oversight of the Committee on Science and Technology, he proposed to create a market for kidneys in the United States in which he would serve as a broker, apparently in a manner comparable to Reddy.[14] His style was so offensive and his scheme so poorly thought out that it appears that his testimony helped seal the support of the law that prohibits a market in organs in the United States.

Recently, reports have surfaced of a black market for human kidneys in the Philippines. Payments of up to $2,500 are the going rate—and the potential donor is not necessarily told of the risks.[15] Rumors even surfaced in September 1999 that someone was attempting to auction a kidney on eBay, with an asking price starting at $25,000.[16] The price was driven up to $5.7 million before eBay stepped in and blocked the deal. It was later claimed that this was a hoax. Hoax or not, such transactions are clearly illegal in the U.S. Since not just anyone can install a kidney and cooperation by competent surgeons is not only implausible, but also risky to their careers, the chances of an illegal transaction in the U.S. seem remote.

The ethics of a market in organs. A well-presented argument in favor of markets for organs is more subtle and difficult to refute. There may well be cases in which people would be so desperate that they would be enticed to sell a kidney or even a liver or lung lobe for a large amount of money. (There may even be some so desperate that they would sell a whole liver or lung or heart, realizing that they would die but that their family would be spared some awful fate, but let us limit our attention, for now, to proposals to sell a single kidney.) Assuming that the vendor is an adult who is mentally competent and has been informed adequately about the risks and benefits of selling a kidney and assuming that person, after careful consideration, comes to the conclusion that it is better to sell the kidney and do something with the money, why should our society prohibit such sales? It cannot be that such persons have always calculated their interests incorrectly. Some people would really be better off with the money than with their second kidney (or they may be able to act more morally with the money—taking care of loved ones in desperate need). If we are going to make such sales illegal, we need an argument that overrules the enlightened self-interest of such sellers. If we are going to do so nonpaternalistically, we need an argument that points to some feature other than the vendor's own welfare.

Moreover, many of the proposals to use markets to encourage organ availability do not rely on sales from living persons. They involve economic incentives to encourage actions to increase the supply of cadaver organs.

Markets for cadaver organs. Various proposals have been put forward to increase cadaveric organ supply.[17] Of course, it would not work to make a payment after procurement to those who are the source of the organ. In the case of cadaver procurement, of course, they are deceased. Some other economic incentive would have to be provided.

One version would pay people to execute donor cards. However, that presents real problems. Because only a small portion of those who execute a donor card actually provide organs suitable for transplant, a very small fee would have to be paid to a great many people. Moreover, we would almost have to acknowledge the right of persons to withdraw consent, and it is hard to imagine a policy that could deal with such withdrawals. Presumably, the one wanting to cancel his or her donation would have to give back the incentive to cancel one's donor card. Moreover, those who really resisted donation might follow a strategy of canceling consent at certain high-risk times of life, such as if they realized they were declining with an illness that could leave them a potential organ source. Relatives who are guardians might also try to change the consent.

A more plausible approach would be to make a payment if and when organs are procured if the donor had previously pledged to donate organs.[18] The income would necessarily go to the estate or to anyone the deceased might name. If payment were made only when an organ was actually procured (or perhaps actually transplantable), the numbers would be much smaller and the payment could be much larger. Anyone who desired to increase the size of his or her estate for loved ones might be enticed by the payment. A similar goal could be achieved by giving anyone a life insurance policy on signing a donor card with the proviso that the insurance would be paid to the beneficiary only if organs were procured.

All of these payments would presently be illegal,[19] but the real question is whether the law should be amended to permit them. The payments could be viewed as an incentive to overcome the inertia of failing to take the steps necessary to actually sign the card making organs available.

Such payments to the estates of those who had signed up for donation would still pose some practical problems. What should happen, for instance, if someone had signed a donor card but turned out to have marginal organs (to someone at the upper limits of the acceptable age, for example)? They, or their family, might demand the right to have the organs procured. Lawsuits for failure to procure could be envisioned. Should the same payment be made to those providing prime organs[20] and those with less desirable ones? Should the same payment be made to those donating only kidneys and those who donate a full set of organs? What about those who donate all organs but yield only a limited number of usable ones? Should family of someone who has ideal organs available be excluded from payment simply because no recipients of certain good organs were available?

The proposals also raise more basic ethical questions. Most Americans find the proposal for a market in organs repulsive. The arguments are complex, however. The debate often starts with the opponents claiming that life and death are too precious to be reduced to market transactions. It is believed that whether one lives or dies should not be a matter of price.

Two market approaches. Two significantly different market arrangements have been considered. One, following the Bombay and Jacobs model, would permit those in need of organs to bargain for an available liver or heart or kidney. That would, in fact, mean that those with the greatest ability to pay would be more likely to live.

We should recognize that many other medical services are allocated by price today. Many wealthy people get a higher quality of medical services because of their ability to pay. Some of us, however, hold to the belief that when it comes to life-and-death interventions, it ought not to be that way. The mere fact that other health services are allocated on the basis of an ability to pay does not mean it is all right for organs to be.

In the United States, however, a second way of linking organ procurement to market forces can be envisioned. We have the possibility of dissociating procurement from allocation. Relying on the market for one does not necessarily mean we have to rely on the market for the other. We could, for example, have a national organ transplant network use money as an incentive to increase the national pool of organs and still have that network allocate organs to transplant candidates without regard to payment. A national insurance for transplants (perhaps modeled on the Medicare funding of kidney transplants) could make organs available from the financially enhanced pool totally on the basis of medical need or predicted medical benefit. That would eliminate discrimination on the allocation side, but we would still be left with the questions about the morality of markets on the procurement side.

It is not as obvious why a market incentive to encourage donation (for either live or cadaveric organ vendors) would be unacceptable provided one could be identified that worked efficiently (avoided payments to those who would end up avoiding procurement and did not spend too much on people who were planning to give anyway).

Coercion and incentives. Some would argue that payments would be coercive, especially to the poor. The difference between incentives and coercion is a complex topic. A coercive force is one that is intended to influence another person by presenting a threat so severe it is irresistible.[21] This immediately makes clear that an offer of an enormous amount of money is not coercive, even if it is irresistible. The money is not a threat; it is an offer. Most analyses of coercion rely on the distinction, limiting coercion to negative sanctions.[22]

Positive incentives that compel action are usually considered to be *offers* or *influences*. The analysis of these positive incentives is more complex. It is quite possible that one might respond affirmatively to a positive incentive (such as a cash payment) without in any way deviating from one's general life plan. Because autonomous actions are those that are in accord with one's life plan, effective positive incentives may be consistent with autonomy. For example, if someone has long thought it would be a nice action—and one that is consistent with her general values—to sign a donor card but had simply never gotten around to it, receiving a modest incentive (either a small payment or an insurance policy of, say, $1,000, payable if organs are procured) to sign the card would not in any way violate her autonomy even though it gets her to engage in a behavior that she had not otherwise had enough motivation to perform. Signing the card is consistent with her general beliefs and values.

Offers generally provide additional options beyond what one would otherwise have. An offer of a 10 percent bonus to change from one work shift to another adds to the range of available choices. It is hard to argue that adding an option violates autonomy. An offer of a 10 percent pay raise to go to work for a competitor likewise increases the employee's options. We normally do not think of such a competitive employment offer as immoral even if the offer is effectively persuasive in getting someone to change jobs.

Two sorts of cases make the analysis still more complicated. These can be called the "unwelcome offer" and the "irresistible offer." An unwelcome offer is one that the recipient would rather not receive. Some offers that increase options are nevertheless ones that people would rather not receive. An offer of a new job at a 10 percent increase in wages may force many additional choices about relocation, separation of the family, and so forth.

If the new job offer not only poses these unwelcome problems but is also an extremely good offer, it may turn out to be irresistible. A 100 percent salary increase for doing similar work may be an irresistible offer. If one prefers to relocate anyway the irresistible offer may be very welcome and quite compatible with one's autonomy. The real issue is how to evaluate an irresistible offer that is unwelcome. Irresistibly attractive offers will force a choice on the employee. If they are nevertheless welcome offers, they are not inconsistent with autonomy, but if the offer is unwelcome, it could force one to abandon a life plan, thereby depriving one of an autonomous life. Such an individual would have more options, but nevertheless feel constrained to abandon his or her life plan.

There is considerable dispute over whether such irresistibly attractive, unwelcome offers are ethical. Offering a large fee to persons to become live "donors" of kidneys probably fits this category provided the individuals are in desperate need for themselves or their families. Some will see such offers as unacceptably controlling and therefore unethical. Others will see them as increasing options and therefore acceptable even though one is forced thereby to abandon a life plan. In organ procurement the fear is that financial incentives may be irresistibly attractive to those who are in desperate situations, thus forcing them to sign a "donor" card or even become a living organ vendor.

One additional variable may prove crucial. Some people who make irresistibly attractive offers of this kind may have the means to address the potential organ vendor's desperate situation using some other means. If they do, they can be seen as exploiting the desperate person's situation. So, for example, I shall suggest in Chapter 12 that if a transplant surgeon could have listed a recipient for a cadaver transplant but refused to do so (perhaps because his staff needed more practice with live donor procurement), thus forcing the potential recipient's spouse into accepting an irresistibly attractive offer to be a donor, that offer would be not only consistent with the spouse's life plan and irresistibly attractive but also unethical because it was exploitative. The surgeon would have forced the spouse to become a donor when he could have solved the problem in another way.

Markets in organs: a summary. This reveals why proposals for markets in organs are so controversial. They are likely to involve offers of money that will have significantly different impacts on people in different positions. The desperately poor may perceive the offer of money for organ donation irresistibly attractive. It may also be exploitative: The ones making the offer may have the resources to and the responsibility for addressing the desperate one's problem in some other way.

For example, if Medicare were to add a financial reward for supplying cadaveric or living organs, the funds would come from the federal government. The people who were sufficiently desperate to view the offer as irresistible may face life-and-death financial crises, but the same federal government that is making the offer may have both the resources and the responsibility for providing a welfare safety net to meet those needs. Fulfilling that responsibility would remove the desperation and thus make the offer no longer irresistible.

The real issue is whether those in authority have it within their power to address the basic needs of a population short of resorting to selling body parts. In the United States it is obvious that there are sufficient resources such that a humane safety-net welfare program should be able to provide enough resources to meet desperate needs for basic welfare without forcing people to extremes. If those who defend markets in organs do so as a way of escaping responsibility for providing for the subsistence of a society's most needy, that is an unacceptable excuse for escaping responsibility.

What, however, if we limit the positive incentives to those that were small enough that they were "resistible"? What if we offered a small incentive to stimulate people to sign the line on the driver's license indicating a willingness to provide organs? What if we offered a $3 reduction in the driving license fee if the donor line were signed—either for or against donation? What if we adopted a policy of paying the estate of the deceased $1,000 if any organs were procured that could be used by the organ procurement organization? It is hard to argue that this would violate autonomy. At least for those who were already willing to donate but simply had not developed the momentum to do so, this would be a welcome offer. It would probably also be resistible, especially if it were modest. It probably could be crafted in such a way that it would not be seen as exploiting the desperate.

Nevertheless, monetizing organ procurement might still be perceived as unseemly. Any positive incentive will appeal more to the more desperate. Anyone who felt strongly attracted by such an incentive might well have basic needs that should be met by the government through other programs.

Payments might also be perceived as unseemly in another way. One of the great advantages of the gift-giving model is that it elevates organ donation to a level of humaneness that seems appropriate for meeting the needs of those with life-threatening medical problems. For some, financial incentives, even modest, resistible ones, change the character of organ procurement from humane gift-giving among fellow members of the human community to a more commercial, business-like transaction.

The bottom line seems to be that some modest level of positive financial incentives may turn out to be justifiable but an approach that should be tried only when all other approaches have been tried and have been found to fail. Thus the critical question is what other compromises are available between the pure donation and salvaging strategies.

Rewarded Gifting

Buying organs is therefore controversial. Some see it as immoral. It is at least a violation of current American law. But the shortage in organs is real. And many people who seem, in principle, willing to donate simply have not found the momentum to do so.

Some have observed that families incur real costs when organs are donated. They propose that, even if we cannot buy organs or pay an incentive, those costs can be reimbursed. Some have gone so far as to coin the wonderfully offensive term *rewarded gifting*,[23] attempting to hold on to the donation model. The implication is that organs will not be bought. Rather they will be given in exchange for which money will be presented as a reward.

These proposals raise subtle complications, however. All hospital costs after death of a patient must be borne by the transplant organization. We cannot play on the fears of families that they will be billed for organ procurement, offering compensation for expenses as a strategy for stimulating them to donate.

What, however, about paying other costs surrounding terminal care? Proposals have been made to pay the funeral costs or pay the family a "reimbursement" for travel, lodging, or meal expenses during the period of the terminal illness or time away from work.

Paying funeral expenses up to a few thousand dollars seems to be the most fashionable proposal. For example, the state of Pennsylvania has recently authorized the payment of $300 to families of organ donors to help cover funeral expenses. But the funeral is normally paid out of the estate. If funeral costs are borne by the transplant agency, the estate increases by that amount. The beneficiaries of estate get that much more. That is almost the same as buying the organs. I say *almost* the same because new deception is involved. The participants—the family as well as the organ procurers—may actually fool themselves into believing they have remained in the gift-giving mode.

There is one way in which the concept of "rewarded gifting" might be appropriate. It is possible that nonmonetary rewards could encourage either live donation or signing of donor cards. Community recognition of and praise for the socially noble character of the organ donor certainly seems appropriate. Even more tangible, nonmonetary rewards might be considered. Live donors, for instance, might be given some special consideration—a few bonus points—should they need organs in the future. That plan has, in fact, been adopted. Four points in the kidney allocation formula are awarded for those with proof that they were previously donors of a kidney, liver segment, lung segment, partial pancreas, or small bowel segment.[24] Giving similar special consideration to those who sign donors cards for cadaver donation is a bit more complicated. People might not perceive the incentive to donate until they are in need of organs themselves. A special consideration limited only to those who have been donors for several years, however, might avoid the problem. These minor, nonfinancial rewards for donors seem appropriate and should be tried more aggressively.

Other ideas in the spirit of noneconomic rewards for willingness to donate organs have been proposed. Richard Schwindt and Aidan Vining have proposed a "mutual insurance pool."[25] According to their plan, an individual in the pool would receive priority for organs from other members if he or she agrees to make organs available in the event of death. Assuming that some control over people joining the pool only when they anticipate needing organs can be developed, this proposal would be essentially similar to giving people bonus points if they have agreed to donate organs.

ROUTINE SALVAGING WITH OPTING OUT

If one feels compelled to move beyond explicit donation without relying on overt market mechanisms or their disguised equivalent, the honest way to do so is to endorse routine salvaging, making it more humane by permitting those who actively oppose organ procurement to be excluded. The policy, called *routine salvaging with opting out*, has its supporters even 30 years after Dukeminier and Sanders made their original proposal.[26] They would take organs without any consent provided individuals have not explicitly rejected procurement. In the next chapter, I shall argue that real problems remain for such a policy. If we take salvaging seriously—with its accompanying notion that the interests of the state take priority over individual choice—physicians would not ask relatives for permission to procure. They would tell the relatives what is going to happen and obtain needed medical information from them.

If we adopt a policy of salvaging (even with opting out), it is possible that the percentage of potentially usable organs that are actually obtained may exceed the percentage actually willing to donate. That may be tolerable, especially if we assume that those who object but do not record their objection probably do not object too strenuously. We should be aware, however, that surveys show that persons of lower education are far less likely to consent to organ donation, yet it is precisely this group of people who would run the highest risk of not knowing the proper procedures for opting out.[27]

The real argument against routine salvaging—with or without opting out—continues to be based on principle. If we are a society that insists on respecting the integrity and autonomy of the individual, we will not assume that something as closely associated with the essence of the individual as his or her body can be appropriated by the state without permission. Even with an opt-out, the assumption that those who do not want their bodies taken must actively register their objection raises serious questions. It seems to get the priorities backward. Preserving the priority of the individual as much as possible seems like a noble and worthwhile goal.

The case for a policy of routine salvaging with opting out nevertheless continues to gather support. It is an honest policy that will be supported by communitarians and others willing to shift the priority away from the rights of the individual in the direction of promoting societal interests. I am not yet ready to make that move, at least until maximum efforts to encourage donation have been tried. The day may come when we are convinced that all good-faith, well-organized efforts to gain organs through the donation model have failed. If that day comes, the society may need to reopen the question of routine salvaging. I would view this as a substantial invasion of the rights of the individual in an area that requires utmost respect for privacy. It should be undertaken only with fear and trembling. In the meantime, there are options worth exploring.

PRESUMED CONSENT

Instead of going through the agony of getting actual donations, we could simply presume the consent of anyone who failed to record his or her objection to organ procurement. The idea of *presumed consent* has captured the imagination of many of those particularly hungry for organs.[28] I shall reserve critical comment on presumed consent to the next chapter. Suffice to say here that I consider "presumed consent" to be the most outrageously unethical of all possible policies for organ procurement. It is not that I am unalterably opposed to taking organs without consent. What is so offensive is the desperate attempt to hold on to the consent and donation model by using the language of consent for what is really a policy of routine salvaging—that is, taking the organs without consent. As I shall argue in the next chapter, the clear truth is that about half the population would not consent to organ procurement if they were asked. To claim that we can presume that someone would consent when the empirical evidence shows that presumption would be wrong half the time is simply dishonest. It dresses salvaging in the flimsy outer garb of the consent doctrine. Far better, if one favors salvaging, to admit it openly.

REQUIRED REQUEST OF NEXT OF KIN

If creating positive financial incentives to encourage vending of organs raises problems, and routine salvaging, even with opting out or disguised as presumed consent, is too much of an assault on our core liberal values, what about simply presenting the option to donate in a more direct way? We might at least consider requiring people to confront the donation question at an opportune moment.

In fact, federal law now requires that families be presented with the option of donating at the time of all appropriate deaths. This includes virtually all who are to be pronounced dead by brain criteria. It may well include others who die based on heart criteria who could become candidates for organ procurement from non–heart-beating cadavers (to be discussed in more detail in Chapter 13). Required request is morally still grounded in autonomy and consent. It would not conscript unwilling donors. It simply asks people and facilitates recording of their reply. It still gives the patient (or next of kin) a chance to donate.

However, the laws that require that the family be asked about donation at the time of the death of their loved ones contain an enormous logical flaw. Not only may the request at this moment of crisis be traumatic for the family, it may be morally suspect as well. The donation model is built on the premise that body parts are the individual's to give. We are striving to respect the autonomy of the *individual*. Any law that requires a request of the family intervenes at too late a point, at least in the case of a person who was once mentally competent and able to formulate his or her own position on organ donation. The one whose autonomy should guide the decision to donate is already dead.

What such required request laws really do is respect the autonomy of the family. It is a clear second best compared with knowing the views that had been held by the deceased. It is that person's wishes that are morally prior. In fact, it would be immoral to ask next of kin *permission* if the deceased's wishes were known. If the deceased is known to have opposed donation, that should settle the matter. If he or she favored donation, the organ procurement personnel should, as I have suggested, politely notify next of kin.

Required request is morally problematic even if patient's wishes are not known. The relatives have a "quasi-property right" in the body, but their wishes should prevail only if there was no reasonable way to know the patient's own wishes.

Proposals to require asking the relatives the donation question may actually function to circumvent the patient's wishes. They may even be designed to do this. Advocates of maximizing organ procurement have known for some time that there is more willingness to donate a relative's organs than one's own—something like 10 to 25 percent greater willingness. Those defending required requests of next of kin appear in some cases to have consciously argued that we should wait until the patient dies and then ask the relatives for permission to increase yield. If that is the reasoning behind the required request laws, they are blatantly offensive to those who ground organ procurement in the right to respect the patient's own wishes. This may be a prudent strategy if the only goal is to maximize organ yield. It will be prudent unless there is a backlash from patients, from health professionals, or procurement personnel. In fact, we may actually be seeing such a backlash in the form of reductions in procurement rates and occasional vitriolic attacks on the organ procurement enterprise.

As an alternative, we might also require that people be asked about organ donation at times when they are healthy. Many states now include such questions on the driver's license. We should at least attempt to maximize the convenience of making the donation commitment before going to secondary decision makers, market-based mechanisms, and routine salvaging.

REQUIRED RESPONSE BY PERSONS WHILE COMPETENT

There may be an even more effective strategy for forging a compromise between the donation and salvaging models. I have previously proposed a policy of what I now call "required response."[29] This policy would go beyond "required request"[30] in that it not only requires that the question be asked but that some answer by given (even if the answer is negative or is "uncertain"). The approach will be presented in Chapter 12, but first we must examine the strategy of presuming consent more carefully. That is the task of the next chapter.

ENDNOTES

1. Jesse Dukeminier and David Sanders, "Organ Transplantation: A Proposal for Routine Salvaging of Cadaver Organs," *New England Journal of Medicine* 279 (1968): 413–19.
2. Charles Marwick, "British Ponder 'Presumed Consent' For Organ Harvesting," *Journal of the American Medical Association* 251 (12, March 23–30, 1984): 1522; Arthur L. Caplan, "Organ Transplants: The Costs of Success, An Argument for Presumed Consent and Oversight" *Hastings Center Report* 13 (Dec. 1983): 23–32;

Arthur J. Matas, and Frank J. Veith, "Presumed Consent for Organ Retrieval," *Theoretical Medicine* 5 (1984): 155–66; Matas and Veith, "Presumed Consent— A More Humane Approach to Cadaver Organ Donation," in *Positive Approaches to Living with End-Stage Renal Disease: Psychosocial and Thanatological Aspects*, ed. Mark A. Hardy et al. (New York: Praeger, 1986), pp. 37–51; William N. Gerson, "Refining the Law of Organ Donation: Lessons from the French Law of Presumed Consent," *New York University Journal of International Law and Politics* 19 (4, 1987): 1013–32; Alan R. Hull, "Dwindling Donations Make Presumed Consent a Proposal Worthy of Consideration," *Nephrology News & Issues* (Oct. 1992): 28–29.

3. For recent discussions of the Nazi research see Arthur L. Caplan (Ed.), *When Medicine Went Mad: Bioethics and the Holocaust* (Totowa, NJ: Humana Press, 1992); and George J. Annas and Michael A. Grodin (eds.), *The Nazi Doctors and the Nuremberg Code: Human Rights in Human Experimentation* (New York: Oxford University Press, 1992).

4. "Nuremberg Code, 1947," in *Encyclopedia of Bioethics*, rev. ed., Vol. 5, ed. Warren T. Reich (New York: Free Press, 1995), pp. 2763–64.

5. Allen E. Buchanan and Dan W. Brock, *Deciding for Others: The Ethics of Surrogate Decision Making* (Cambridge: Cambridge University Press, 1989), pp. 128–29; Robert S. Olick, *Deciding for Incompetent Patients: The Nature and Limits of Prospective Autonomy and Advance Directives*, Ph.D. dissertation, 1997, Georgetown University, Washington, DC.

6. Ronald Dworkin, *Life's Dominion: An Argument about Abortion, Euthanasia, and Individual Freedom* (New York: Vintage Books, 1994), pp. 201–04.

7. David W. Meyers, *The Human Body and the Law* (Chicago: Aldine, 1970), pp. 128–29.

8. Laura A. Siminoff, and Kata Chillag, "The Fallacy of the 'Gift of Life.' " *The Hastings Center Report* 29 (6, Nov.–Dec. 1999): 34–41.

9. Data from United Network for Organ Sharing (UNOS) Website at <http://www .unos.org/critical data/waiting list> (April 1999).

10. The medical examiner is presently given the authority to veto organ procurement. This will occur if the medical examiner is concerned that the deceased may be a victim of a crime and that organ procurement could make evidence problematic. Some medical examiners routinely block organ procurement from infants because they want to investigate possible child abuse. Giving the medical examiner priority over organ procurement reflects a societal value choice. If it wanted to, the society could change the priority giving the organ procurement organization first access to the body. This could jeopardize an occasional prosecution of a crime, but it could provide several life-saving organs. Sometimes the choice is not as clearcut. For example, a medical examiner may prohibit organ recovery of thoracic and

abdominal organs from a victim of what appears to be a gunshot wound to the head on the outside chance that a full autopsy of the thorax and abdomen could reveal some unexpected cause of death. A good case can be made that society should change its priories and permit organ procurement in such cases even if our confidence in the cause of death is lessened somewhat.

11. Roger W. Evans, Carlyn E. Onans, and Nancy L. Ascher, "The Potential Supply of Organ Donors: An Assessment of the Efficiency of Organ Procurement Efforts in the United States," *Journal of the American Medical Association* 267 (1992): 243–45. This estimate is consistent with the finding of the 1993 Gallup survey prepared for the Partnership for Organ Donation in 1993 that found that 37 percent were very likely to donate and another 32 percent somewhat likely.

12. The Gallup Organization, Inc., "The American Public's Attitudes toward Organ Donation and Transplantation," conducted for The Partnership for Organ Donation, Boston, MA, Feb. 1993, pp. 4, 15.

13. David A. Peters, "Marketing Organs for Transplantation," *Dialysis & Transplantation* 13 (Jan. 1984): 40–41; Thomas G. Peters, "Financial Incentives in Organ Donation: Current Issues," *Dialysis & Transplantation* 21 (5, May 1992): 270–73; Jeffrey Prottas, "Encouraging Altruism: Public Attitudes and the Marketing of Organ Donation," *Milbank Memorial Fund Quarterly/Health and Society* 61 (2, 1983): 278–306; David E. Chapman, "Retailing Human Organs under the Uniform Commercial Code," *John Marshall Law Review* 16 (2, Spring 1983): 393–417; American Medical Association, Council on Ethical and Judicial Affairs, "Financial Incentives for Organ Donation," *Archives of Internal Medicine* 155 (March 27, 1995): 581–89; J. Harvey, "Paying Organ Donors," *Journal of Medical Ethics* 16 (1990): 117–19; Andrew H. Barnett, Roger D. Blair, and David L. Kaserman, "Improving Organ Donation: Compensation versus Markets," *Inquiry* 29 (1992): 372–78.

14. Barry H. Jacobs, "Statement before the Subcommittee for Investigations and Oversight of the Committee on Science and Technology," *Procurement and Allocation of Human Organs for Transplantation: Hearings before the Subcommittee on Investigations and Oversight of the Committee on Science and Technology*, U.S. House of Representatives, 98th Congress, Nov. 7, 9, 1983 (Washington DC: U.S. Government Printing Office, 1984), p. 259.

15. "Organ Harvesting for Profit," <www.toledoblade.com/editorial/edit/9i03ed3.htm>, Sept. 3, 1999.

16. "Ebay Stops Kidney Auctions," <www.usatoday.com/life/cyber/tech/ctg022.htm>, Sept. 7, 1999.

17. United Network for Organ Sharing, Ethics Committee, Payment Subcommittee, *Financial Incentives for Organ Donation*, unpublished paper available at <www.207 .87.26.13/cinetpub/wwwro. . .ethics%5Fwhitepapers%5Ffinance.htm>, Dec. 16, 1998; American Medical Association, Council on Ethical and Judicial Affairs,

"Financial Incentives for Organ Donation," *Archives of Internal Medicine* 155 (March 27, 1995): 581–89; Thomas G. Peters, "Financial Incentives in Organ Donation: Current Issues."

18. See, for example, John B. Dossetor and V. Manickkavel, "Commercialization: The Buying and Selling of Kidneys," in *Ethical Problems in Dialysis and Transplantation*, ed. Carl M. Kjellstrand and John B. Dossetor (Boston: Kluwer Academic, 1992), pp. 61–71.

19. National Organ Transplant Act, Public Law No. 98-507, 98 Stat. 2339 (1984).

20. The term suggests that the butcher shop metaphor would be quite precise for markets in human flesh.

21. Ruth Faden and Tom L. Beauchamp in collaboration with Nancy N. P. King, *A History and Theory of Informed Consent* (New York: Oxford University Press, 1986), pp. 339–40.

22. See, for example, Robert Nozick, "Coercion," in *Philosophy, Science and Method: Essays in Honor of Ernest Nagel*, ed. Sidney Morgenbesser, Patrick Suppes, and Morton White (New York: St. Martin's Press, 1969), pp. 440–72.

23. For uses of the term see A. S. Daar, "Rewarded Gifting," *Transplantation Proceedings* 24 (Oct. 1992): 2207–11; J. B. Dosseter, "Rewarded Gifting: Is It Ever Ethically Acceptable?" *Transplantation Proceedings* 24 (Oct. 1992): 2092–94; Alexander, J. Wesley, "Pro: Rewarded Gifting Should Be Tried," *Transplantation & Immunology Letter* 8 (1, March 1992): 4, 6; Thomas H. Murray, "The Moral Repugnance of Rewarded Gifting," *Transplantation & Immunology Letter* 8 (1, March 1992): 5, 7; Barry D. Kahan, "Rewarded Gifting–PRO and CON: Bringing the Arguments into Focus," *Transplantation & Immunology Letter* 8 (1, March 1992): 3.

24. UNOS Policy 3.5.9.6, as posted on the UNOS Web site, <www.unos.org>, May 27, 1999.

25. Richard Schwindt and Aidan Vining, "Proposal for a Mutual Insurance Pool for Transplant Organs," *Journal of Health Politics, Policy and Law* 23 (1998): 725–41.

26. James L. Muyskens, "An Alternative Policy for Obtaining Cadaver Organs for Transplantation," *Philosophy & Public Affairs* 8 (Fall 1978): 88–99; Arthur J. Matas, John Arras, James Muyskens, Vivian Tellis, and Frank J. Veith, "A Proposal for Cadaver Organ Procurement: Routine Removal with the Right of Informed Consent," *Journal of Health Politics, Policy and Law* 10 (2, Summer 1985): 231–44.

27. *Organ Donation Study*, United Network for Organ Sharing Executive Summary, Feb. 15, 1992.

28. Charles Marwick, "British Ponder 'Presumed Consent' for Organ Harvesting," *Journal of the American Medical Association* 251 (12, March 23–30, 1984): 1522; Arthur L. Caplan, "Organ Transplants: The Costs of Success, An Argument for Presumed Consent and Oversight"; Arthur J. Matas and Frank J. Veith, "Presumed

Consent for Organ Retrieval"; Matas Veith, "Presumed Consent—A More Humane Approach to Cadaver Organ Donation"; Alan R. Hull, "Dwindling Donations Make Presumed Consent a Proposal Worthy of Consideration."

29. Robert M. Veatch, *Death, Dying, and the Biological Revolution* (New Haven, CT: Yale University Press, 1976), p. 272. The more developed formulation appears in the revised edition of that book in 1989 and in Veatch, "Routine Inquiry about Organ Donation—An Alternative to Presumed Consent," *New England Journal of Medicine* 325 (17, Oct. 1991): 1246–49, a revised version of which appears as Chapter 12.

30. Arthur L. Caplan, "Ethical and Policy Issues in the Procurement of Cadaver Organs for Transplantation," *New England Journal of Medicine* 311 (15, Oct. 11, 1984): 981–83; New York State Task Force on Life and the Law, *The Required Request Law: Recommendations of the New York State Task Force on Life and the Law,* March 1986.

Ten

The Myth of Presumed Consent: Ethical Problems in New Organ Procurement Strategies

Robert M. Veatch and Jonathan B. Pitt

THE ACUTE SHORTAGE of organs for transplantation has led to considerable interest in laws that are designed to increase the number of organs procured. These laws are often referred to as *presumed consent* laws. Such laws are alleged in many popular and scholarly articles to exist in several European countries and Singapore, among other places. The reasoning behind recent arguments in favor of adopting a so-called presumed consent law in the United States is that if we can presume the consent of the deceased to organ procurement there will be a substantial increase in the yield of organs.

The Difference between Presumed Consent and Salvaging

The problem with this approach, however, is that, with a few exceptions, the existing laws never actually claim to presume consent, nor can they rightly be said to do so. They simply authorize the state's taking of the organs without explicit permission. It therefore seems wrong to call them presumed consent laws. They are, in effect, what, as we saw in the previous chapter, used to be called *routine salvaging* laws.[1] We believe that the time has come to be more careful in distinguishing between policies of *presumed consent* and those of *routine salvaging*. Although the net outcome may be the same under either kind of policy, the underlying assumptions about the relation of the individual to society are radically different.

It is our hypothesis that those who support a societal right to procure organs without consent find it embarrassing to speak bluntly about taking organs without consent, hence they adopt the *language* of presuming consent even when there is no *basis* for such a presumption. In doing so, they preserve the appearance of the preferred gift mode and the guise of respect for individual choice. (This desire for euphemistic language is also seen in the persistent practice of referring to persons from whom organs are taken as *donors*, even in cases, such as small children, in which these people could never have actually made a gift or donation.) We shall suggest that important matters of societal relationships are at stake in distinguishing between policies that allow procuring organs on the presumption that people would consent and those that simply take organs without consent. One form of society gives central place to the individual, holding that his or her person can be used by the state only with some form of consent. That has been the society of liberal Western culture, particularly the United States. This philosophy underlies the gift mode and the doctrine of consent that has been central, not only to organ procurement but to the practice of medicine in general, for decades.

Another form of society gives more central authority to the community or state, authorizing it to use the individual for important societal purposes even without individual consent. It underlies routine salvaging, or the taking of organs without consent. For the purposes of this chapter, we are not pressing for one form of policy or the other. It is possible that the time has come for elevation of the state by adopting a routine salvaging law, at least in some societies. That seems to be the rationale behind new movements toward enhancing communitarianism and stressing the common good in social policy.[2] It is also possible that the importance of the individual continues to require procuring organs in the gift or donation mode in which organs may be taken only with proper permission. The conflation of these two is, we shall suggest, a dangerous prospect indeed.

The State of the Law

The current laws in various jurisdictions that authorize procuring organs without consent come in two forms. The vast majority authorize routine salvaging without presuming consent. Only rarely does a law or a proposed law actually presume consent.[3]

Countries with Routine Salvaging Laws (With No Claim of Presuming Consent)

It is striking that it is so common for commentators to refer to these laws as "presumed consent" laws. For example, according to Gerson, the French law on organ procurement adopted in 1976 is one that presumes the consent of persons who do not, during their lifetime, expressly refuse to have their organs taken on their death.[4] However, on examining the law itself, one is hard-pressed to find any mention of presuming consent, overt or implicit. The law states that "an organ to be used for therapeutic or scientific purposes may be removed from the cadaver of a person who has not during his lifetime made known his refusal of such a procedure."[5] Although the law offers a provision for those willing and able to record their dissent, it is not clear why we should conclude that the rationale behind the opting-out system it establishes is based on the presumed consent of the decedent rather than the primacy of the state. Gerson, citing a 1984 *Transplantation Proceedings* article by Cantaluppi, also attributes presumed consent laws to Austria, Belgium, (the former) Czechoslovakia, Finland, Italy, Norway, Spain, and Switzerland, among other countries.[6] However, *not one* of these laws mentions anything about presuming consent, directly or indirectly.[7] Among the other countries that have laws authorizing organ procurement without claiming to presume consent are Cyprus,[8] Hungary,[9] Singapore,[10] Syria,[11] and the former Yugoslavia.[12] Some of these have been referred to in the literature as countries with presumed consent laws, yet none of them actually claims to presume consent in its legislation.

Laws with an Explicit Presumption of Consent

By contrast we have located a few laws and proposed laws that do actually state a presumption of consent or its equivalent. For example, the Colombian law on organ procurement states that, ". . . there shall be a legal presumption of donation if a person during his life time [sic] has refrained from exercising his right to object to the removal from his body of anatomical organs or parts during his death. . . ."[13]

Within the United States at least two states have considered laws that would, if enacted, have properly been called presumed consent laws. In Maryland, a bill proposed on March 10, 1993, had it not been defeated, would have allowed for the presumption of consent of those who did not opt out. It read, "In the absence of specific objection by an individual expressed during that individual's lifetime, or by any of the individual's next of kin immediately following the individual's death, the individual is deemed to have consented to the donation of the individual's body or any part of the individual's body for and of the purposes specified. . . ."[14] In Pennsylvania, a subchapter titled, "Presumed Anatomical Gifts," of a proposed amendment to an act, reads, "Organs and tissues may be removed, upon death, from the body of any Commonwealth resident by a physician or surgeon for transplantation or for the preparation of therapeutic substances, unless it is established that a refusal was expressed. . . ."[15] Both of these proposed law changes adopt the language of presuming consent. This, of course, begs the question of whether consent can actually be presumed in these jurisdictions at all.

Why Consent Cannot Validly Be Presumed

Although the difference between the European laws that do not presume consent and the New World laws and proposals that do presume it may seem small, matters of fundamental importance are at stake. It is important to see why consent cannot validly be presumed in the present cultural environment.

To presume consent is to make an empirical claim. It is to claim that people *would consent* if asked, or, perhaps more precisely, that they would consent to a policy of taking organs without explicit permission. The reasoning behind true presumed consent laws is that it is legitimate to take organs without explicit consent because those from whom the organs are taken would have agreed had they been asked when they were competent to respond.

That, however, is a claim that, if it is to be made with authority, must be corroborated with empirical evidence. Social survey evidence makes clear that if we assume people would agree to having their organs procured if they were asked, we would be wrong something like 30–50 percent of the time. A 1993 Gallup poll shows that only 37 percent of Americans are "very likely" to want their organs transplanted after their death, and only 32 percent are "somewhat likely." Furthermore, only 55 percent are willing to grant formal permission for organ removal. It should also be noted that although 55 percent are *willing* to grant permission, only 28 percent have *actually* done so.[16] In other words, only about half of the Americans who are willing to grant permission have taken the proactive steps necessary to do so, creating a large number of *false negatives*. We might expect that if the United States's were an opting-out system, we might also see a large number of *false-positives*. Based even on the larger figure of 69 percent who would be either "very likely" or "somewhat likely" to want their organs to be transplanted, it is clear that there can be no basis for presuming consent. Claiming such a presumption is an ill-informed notion at best; it is an outright deception at worst.

Perhaps even more pertinent to this discussion are the relative proportions of Americans who would agree to the system of presumed consent itself, as the ethos of the presumed consent mode would seem to demand. One recent survey shows that only 38 percent of Americans agree with presumed consent, defined as a system in which doctors routinely remove organs from deceased persons unless the person indicated a wish to the contrary while alive.[17] Another survey shows that number to be only 7 percent.[18]

To gain a better understanding of the issues involved, a comparison with the presumption of consent to treatment in an emergency room is helpful. When people suffer accidents or heart attacks that render them incapable of consenting to medical treatment, they are rushed to an emergency room where they are treated by the hospital team. They are treated without explicit consent. This policy is defended on the grounds that consent is presumed.[19] Under these circumstances such a presumption allows us to preserve the notion that people can receive medical treatment only with their consent.

In the case of the emergency room treatment of the patient incapable of giving explicit consent, the presumption of consent is surely valid. Were we to conduct a survey of the population asking its members whether they would want such a presumption made, agreement would be close to unanimous. To be sure, some small group would object. A patient who is a Jehovah's Witness, for example, may refuse blood products; a Christian Scientist may refuse treatment altogether. This reveals that on occasion the presumption of consent in the emergency room may be an erroneous presumption (it will, on occasion, yield *false-positives*). But it will be accurate an overwhelming percentage of the time, and the presumption is therefore justified.

By contrast if we presume consent in the case of organ procurement, we will be wrong at least 30 percent of the time. It is interesting to ask exactly what percentage of people would have to agree to a policy when surveyed before we can presume that individuals being treated by that policy would have consented. One's first instinct might be to assume that a majority must indicate endorsement of the policy, but that surely is wrong. It would lead to erroneous presumption of consent as much as half the time. One possibility is to take a figure of 95 percent approval in a survey as sufficient to presume that any one individual would have consented, if asked. That would mean 5 percent of the time we would have erred in presuming the individual would have consented. (Even then the rights of individuals would be violated 5 percent of the time.) In a society that affirms the right of the individual not to have his or her body invaded without appropriate consent, procuring organs on the basis of a presumption of consent will violate that right at least 30 percent of the time.

What Is at Stake

What is at stake is something very fundamental: the ethics of the relation of the individual to the society. A pioneer in the study of contemporary medical ethics, Paul Ramsey, introduced the issue in distinguishing between organ procurement in the modes of "giving" and "taking."[20] In liberal Western society certain rights are attributed to the individual. Among these is the right to control what is done with one's body. Hence in Western culture medical treatment is acceptable only with the consent of the individual or the individual's appropriate surrogate. Research on a human subject is ethically acceptable only when consent is obtained. According to the Nuremberg Code, such voluntary consent is absolutely essential. An individual is in a position whereby he or she has the authority to give to society by authorizing medical research and now by authorizing procurement of organs for transplant, research, therapy, and other purposes.

The alternative is the mode of "taking" or what in previous chapters, following Dukeminier and Sanders, is called "routine salvaging." In this model the central authority has claims over the individual without relying on the individual's consent or approval. In the model of presumed consent, the individual is prior to the state; in the alternative the individual is subordinate. This underscores the problems associated with casual misuse of the term "presumed consent." Many authors merely confuse routine salvaging for presumed consent, claiming that they are the same thing.[21] Others have implied that their versions of so-called *presumed consent* can be justified by the concept of eminent domain.[22] However, eminent domain involves the taking of private property for public use and has no bearing on questions of consent. Clearly a system that validly presumes the consent of persons does not—cannot—rely on notions of eminent domain.

Choosing the language of legitimating organ procurement is, in effect, choosing how we want to see the individual in relation to the state. Those who use the language of presumed consent are trying to hold on to the liberal model in which gift-giving is the foundation of organ procurement. In cases in which consent can validly be presumed, presumed consent seems consistent with such an orientation. However, in cases in which the evidence makes clear that consent cannot be presumed, this language is simply a disguise for the less acceptable reality of state authority over the individual.

This in itself, of course, does not make routine salvaging wrong; it is, however, deceptive if one advocates such a relationship in the name of the more liberal mode of gift-giving and consenting. Such deception is a moral affront to members of a society built on respect for the rights of the individual.

It is worth speculating on why there is this strong propensity to use the language of presuming consent when the apparent intention is to take organs without consent. One possibility is that, at least in countries reflecting liberal political philosophy's affirmation of the rights of the individual, it is more comforting to use the language of gift-giving and consent. It leaves the impression of the priority of the individual. Thus there is a strong tendency to use the language of the gift mode, even in cases in which the source of the organs may be a small child who never could have made an actual donation and in cases in which a medical examiner rather than the individual whose organs are being taken is the one approving the procurement. The language of consent is a more comfortable language, one that may be necessary to win approval of policies that de facto authorize procurement without donation.

Endnotes

1. Jesse Dukeminier and David Sanders, "Organ Transplantation: A Proposal for Routine Salvaging of Cadaver Organs," *New England Journal of Medicine* 279 (1968): 413.

2. Daniel Callahan, *What Kind of Life: The Limits of Medical Progress* (New York: Simon and Schuster, 1990).

3. The authors gratefully acknowledge the help of the following persons, consulted regarding foreign legislation: Dr. Francesc Abel S.J., Dr. Edwin Bernat, Fr. Antonio Puca, Dr. Knut W. Ruyter, and Dr. Paul Schotsmans.

4. William N. Gerson, "Refining the Law of Organ Donation: Lessons from the French Law of Presumed Consent," *New York University Journal of International Law and Politics* 19 (4, 1987): 1013.

5. J. A. Farfor, "Organ for Transplant: Courageous Legislation." *British Medical Journal* (Feb. 19, 1977), 1: 497–98.

6. William N. Gerson, "Refining the Law of Organ Donation: Lessons from the French Law of Presumed Consent," 1019, n. 35.

7. *International Digest of Health Legislation*, 37 (1, 1986): 332–33 (Austrian Law of June 1, 1982); *IDHL* 38 (1987, 3): 523–27 (Belgian Law of June 13, 1986); *IDHL* 3 (1982, 3): 477–79 (Czechoslovakian Mandatory Directives of Feb. 27, 1978); *IDHL* 36 (1985, 4): 971–72 (Finnish Law of April 26, 1985); *IDHL* 28 (1977, 3): 621–27 (Italian Law of Dec. 2, 1975); Antonio Puca, *Trapianto di Cuore E Morte Cerebrale del Donatore* (Torino, Italy: Edizione Camilliane, 1993), pp. 128–33; 201–24; *Lov om tansplantasjon og avgivelse av lik m.m.*, Feb. 9, 1973; *Ley de Octubre 1979*, no. 30/79, art. 5.3; *IDHL* 36 (1985, 1): 50 (Swiss Regulation of Sept. 17, 1984).

8. *IDHL* 40 (1989, 4): 836–38 (Cyprus Law of May 22, 1987).

9. *IDHL* 40 (1989, 3): 588–90 (Hungarian Law of Feb. 17, 1988).

10. Republic of Singapore, "Human Organ Transplant Bill," *Government Gazette Bills Supplement* (Oct. 31, 1986): 1–10.

11. *IDHL* 38 (1987, 3): 530 (Syrian Law of Dec. 20, 1986).

12. *IDHL* 42 (1992, 1): 46–51 (Yugoslavian Decree of Oct. 18, 1990).

13. *IDHL* 41 (1990, 3): 436–37 (Colombian Law of Dec. 20, 1988). See also the Argentinian law: *Trasplantes de órganos y materiales anatómicos Actos de disposición. Prohibiciones. Profesionales. Servicios y establecimentos. Procedimiento judicial especial.* (Ley 24.193, Art. 62, March 24, 1993).

14. Maryland State Senate Bill 428, § 4-509.2.

15. General Assembly of the Commonwealth of Pennsylvania, proposed amendment to Title 20, Chapter 86, Subchapter C.

16. Gallup Organization, "The American Public's Attitudes toward Organ Donation and Transplantation," conducted for The Partnership for Organ Donation, Boston, Feb., 1993, pp. 4, 15.

17. *Organ Donation Study*, United Network for Organ Sharing Executive Summary (Feb. 15, 1992).

18. Diane L. Manninen and Roger W. Evans, "Public Attitudes and Behavior Regarding Organ Donation." *Journal of the American Medical Association* 253 (21, June 7, 1985): 3111.

19. Paul S. Applebaum, Charles W. Lidz, and Alan Meisel, *Informed Consent: Legal Theory and Clinical Practice* (New York: Oxford University Press, 1987), pp. 66–69.

20. Paul Ramsey, *The Patient as Person* (New Haven, CT: Yale University Press, 1970).

21. Theodore Silver, "The Case for a Post-Mortem Organ Draft and a Proposed Model Organ Draft Act." *Boston University Law Review* 68(4): 681–728; Aaron Spital, "The Shortage of Organs for Transplantation." *The New England Journal of Medicine* 325(17): 1243–46.

22. Donald R. McNeil, "The Constitutionality of 'Presumed Consent' for Organ Donation." *Hamline Journal of Public Law and Policy* 9(2): 343–72; Frank P. Stuart, Frank J. Veith, and Ronald E. Cranford, "Brain Death Laws and Patterns of Consent to Remove Organs for Transplantation from Cadavers in the United States and 28 Other Countries." *Transplantation* 31(4): 238–44.

ELEVEN

REQUIRED RESPONSE: AN ALTERNATIVE TO PRESUMED CONSENT

IT IS UNDERSTANDABLE that some people are growing impatient with the donation model reflected in the Uniform Anatomical Gift Act that has been in place now for more than three decades.[1] We have seen that, in particular, the idea of presuming the consent of the deceased to the use of his or her organs for life-saving transplant is getting new, more serious attention. Although that sentiment is understandable, we saw in the previous chapter that good moral and practical reasons exists why the presumed consent approach is fatally flawed. Indeed, it is routine salvaging in disguise, and I have suggested that salvaging is an idea whose time has not come, but presumed consent, which is deceptively disguised to retain the garb of the donation mode, is even more offensive. Other approaches, including a truly systemic routine inquiry to individuals while alive and competent, are better, more morally defensible, and perhaps even more effective. Existing routine-inquiry policies, however, are defective because they either occur at the wrong time or make it too easy to escape serious efforts to respond. They may pose the donation question of relatives after the patient whose organs might be procured has deteriorated to the point that he or she is beyond responding. Or they may pose the question to individuals about donating their own organs in a manner in which they can avoid thinking about what for many turn out to be hard questions.

If that inquiry were presented at a time when the individual could form his or her own moral stance about organ donation and were combined with the requirement that the individual respond in some fashion, the large gap between those who say they would be willing to donate and those who have actually executed a written record of their willingness to donate could be eliminated. The result could be an accurate record of everyone who wanted to donate without sweeping in those who have some objection to the process. Real, active choice by decision makers would be the result. I call this approach *required response*.

Since the late 1960s in the United States, public policy regarding procuring organs for transplant has rested, as we saw in Chapter 9, on a model of donation. The donation model has focused on consent of the donor for organ procurement. Organs and tissues of deceased humans do not belong to the state, the hospital, or any other group to be used for its own purposes without permission. The model of routine salvaging of organs has been found to be incompatible with basic premises of a free, liberal society. Although neither the living individual nor the next of kin of the deceased technically "own" the body parts, they can be thought of as having "quasi-property rights" in them. This is perhaps better thought of as a duty—the duty to dispose of body parts in a responsible manner with the discretion to choose among reasonable courses of action. For many years in the United States and many other countries this has included the right to donate organs and tissues for transplant and other uses (education, research, and therapeutic uses other than transplant). It has also included the right to refuse to donate.

This right of refusal rests first with the individual while competent. In Western culture it is the individual him- or herself who is most responsible for choosing a life plan. That has included the right and responsibility to shape the disposal of assets after death through a legally binding will. It now also includes a first priority for the individual's own will regarding disposal of the body and the use of body parts for medical purposes. Thus any law requiring routine inquiry of the next of kin of patients who are dead by brain criteria or are approaching that diagnosis come too late in the process. At best we get a substituted judgment, with family members attempting to convey what they believe would have been the patient's wishes. Often what we get is the relative's personal value judgment based on their beliefs and values—not the values of the one whose organs are under consideration. Absent any wishes about disposal of body parts expressed by the individual while competent, the next of kin has been given the discretion to donate or refuse donation, but it is hard to see why the relative's moral, religious, and philosophical position is morally relevant. At best, it is the second alternative for decision making in a liberal society.

The Inadequacy of Alternative Proposals

Now, as we saw in the previous chapter, some are proposing that consent simply be presumed.[2] Often this includes an "opting-out" provision so that individuals while competent (and perhaps their next of kin as well) would have the right to record an objection, but unless such an objection were recorded, the consent of the individual to the use of his or her organs would be presumed. It is believed that such a presumption would significantly increase the number of organs procured.[3]

Although presumed consent is a legal and moral doctrine that has existed in medicine in other contexts, such as in treatment of unconscious or incompetent patients in emergencies, that presumption rests on empirical claims that are not warranted in the case of organ procurement. The presumption of consent would be factually wrong something like 30–50 percent of the time.

Empirical data make clear that, whatever the reason, a substantial fraction of the American population would not consent to having their organs and tissues used for transplantation.[4] It is not even clear that presuming consent would increase the yield of organs. We must take into account that some standing in the tradition of liberal respect for the individual who are not otherwise opposed to organ *donation* may be sufficiently offended by presumed consent that they will turn against the organ procurement system and record their objections to the whole process.

At their best, the proposals for presuming consent are muddled thinking; at their worst they are deceitful attempts to circumvent the fact that we know a significant percentage of people would not consent. Ethically, it is simply wrong to presume that the deceased or the next-of-kin would consent to use of the organs. As a practical matter it will not work and could jeopardize an already fragile system.

The case against presuming consent is strengthened when we examine the alternatives. First, and most obviously, there are many things that could and should be done to maximize the actual consent of the individual while competent or, absent some expression from the individual, the actual consent of the next of kin.

We are learning a great deal about who should ask about procuring organs and how the request should be made. Some organ procurement organizations (OPOs) report that inexperienced clinicians frame the request inappropriately in such a way to discourage donation. We are just beginning to understand why people might resist donation. Some reasons are based on faulty logic or on an inaccurate grasp of the facts; others require serious attention. Some resistance comes from the fact that patients and families lack adequate trust of the procuring institution. The way to deal with such problems is not to presume consent but to have the institution act in such a way to deserve to be trusted. Other times, persons may decline to donate out of mistaken beliefs. As we saw in Chapter 1, no major Western religious tradition decisively objects in principle to organ procurement. Some, for example, Judaism, consider donation one's moral duty when the donation can save an identifiable life. We have not invested adequately in maximizing actual donation through the execution of Uniform Anatomical Gift Act cards or by relying on next-of-kin to donate.

Almost all states now have required request laws mandating that someone ask the next of kin for permission to procure organs in cases in which usable organs may be obtained. In addition, at the federal level the Omnibus Reconciliation Act of 1986 requires hospitals to comply with United Network for Organ Sharing (UNOS) rules, including having written protocols for identifying potential donors and "assuring that families of potential donors are made aware of the option of organ and tissue donation and their option to decline."[5] Although the results have not as yet been encouraging, there is a great deal that could be done to improve the quality of the request, including some of the strategies mentioned previously. Nevertheless, this routine inquiry of relatives comes too late in the process and asks the question of the wrong person. One of the flaws with the current required request laws is that they ignore the first responsibility of the individual and focus attention only on the substitute surrogate decision maker.

Required Response of Competent Persons

A more defensible alternative is to systematize inquiries to individuals while they are competent to encourage them to make decisions about how they would want their bodies used on their deaths *and then to require that they respond.*[6] Under such arrangements required requests of next of kin would be a fallback position used only when the deceased had never recorded a decision while competent to do so, either because he or she did not have access to the forms and the knowledge about how to execute them or because the individual found thinking about such matters too unpleasant.

Even if we maintain the donation mode of thinking about procuring organs, it is not too much to say that morally one ought to at least make the effort to think enough about this difficult subject to decide whether one wants to be part of the life-saving project of organ donation should that be feasible on one's death. As a corollary I believe the time has come to adopt as social policy a series of efforts to ask people whether they are willing to donate their organs and tissues on their deaths and to expect them to think through the question sufficiently to give a response.

Some of these inquiries should be informal in settings in which the inquiry is not required legally but should be encouraged morally. Of these, many could occur in medical settings. For example, it seems only reasonable that a query about one's wishes about organ procurement should become a routine part of every physician's history and physical. Physicians are learning that they cannot provide good and proper medical care for their patients if they do not have an idea in advance of their patients' preferences. We are routinizing discussions of "living wills," decisions about CPR, and who should be one's surrogate decision maker; we should also make discussion of organ donation a routine part of the history and physical. The physician whose patient fails to provide an adequate response should feel that the record is incomplete. He or she should respond with a distress similar to that when the patient fails to give a clear answer to other queries in the history taking. Although the physician cannot literally *demand* an answer, he or she should convey that high-quality medicine requires that the record be as complete as possible. Also, queries about willingness to donate organs should become a routine part of every hospital admission as required by both state and federal law.

It might be objected that this is too macabre a subject for a physical exam or hospital intake interview. It might even be seen as bad public relations, suggesting to a patient that death is a likely outcome of the encounter. But surely there are already questions posing problems of diplomacy incorporated in such sessions. Physicians ask about sexual histories; hospital intake interviews include questions about who will pay the bills. Skilled professionals learn how to pose these questions diplomatically. If these discussions occur in all routine physical exams and intake interviews, both patients and clinicians will grow accustomed to them. They will provide a good opportunity for repeated reflection.

Perhaps as promising would be opportunities for routine inquiry outside the health care context. Routine inquiry should become a part of other social encounters, such as in religious and fraternal groups. At a more formal, legal level, many states now ask people about organ donation during drivers' license renewals. It would be a small additional step to require in some of these settings that the question be answered. Of course, persons would not be required to answer in the affirmative. They could even be given an opportunity to answer, "I don't know" or "undecided" to the donation question. (In that case, the surrogate decision-making provisions of the Anatomical Gift Act would come into play.)

Although some might see this as an offensive intrusion of the state into private matters, it seems little to ask for what could have a significant life-saving impact. All that would be asked is that one think enough about the life-saving potential of a donation to decide one way or another, not that a *particular* decision be made. Our obligation to the community surely goes far enough to permit a requirement that the question at least be addressed.

In some settings, such as the driver's license application, it would not be difficult to require that the question be answered. An unanswered question would be considered an incomplete application. That, after all, is what happens when other questions are not answered, such as questions about one's automobile insurance.

There are other nonmedical ways that routine inquiry with required response could take place. One of the most practical would be to have an organ donation question on the income tax return. The form is completed by virtually all adults;

it is updated yearly; the data could easily be entered into a central computer at the same time other tax data are. This means that there would be a single national registry rather than a separate database in each state as occurs with drivers' license information. A tape of the data for just that question could be sent to UNOS or any central organ procurement agency, thus facilitating privacy protection. As long as negative answers and opportunities for expressing uncertainty are provided for, such required responses seem well within the model of affirming the primacy of the individual and the donation model. Other potentially sensitive questions, such as willingness to make political and charitable contributions, now appear on federal and state tax forms. Although undoubtedly some will object, these nontax queries have generally been accepted by legislatures and the general population and have been found workable. Thousands of organs—and therefore thousands of lives—hang in the balance. We know that many people are, in principle, willing to donate these organs, but have simply never had the resolve— or the opportunity—to record their donation in an effective way. If we can be asked to contribute to a political party on a tax form, certainly we can be asked to record our willingness to save lives through organ donation.

Other ways to connect routine organ donation inquiries to existing computerized data banks might be possible as well. The health insurance industry maintains a centralized database of insurance records through the Medical Insurance Bureau. It could systematically include organ donation data, even making absence of such data be classified as an incomplete record. There is, however, already substantial suspicion among those who know of its existence that that database constitutes an unacceptable breach of confidentiality. It might not be the ideal mechanism for required response. The census compiles a national database, which could include queries about organ donation, but that survey, even though it is national, occurs only once a decade, not sufficiently frequent to keep an accurate record of individual decisions about donation. The state driving license database and the federal income tax records seem to be the most feasible locations for this information. If we can bring ourselves to be concerned enough about a few thousand of our fellow citizens whose lives and well-being hang in the balance, the federal income tax seems to be the ideal place to require a response to the organ donation question.

ENDNOTES

1. Alfred M. Sadler, Blair L. Sadler, and E. Blythe Stason, "The Uniform Anatomical Gift Act," *Journal of the American Medical Association* 206 (1968): 2501–06.

2. Frank P. Stuart, Frank J. Veith, and Ronald E. Cranford, "Brain Death Laws and Patterns of Consent to Remove Organs for Transplantation from Cadavers in the United States and 28 Other Countries," *Transplantation* 31 (April 1981): 238–44;

Arthur L. Caplan, "Organ Transplants: The Costs of Success, An Argument for Presumed Consent and Oversight," *Hastings Center Report* 13 (Dec. 1983): 23–32; Thomas E. Starzl, "Implied Consent for Cadaveric Organ Donation" (editorial), *Journal of the American Medical Association* 251 (1984): 1592; A. J. Matas and F. J. Veith, "Presumed Consent for Organ Retrieval," *Theoretical Medicine* 5 (1984): 155–66; Arthur J. Matas and Frank J. Veith, "Presumed Consent—A More Humane Approach to Cadaver Organ Donation," in *Positive Approaches to Living with End-Stage Renal Disease: Psychosocial and Thanatological Aspects*, ed. Mark A. Hardy et al. (New York: Praeger, 1986), pp. 37–51.

3. T. Randall, "Too Few Human Organs for Transplantation, Too Many in Need . . . and the Gap Widens," *Journal of the American Medical Association* 265 (1991): 1223.

4. Omnibus Reconciliation Act of 1986, 42 U.S.C.§ 1320b-8.

5. Ibid.

6. Robert M. Veatch, *Death, Dying, and the Biological Revolution*, rev. ed. (New Haven, CT: Yale University Press, 1989).

Twelve

Live-Donor Transplant: Including the Permanently Unconscious and Paired- and Live-Donor/Cadaver Exchanges

IN THE EARLY days of kidney transplantation, organs were routinely procured from people who were living donors. However, since the almost universal adoption of brain-based criteria for pronouncing death beginning in the late 1960s, virtually all countries that do transplants have relied extensively on organs from sources who are neither living nor donors. Although their body functions are being maintained through ventilatory support, they have been legally pronounced dead; they are merely respiring cadavers. Moreover, generally these deceased organ sources are not really donors; it is the next of kin who make such donations.

There are a few cultures where this is not the case: As discussed earlier in the book, certain East Asian cultures have to this day not accepted brain criteria for pronouncing death. This was true of Japan until recently,[1] and still few cadaver organs have been procured there. They rely almost exclusively on living people to provide kidneys and, now, certain other organs such as liver or lung lobes. Scandinavian countries, because of human lymphocyte antigen (HLA) compatibilities and unavailability of cadaver organs, also place great emphasis on live donors. But all countries continue to suffer from a severe shortage of cadaver organs. In the future, at least until there is further progress in immunosuppression, xenotransplant, or artificial organs, significant numbers of organs will have to be obtained via donations from living people.[2] It is estimated that of the 300,000 kidney transplants done to date worldwide, about 70,000 have come from living donors.[3] In the United States approximately 30 percent of kidney transplants were from living donors in 1998, and that percentage is increasing. In addition, small numbers of organs were procured from living donors of liver lobes (49 cases in 1998), lungs (17), and pancreata (2).[4]

Two major ethical questions arise in organ procurement by donation from the living:[5] (1) Under what circumstances can organs be procured from the living? (2) What approvals or consents are necessary to procure the organs?

The Dead Donor Rule

Transplant is generally premised on the dead donor rule. The general rule is that the source of organs must be dead before organs are procured.[6] For unpaired life-preserving organs (organs like the heart and liver rather than the kidneys) that rule has always, at least until very recently, remained firm. But there is an immediate ethical confusion. Most sources of organs are not donors. They have never donated their body parts for any purpose, let alone transplant. No infants and children have made a legal donation. Most adults have not either. The donations are made by family members, legal guardians, or surrogates. I refer to those from whom organs are procured as *organ sources*, whether the source of the organ did the donating or someone else did. This term would also apply to paid organ sources, who, of course, can never accurately be called donors.

The dead donor rule led to the original debate over changing to a brain-oriented definition of death. Under the dead donor rule, if and only if the patient is dead can life-prolonging organs be procured. Recently, however, several new developments have made the application of the dead donor rule more complicated. There are increasingly ambiguous cases in which it is not clear whether the organ source is really dead. In particular, the permanently unconscious (such as anencephalic infants and fetuses and individuals in a permanently vegetative state) have been considered potential sources of organs even though they may retain certain brain functions. Two separate interpretations have been proposed. Some have claimed that the definition of death should be further amended to what in Chapters 5 and 8 I called the higher-brain definition, under which those who have permanently lost all higher-brain functions—usually related to capacity for consciousness—are considered dead.[7] In that case organs could be procured from such formerly living persons without violating the dead donor rule. Those who hold this position sometimes claim that the meaning of the word *death* for social and public policies purposes means nothing more than that there has been a quantum change in the moral status of the individual such that certain behaviors normally associated with dead people (such as procuring organs) are acceptable. Others who favor procuring organs from the permanently unconscious claim that the definition of death need not be changed but that, under certain conditions, it would be acceptable to procure organs from still-living individuals.[8] In this case, we could say that these individuals are "living donors" or at least living sources of organs. In that case, the dead donor rule would have been abandoned, or at least exceptions would have been created.

This is just one new class of living organ donors or sources. Others include some non–heart-beating donors, living unrelated donors, paired living donors, live donors who exchange their organs for a cadaver organ, and what I shall call *purely altruistic donors*—that is, those who donate solid organs without designating a relative or friend to receive them. After categorizing the various types of living donors or sources of organs, I will review in this chapter the new ethical issues raised by these organ procurements from living people.

New Living Donor Cases

In addition to the traditional living related donor, several new groups are emerging including some sources who are at the margins of life and several classes of people who donate to persons to whom they are not related.

Organ Donors and Sources at the Margins of Life

Non–heart-beating donors, anencephalic infants and fetuses, and persistent vegetative state patients are sometimes considered living donors. To the extent that they are living, they are what could be called organ donors and sources at the margins of life.

NON-HEART-BEATING DONORS

Organs are being procured from what are called non–heart-beating cadavers.[9] However, there is real debate about whether all these people are truly dead. In cases in which living, critically ill persons have decided to forgo life support and wish to donate organs, a University of Pittsburgh protocol permits purposeful stopping of life support in the operating room so that organs can be procured immediately.[10] Death is pronounced 120 seconds after asystole, which many argue is before the actual moment of death. If these persons are not truly dead, they may be a whole new class of living donors. The subject of non–heart-beating organ donors is the focus of the following chapter. I shall argue there that organs can be procured from non–heart-beating cadavers in such a way that they really are dead.

ANENCEPHALIC INFANTS

The dead donor rule is also being challenged by recent efforts to attempt to treat anencephalic infants as organ sources. Many are still living by any current legal definition of death. Their hearts are still beating and considerable brain function remains intact. Nevertheless, some people advocate procuring organs from these infants while they are still legally alive. These issues are the subject of Chapter 14, where I will argue that, with proper permission from next of kin, it is acceptable to procure organs from these infants after they die but not while they are living. These cases will not be further considered here.

PERMANENT VEGETATIVE STATE PATIENTS

The permanently vegetative individual is not brain dead.[11] Such an individual, however, is permanently unconscious and free of all sensation. Some have proposed procuring organs from these patients. With proper advance consent or surrogate permission, organs might be procured, perhaps as a part of a series of actions to end life support based on an advanced directive. Most commentators, however, seem unprepared to endorse procurement of life-prolonging organs before death. It appears that the more accurate account of these proposals would be that their advocates, among whom I include myself, really are putting forward a proposal for further modification of the definition of death. They are proposing a higher-brain concept of death in which permanently vegetative individuals—who, by definition, can never again be conscious—would be treated as deceased. Of course, if they are dead, then organ procurement would not violate the dead donor rule.

I think all the cases I have discussed thus far—non–heart-beating donor, anencephalic infants, and permanently unconscious individuals—are (or should be) really proposals to apply the dead donor rule curatively, pressing the limits of the borders between life and death.

The Living Related Donor

One clear exception to the dead donor rule is the more traditional living, related donor who offers solid organs in a way that is not life threatening to the donor. We have for many years accepted donation of a kidney or other non–life-preserving organs from live, genetically related donors.

The traditional wisdom was that it was acceptable to procure organs or tissues for transplant to a genetically related person if the organ is *renewable* and there was only minimal risk provided there was adequately informed consent. This would include blood and probably bone marrow as well as sperm. Recently, support has been found for limited donation of organs and organ parts that were not renewable, provided the donor can be expected to survive with the parts that remain.[12] This has included transplant of a single kidney, a lobe of the liver[13] or lungs,[14] and possibly also pancreata.[15] There is an advantage of living donation over cadaver organs from genetic (and therefore HLA) compatibility, including being able to plan the timing of the organ procurement and perhaps other factors. This advantage is decreasing, however, with greater success of immunosuppression drugs that make organs from nonrelated donors more viable.

It has obviously been considered unacceptable to transplant unpaired, non-renewable life-prolonging organs. This remains the current conclusion for practical purposes, although some theorists, particularly libertarian theorists, debate whether this prohibition should be absolute. Consider, for example, a person dying from a condition for which an unaffected organ can be salvaged. In the era of Jack Kevorkian, the American physician promoting assisted suicide, and increasing use of medical execution, procuring life-prolonging organs before death may not be forever out of consideration. It is explicitly endorsed by Kevorkian.[16] I once corresponded with a death row inmate who wanted to be executed in such a way that his organs could be procured.[17] Surgeons, however, will overwhelmingly refuse to cooperate in such lethal organ procurements from living donors even if the quality of their consent is impeccable and the potential donors are inevitably going to die soon (from disease, forgoing of life-support, or execution) regardless of organ procurement.

Living Unrelated Donors

We are now entertaining the possibility of organ gifts from donors who are not genetically related. The concept of a living, unrelated donor is ambiguous.[18] "Related" is often taken by transplant teams to mean "genetically related." This does not include spouses or stepparents or stepchildren. We now speak of (1) genetically related, and (2) legally but not genetically related relatives (spouses, in-laws, and steps). We could also identify intermediate cases (such as genetically more distant relatives). We can further contemplate living donation from those who are neither genetically nor legally related: (3) close friends (including live-in lovers and gay couples) and (4) strangers.[19]

Transplant surgeons have resisted such transplantation. Genetically related individuals share human lymphocyte antigen (HLA) to some degree (from a full six-antigen match for identical twins and some other siblings to lesser degrees for more distant relatives). Surgeons have condoned genetically related organ donation because of the better match and the related higher likelihood of graft survival. The added advantage of the genetic relation is, however, rather marginal. Some cadaver transplants may involve better matches than some of those involving genetically related donors. Moreover, some emotionally related persons (spouses and other persons related by marriage and friends) may be more urgently committed to the well-being of the one needing the organ and therefore to the donation of the needed organ. Increasingly, there is support for donation by those who are only emotionally related persons if they are adequately informed and sufficiently autonomous to give adequate consent.[20]

Paired, Live-Donor Exchanges

We are also beginning to explore new and unconventional means of increasing the number of live donor organ procurements. One strategy would involve facilitating paired exchanges between two donor-recipient pairs.[21] This strategy could be used in cases in which there are two willing living donors who each turn out to be incompatible with their desired recipient but compatible with the other donor's desired recipient. Normally, this would involve ABO (blood type) incompatibilities, but could also occur for other reasons (such as positive T-cell cross-matches or size incompatibilities). The results would be transplants to genetically unrelated individuals, but the motivation of the donor would be to serve the interests of a potential recipient who may be either genetically or emotionally related. I refer to this type of live donor exchange as "living-donor paired exchanges."

Theorists have even considered variants that are more controversial.[22] First, at least in theory, one might be able to find two persons, each of whom needed an organ part that could be procured without ending the life of the donor (a kidney, liver lobe, lung lobe, or pancreas portion, for example). If the two persons needed different organs or organ parts, they could theoretically each serve as the other's donor. Of course, this scheme would raise complicated technical questions: whether the organ parts procured would be sufficiently healthy if they came from a person in serious organ failure from another organ and whether the parties could survive surgery at two sites simultaneously. Certainly, such persons would be highly motivated and would be able to understand the burdens from both the donor and recipient point of view.

Second, a more controversial proposal would be to identify a group of persons, each of whom were in organ failure for a single organ but whose other organs remained healthy. These might involve persons needing a liver, lung, heart, pancreas, and so forth. (Presumably, considering what is contemplated, kidney recipients would not be interested because they could remain alive with dialysis.) This small group, after being educated to the fact that they were all dying soon without organs, could be asked whether they wished to volunteer for a lottery in which the loser would be anesthetized and have all his or her usable organs removed for the benefit of the others in the lottery. This would involve living, nonrelated donation that would actively cause the death of the lottery loser.

One can see that if people were facing rapid certain death without such an arrangement, the lottery could be perceived, from the perspective of all parties before they know who the loser in the lottery was, as being in the rational interests of all involved. On the other hand, this would be a clear violation of the dead donor rule. The surgeon procuring the organs would be guilty of an illegal act, a murder. The fact that the murder was humane, rational, and consented to by the parties would not exonerate the murderer under current law. Some, especially those who already favor legal changes to support voluntary euthanasia and assisted suicide, would probably favor legalizing such lotteries. In fact, in a state such as Oregon in which assisted suicide is currently legal, this lottery could probably already take place if the proposal were modified so that the loser chose physician-assisted suicide and the organs were procured after the death of the donor. (If the non–heart-beating cadaver protocol were used, of course, the heart recipient would have to drop out of the lottery because, by definition, the lottery loser's heart would be irreversibly stopped.)

Almost everyone would probably find such life-ending organ donation by lottery morally repulsive. It would be a frontal assault on the dead donor rule (unless the assisted-suicide variant were used, which would "waste" one of the organs, assuming the death occurred because of heart stoppage). What is striking is that such a scheme seems clearly to be in the self-interest of those who would play the lottery and all but one clearly come out better while the loser is only a little worse off. Moreover, this scheme is not far removed from the non–heart-beating-cadaver protocols (which we will discuss in the next chapter). The opposition to legalizing such a scheme must rest on the core ethical premise of the dead donor rule: There is something morally wrong with actively and intentionally killing another human being, at least one who is innocent and wants to live. Unless we are willing to create a critical exception to the dead donor rule, such survival lotteries will have to remain illegal.

Live Donor/Cadaver-Paired Exchanges

An additional live donor scheme is closely related to the original paired living-donor exchanges already described. A donor who is incompatible with a desired recipient (a spouse or relative, for example) might donate an organ in exchange for priority on the waiting list for cadaver organs for the donor's chosen recipient. These I shall refer to as *live donor/cadaver-paired exchanges*. Once the donor had had a kidney removed, for example, it would be placed in the pool to be allocated to a stranger according to normal allocation rules. In exchange, the person designated by the donor would be elevated to the top of the cadaver recipient waiting list to receive the first compatible organ. Everyone else on the waiting list would be as well-off or better off than they were before. (They might be considered slightly better off because one person would have been removed from the waiting list, improving the situation of each other person waiting.) To my knowledge, there is no place in the world where this has been attempted. The Washington Regional Transplant Consortium (WRTC) has endorsed the idea in principle, but because it would involve modifying the standard allocation algorithm of the United Network for Organ Sharing, a variance would have to be granted. Initial plans for a request for a variance are in the works.[23]

Purely Altruistic Live Donors

Finally, some transplant programs are beginning to consider purely altruistic live donors of kidneys to strangers in which the donors have no expectation of any reward beyond the satisfaction of helping another human being in need. These I refer to as *purely altruistic live donations*. The WRTC has recently endorsed in principle this type of donation as well as the paired and live donor–cadaver exchanges. Several organs can be procured without jeopardizing the life of the donor: bone marrow, kidneys, and now liver lobes, lung lobes, and pancreatic tissue. The dominant organ of concern, however, is the kidney, and I shall deal primarily with the kidney in this review of the ethics of live donation of organs.

Two Approaches to the Ethics of Live Donation

There are two major ethical approaches to these problematic cases. One focuses on benefits and harms to the recipient and the organ source. The other focuses on autonomy and whether donation is truly voluntary.

Benefits and Harms

The United Network for Organ Sharing (UNOS) ethics committee has endorsed living-donor transplant, including those involving genetically unrelated individuals.[24] The members of the committee began this discussion deeply divided. The transplant surgeons were very concerned about risks to donors, including physical risks. For kidneys, that issue would be essentially the same whether the donor was genetically related, unrelated, or involved in a paired exchange. The main difference is that benefit to the recipient may be somewhat less with a donor who is not genetically related because of somewhat lower graft survival. With advances in immunosuppression, that difference is shrinking.[25] The rejection risk for the nongenetically related donor today is less than for the genetically related donor of the 1950s or 1960s. The risks also include psychological risk to the donor if the graft is rejected or if the recipient dies.

On the other hand, the nonclinicians focused on harms to the potential donors if they were *not* permitted to donate: the devastating sense of loss and the anger at the system that will not let an individual save his or her spouse or stepchild. The consequences to the potential donor could be devastating.

The risks and benefits of paired exchanges or of live donor gifts to the cadaver waiting list in exchange for priority placement of a recipient involves risks and benefits that are almost the same as direct donation to a genetically unrelated relative or friend. The only issues would involve differences in the timing of the transplant and possibly, when recipients are in two different hospitals, the need for the donor to have his or her organ procured in an institution that is not the one he or she might otherwise have chosen. (Paired exchanges involving two different hospitals must involve either the transport of the procured organs or the movement of either donors or recipients to the second hospital.) It has been observed that a transplant surgeon who believes his or her institution is superior in its skill in living donor nephrectomy might face the awkward situation of having to advise the donor that having the surgery in the hospital of the paired recipient would pose an added risk to the donor.

A true utilitarian would consider net utility all things considered.[26] There appears to be a clear expected benefit to the recipient or recipients. Arguably there would be a net benefit to the organ sources as well. In the end, the UNOS ethics committee chose to accept living donation, including emotionally related donors.[27]

Nonconsequentialist Ethics

Those who consider moral factors other than consequences focus on the rights and responsibilities of the parties involved. They hold that ethics is not exclusively a matter of benefiting the patient and protecting the patient from harm. The old Hippocratic ethics was grounded in the benefits and harms approach.[28] It was pure paternalism. But that consequence-based ethic could theoretically justify procuring organs from living sources without consent—in cases in which a physician believed the patient would be harmed more by refusing to donate. A more social–ethical approach would also consider the benefits and harms to other parties involved including the recipient, which could easily make procurement from living organ sources acceptable, even mandatory—theoretically the surgeon would be expected to procure organs for such transplants even without the organ source's consent. Those who insist that there is more to ethics than maximizing good consequences will consider other factors morally crucial.

COMPETENT ADULTS

The arguments proceed rather differently when nonconsequentialists consider competent adults and incompetents persons. Let us consider those who are competent first.

The autonomy-based right to consent to donation. Ethics is, according to this second view, a matter of rights and responsibilities, not mere benefits and harms. This is the approach of Immanuel Kant and the rights-oriented tradition of liberal political philosophy. In exploring how nonconsequentialists handle the rights and responsibilities of living organ procurement, let us focus first on competent adults.

Does a consenting adult have a right to make decisions about his or her own body—for example, does such a person have a right to refuse medical treatment? In a liberal society the answer is surely "yes." This is the ethical basis for decisions of people to refuse life-sustaining medical treatment. The right is usually understood to be only a liberty right—that is, a right to refuse to be touched without one's permission. It has not normally been understood to entail an entitlement right—that is, a right of access to a medical procedure and the means to obtain that procedure. Hence traditionally a person would have the right to consent only in cases in which a provider is willing to cooperate. This is the basis for participation in research involving human subjects. It is also the ethical basis for living, genetically related donation. It could be the basis for living, nongenetically related donation from relatives, friends, and even strangers, as well as paired exchanges and donations to the cadaver pool. If potential donors are substantially autonomous agents, they have the right to consent or refuse consent to medical procedures that are consistent with their freely chosen life plans. At least until very recently, it has not been suggested that one has a right to be a donor if a surgeon is not willing to cooperate, but assuming a willing surgeon, a source of funding, and so forth, the willing donor's consent is the basis for legitimating the donation.

Opposition to autonomy as the basis for live donation. One objection to grounding the ethics of live donation in the autonomy of the substantially competent adult is that consent requires that the parties be adequately informed and that providing such information may put pressure on the potential donor to provide the organ. Some transplant surgeons have cooperated in creating "outs" for family members who really would rather not donate but perceive that a straightforward refusal will damage their relationship with the potential recipient. Surgeons have been known to claim a "medical incompatibility." The consent doctrine requires that information be provided accurately, thus undercutting this scheme for protecting the donor–recipient relationship. Of course, the physician involved could inform the potential donor of the compatibility, leaving it to that person to decide whether to deceptively claim a "medical incompatibility." It is normal, however, for the surgeon to communicate to the recipient if there is such an incompatibility. Insisting that the donor's condition can only be presented to the recipient would be unnatural and would risk having the truth discovered.

This plan to mislead the recipient, of course, is an equivocation at best and an outright lie at worst. It is a statement intended to mislead the recipient into believing a physiological reason exists for why the organ donation cannot take place when, in fact, the reason is rooted in the will of the donor. Kantians and other nonconsequentialists who consider lying and equivocation prima facie ethically wrong will find reason to criticize such practices.

A second problem with grounding the ethics of live donation in autonomy and consent is that some would consider the offer to be an organ donor for a spouse or close friend irresistibly attractive. Recently, for example, parents have not only offered, but have actually provided liver lobes to their children who would surely die if the parent did not intervene. In fact, a prisoner in the California

State Prison in Sacramento, one David Patterson, attempted donate both his kidneys to his 13-year-old daughter.[29] After the first kidney he donated to her failed, he wanted to provide his second. Presumably, he would have to be maintained on dialysis. Officials decided against permitting the donation.

Offers to parents to engage in an act that will save a child's life may be impossible to reject, an "offer one can't refuse." The availability of paired exchanges and donations to the cadaver pool simply increases the potential problem because familial donors will have less excuse for failing to donate. If the offer to donate were considered irresistibly attractive, so the argument goes, it would no longer permit an autonomous choice by the potential donor.

The problem of irresistibly attractive offers was encountered in Chapter 9 when we were considering markets in organs and whether money payments for organs would be coercive to poor individuals who might be forced to sell their organs to meet desperate needs for income. There we saw that *coercion* may not technically be the correct term. The most careful definitions of coercion include the requirement that coercion involve a "threat" rather than an "offer" and that the threat be irresistible and intentional.[30] Moreover, coercion must be distinguished from pressure or manipulation. The core issue, for our purposes, is whether the offer, whatever it is called, renders the decision maker substantially nonautonomous.

Autonomous actions are actions that one chooses based on one's own life plan—according to one's own beliefs and values. Just as accepting money payments for an organ may be consistent with one's life plan, so might deciding to become a live donor. Choosing to make a modest sacrifice of one's own health for the benefit of one's spouse or stepchildren is plausibly consistent with one's life plan. Likewise, making such an offer to a close friend can be consistent with one's own life plan. Even making such an offer to a stranger might be for some competent adults. Offers cannot violate autonomy simply by being terribly attractive.

That does not mean that all offers that are attractive are ethical. We saw in Chapter 9 that we also need to consider whether the offer is "unwelcome" and "exploitative." Whether an irresistibly attractive offer is ethical will depend on the mind-set of the potential donor as well as on the state of the one making the offer. In this case the offer to a relative to become a candidate for live donation may or may not be welcome. A spouse, for example, may truly be eager to do "anything" to save a husband or wife and not concerned that the offer is made, whereas other relatives may find the offer quite unwelcome even if that relative perceives there is no way to refuse.

It is usually not the case that the offer to become a live donor is exploitative. Normally, the health professional presenting the live donor option will discuss the alternatives of dialysis and cadaver donation and not try to take advantage of the potential donor's desire to help the recipient. One could imagine a case in which a surgeon would try to exploit the potential donor, say, because the surgeon needed practice at doing live donor procurement, but that would surely be an exceptional situation.

Consider an analogous case. Saul Krugman, a researcher in New York, conducted a series of experiments to develop a hepatitis vaccine.[31] Part of his plan involved administering hepatitis to institutionalized mentally retarded children who were residents at Willowbrook State School, a New York institution for retarded individuals. At this institution at the time, sanitation was notoriously poor, so poor that children would almost certainly get hepatitis anyway. Krugman took advantage of that fact to make an offer to the parents of these children that would spare them uncontrolled exposure to hepatitis and living in squalid conditions. If the parents would agree to have him give hepatitis to their children as part of a research protocol, he would see that they received high-quality medical care in a pleasant and clean facility. Because, it was argued, the children were inevitably going to get hepatitis one way or another, parents might have found the offer irresistible—if this were the only choice.

The moral controversy surrounding this case raised the question of whether the offer to the parents was irresistible because it was so attractive and if it was immoral because of its power. Although many people concluded that the offer would plausibly be irresistible and that making the offer was immoral, it does not follow that it is immoral *because* it is so attractive.

Parents who were autonomous agents were devoted to the welfare of their children. They could autonomously choose to place their children in the study because it clearly promoted the children's welfare compared to the alternatives available to the parents. Even though the offer was much more attractive than the alternative, that does not, by itself, make the offer a violation of autonomy. If the parents' choice was consistent with their life goals of promoting their children's welfare, then even if it was a forced choice, it was one consistent with their autonomy.

The real problem with the Krugman experiment was that the one making the offer might have had other options to address the poor conditions in the institution's regular buildings. Krugman was a powerful figure in a medical facility associated with that institution, and perhaps he could have devoted his energies to improving the sanitation so that hepatitis would no longer have been endemic. It was the fact that the one making the offer to the parents had other options available that make the offer unethical, not the fact that the offer, once made, was irresistibly attractive to the parents. Krugman, in effect, took advantage of their miserable situation when he could probably have done something about that situation.

By analogy, when transplant surgeons offer living donation to a friend or relative of someone in kidney or liver failure, it would be unethical if they made that offer only after they had withheld an available cadaver organ. If a surgeon were to withhold a cadaver organ to gain practice in procuring from live donors, that would, of course, be unethical. It would force the family member to become a live donor. But assuming the living donation is being considered because the surgeon has nothing else to offer (short of a long and perhaps fruitless time on a waiting list), then the mere fact that the offer seems powerfully attractive to the potential donor cannot by itself make the offer immoral any more than offering painful cardiac surgery to a critically ill heart patient would be considered unethical because it was so attractive an offer compared to the available alternatives.

If Krugman had a realistic alternative for improving the medical welfare of his research participants, then taking advantage of the poor conditions was unethical. If he had no reasonable alternative, then arguably his behavior was ethical. Likewise, if there is no plausible alternative to transplanting from a living donor, then there is nothing unethical about making overpoweringly attractive offers to potential donors.

The problem of perceived pressure to donate is just as great for living genetically related relatives as for nongenetically related relatives. In fact, strangers, by this analysis, are the least likely to be pressured into consenting. The focus on respect for autonomy provides an argument for accepting volunteers who are strangers, at least for bone marrow and, arguably, for kidneys as well. What might be thought of as the "coerciveness" of an offer to donate is merely an offer that is terribly attractive given some relatives' commitment to their loved ones' survival. It is not unethical because it "coerces" the "donor," and therefore violates the donor's autonomy, unless it exploits the commitment to the recipient to force the donor's behavior when other options were available that were not fairly presented.

INCOMPETENT ORGAN SOURCES

Although this analysis seems to provide moral support for adults who autonomously choose to donate organs (regardless of the degree of kinship), it says nothing about the use of small children, infants, or mentally incompetent individuals as organ sources. Autonomous donation is a meaningless term in cases of incompetent potential organ sources. The question of minors and other incompetent persons as sources of organs will be addressed in more detail in Chapter 15 but should be examined here as well. I have already built the foundation for a very limited justification of procuring organs and tissues from infants, children, and others incompetent to donate. We view children as part of moral communities.

As such they are the bearers of rights. However, they also have very limited responsibility to contribute to the community. For instance, we acknowledge the legitimacy of involving them in minimal-risk research.[32] We impose the condition of parental consent to protect against abuse, but with proper consent and other standards *minimal* imposition of social service on incompetent individuals is morally tolerable, perhaps even essential to nurturing a responsible citizen.

Probably children have a greater obligation to their family members than they do to participate in minimal-risk medical research, so marginally more risk is probably acceptable. Several court cases in the United States have supported this conclusion regarding procuring organs for transplant from living incompetent siblings. The more philosophical question is on what basis such approval might be given. Two arguments have been put forward in favor of procurement from certain minors.

Benefit to the child supplying the organ. One legal case developed the notion that it can actually be in the interests of the donor to donate a kidney. Although the potential organ source was an adult, his mental retardation rendered him like a child in all relevant respects. By contrast a second case suggests some moral limits on the use of this argument.

In *Strunk v. Strunk*, a Kentuckian named Tommy Strunk, a 28-year-old married employee of the Penn State Railroad and a part-time student, was suffering from chronic glomerulus nephritis.[33] His dialysis treatments were reaching the point at which they could not continue much longer. He needed a transplant. His mother, father, and a number of collateral relatives were tested and found incompatible. His brother, Jerry, however, was found "highly acceptable." The problem was that Jerry was a 27-year-old who was committed to the Frankfort State Hospital, a state institution for the "feebleminded." He had an IQ of approximately 35 and was further handicapped by a speech defect, making it difficult for him to communicate. The mother of the two men petitioned the court for authority to proceed with the transplant.

Although Jerry was not a minor, he was described as having a mental age of 6 years. The court concluded that it was actually in Jerry's interest that his brother receive his kidney. Jerry was described as "greatly dependent upon Tommy, emotionally and psychologically, and . . . his well-being would be jeopardized more severely by the loss of his brother than by the removal of a kidney."[34]

The moral logic was identical to that of a parent offering permission or "proxy consent" for a therapeutic treatment for their child. The transplant was obviously therapeutic for Tommy, the recipient. But the court took the view that the transplant was also "therapeutic" for Jerry as well. It offered Jerry the benefit of increasing the chances of his brother's survival and capacity to provide support for Jerry. If that is true, then this is not a case of using the incompetent sibling solely for the benefit of the mentally healthy brother. It is a case of acting to benefit the incompetent one.

Although the court accepted this "patient-benefit" argument, it seems clear that it would not apply in all cases of obtaining organs from children or other incompetent organ sources. A second case suggests an interesting contrast. Four years later *In Re Richardson*, which involved a similar set of circumstances,[35] was heard in the Louisiana courts. Thirty-two-year-old Beverly Jean Richardson was in need of a kidney transplant. She had only months to live. (The reasons why dialysis would not be successful in bridging until a cadaver organ could be obtained are unclear.) The most acceptable organ source was her brother, 17-year-old Roy. He, however, was, in addition to being a minor also severely retarded, having a mental age described as that of a 3- or 4-year-old.

Richardson's parents relied on the *Strunk* case, attempting to argue that it was in Roy's interest to provide a kidney for his older sister. The court did not accept the argument, concluding that "such an event is not only highly speculative, but in view of all of the facts, highly unlikely."[36] The reasons are not spelled out, but reports about the case suggest that the sister was not close to the institutional-ized young man. The fact that he had been institutionalized suggests that he was not likely to be dependent on his sister. Moreover, the court observed that Roy's condition gave him a short life expectancy. The facts of this case fail to support the claim that it would be in Roy's interest to be the source of an organ for his sister taking into account the medical risks and discomfort of the organ-procurement surgery.

Duty of incompetents to others. This suggests the second kind of argument that has been brought forward to support procuring of organs and tissues from minors and other incompetents. Some people have observed that it is a bit of a stretch to defend such procurements solely on the grounds of benefit to the source of the organ but that this may be an unnecessary standard in any case. In the sphere of human subjects research, many now reject the standard that experimental treatments may be undertaken for incompetents only when it is in their interest to do so. Surely, the welfare of children and other incompetents is a very high priority, but, it is argued, even children are part of larger social communities and have some limited obligations to be altruistic toward other members of this community. Risk-free research seems justifiable provided other obvious conditions are met: that the research cannot be carried out on competents who consent, that parents give their permission, and that older minors who are able to do so give their assent. Under the most rigorous standards that legitimate research only when it is for the benefit of the subject, even risk-free research could not be permitted when it does not promise some benefit to the subject.

If risk-free research is permissible, it must be because even incompetent minors owe something to the communities of which they are a part. That debt to the community might even justify research with minor risks—such as a needle stick or wearing of electronic monitoring equipment to measure heart rate. For these kinds of reasons, federal regulations permit children to participate in research offering minimal risks and even greater than minimal risks under certain special circumstances.[37]

If such bonds of community permit imposing minor risks on children who cannot consent merely to benefit strangers, it might be plausible for somewhat more serious risks to be imposed on children to benefit other members of their immediate families. In families in dire straights from poverty or natural disaster, we assume that the parent's duty to do whatever is beneficial for the child is attenuated by the critical limits placed on the family. Although parents are expected to make extreme sacrifice for the welfare of their children in such circumstances, they are not expected to make total sacrifice. They must pay at least some attention to their own needs (if for no other reason than that it is in the child's interest that the parent remain capable of providing continuing care). It is even more obvious that the parents may sacrifice one child's interest for the benefit of other children. Even in more ordinary circumstances we might expect parents to require children to make some modest contribution to others—as part of the child's socialization into the role of responsible moral citizen. In the same way children may be expected to contribute a portion of an allowance to charity or church. They may be required to sacrifice their own interests as part of the process of learning altruism. Many would consider that children have some limited form of a duty to make personal sacrifice to benefit others, especially those in greater need or those who are part of the child's family. Being part of a family requires some form of limited duty to others even for minors who cannot be said to be substantially autonomous and capable of choosing to be altruistic. It is this reasoning that has been offered to support organ and tissue procurement from children and other incompetent individuals.

It is not clear exactly what the limits should be on imposing such family-serving risks. Surely the risks should not be as great as we would permit a competent adult to accept. Procuring a pint of badly needed blood from an older child to be transfused into a needy sibling when no other source was available seems well within these limits. A hospital ethics committee on which I serve used this argument to justify a bone marrow procurement from a living 9-month-old infant sibling who was the only feasible source of marrow for a brother suffering from leukemia. The infant would be at risk of needing a blood transfusion if she were a bone marrow source. We were concerned about possible hepatitis or HIV transmission to the infant as well as the pain. After much deliberation, we thought the risk was justified. The procurement proceeded without adverse consequences.

Procuring a kidney is a step beyond procuring bone marrow. The kidney will not regenerate and the surgery is much more substantial. It seems reasonable that the presumption should be against such procurements unless there is no other alternative, there is judicial review, and the parents can make the case that the recipient is an integral part of the family unit. If such requirements are met, procuring a kidney for transplant to a family member who has no other source for an organ and who can no longer be maintained on dialysis may possibly be within the limits of what we can impose on a child or an incompetent person. Doing so would surely be controversial. Reasonable people may differ on whether imposing such contributions on nonconsenting minors goes too far.

Probably the kidney is as far as it can go. Lung lobe procurement even from consenting adults raises serious problems because of the greater risks of the surgery to remove it.[38] It is surely more than we should ask of minors and other incompetents. If we ask the question, "What does one human being owe to others," we will frame the question properly. Competent potential donors can then have considerable leeway to decide to donate, providing any organs donated are not considered life prolonging. From incompetent patients, we should be severely limited in what we can expect. Surely, we do not expect incompetents to provide organs whenever the benefits to others will be greater than the harm expected for the one who is the source of the organs. But some modest contribution may be morally tolerable. From the nonconsequentialist perspective, it is not the risk and benefit that is critical, it is what we have a right to expect of the incompetent.

Paired Exchanges

The ethics of paired live-donor exchanges add only modest complications to the analysis. A paired exchange leads to organ transplants to genetically unrelated individuals, so the risks and benefits are comparable to living emotionally related donation. We have seen that this is increasingly considered acceptable. The motivation of the donors is certainly understandable. It is precisely the same as donating directly to one's relative.

The timing of paired exchanges poses some additional problems. It is rare enough that we will find two donors, each of whom is willing to donate but incompatible with their desired recipient while they are compatible with the paired recipient. The most obvious case will be a pair involving a donor from an A blood group and a recipient from a B blood group who can cross-exchange with a donor from the B group paired with a recipient of an A blood type. Often for various technical reasons the ideal time for transplant for the two recipients and two donors may not be the same. However, if one donor contributes a kidney to the other donor's desired recipient before the time of the second nephrectomy, some guarantee would have to be in place that the second donor would not change his or her mind. Yet it is hard to imagine how such a compulsory, uncancellable pledge to donate would be ethical or legal. This would probably mean that the pair of transplants would have to occur simultaneously, even if the timing was not ideal for some of the parties.

Paired exchanges could involve kidney patients of the same surgeon. If so, and if organs are procured simultaneously, presumably one of the transplant recipients would have to accept someone other than his or her chosen surgeon. If different surgeons are involved this problem would be avoided, but that would mean one of the patients would have to accept a "substitute surgeon." If they are at different institutions, then either the donors or the recipients would have to travel to another hospital (unless the organs are transported, which is less than ideal medically). If the recipients each travel to the other's hospital, we face the problem mentioned previously. If one of the surgeons who originally evaluated the donor believes the other hospital is inferior in quality, presumably that surgeon would have to inform the recipient of that fact—creating a complicated situation for all involved.

These problems can presumably be overcome, at least in some cases, making paired live donor exchanges essentially comparable to living emotionally related donation. Those who would accept such donation will probably accept paired exchanges as well.

Live-Donor–Cadaver Exchanges

Placing the live donor's organ in the cadaver organ pool in exchange for first priority for a suitable organ for one's desired recipient is, in many ways, a much more efficient scheme. It would avoid the problems of arranging simultaneous donations in paired exchanges and eliminate the problem of a surgeon who believes another hospital is inferior. Most important, it would make live donation available in many more cases. The donor–recipient pair would not be restricted to the rare instances when a suitable cross-exchange can be arranged. For example, if blood type is the basis for the donor–recipient incompatibility, no paired exchanges would ever take place for AB-blood-type recipients or O-blood-type donors. There will be no case in which another donor will be more suitable in terms of blood group. However, the donor in each case could donate to the cadaver pool. In virtually all cases, someone on the cadaver organ waiting list would be able to use the organ.

This raises a new set of ethical issues, however. First, although no one on the cadaver waiting list will be made worse off by these exchanges, it is not clear that all parties on the waiting list will understand this. They will see someone taken from a lower position and given highest priority. That person will have been responsible for adding an organ and reducing the waiting list by one, thus creating a small benefit for everyone else on the list, even though he or she moves to the head of the list. Those on the waiting list in more favorable positions will be in exactly the same spot as before; those in less favorable positions will be in a slightly better spot. However, if those on the list do not understand the reasoning, damage to the overall transplant program could result.

A second issue is whether these exchanges would be fair to certain people on the waiting list. Consider, for example, O-blood-group persons who have no suitable friends or relatives who could make a live donation. It is likely that many of the live donors contributing under this scheme would be acting to support friends or relatives with O blood type while they themselves have some other blood group. (A similar problem would occur to a lesser degree for A- and B-group recipients whose donors are AB.) These recipients will end up taking O-blood-group organs from the cadaver pool, making it even harder for other O-group recipients to get suitable organs. This may require reassessing the point assignments for these recipients so that they can compete more aggressively for compatible organs that they might otherwise lose to people of other blood groups who have longer waiting times or other sources of allocation points. If a live donor/cadaver exchange is established, the impact on waiting times for potential recipients on the list should be monitored carefully, making adjustments as necessary.

The Right of Persons to Become Donors

There is one final problem worth addressing. If competent persons may donate organs to family, friends, and perhaps even strangers as an act of charity without violating any moral principles, and incompetents may have a very limited altruism imposed on them for the welfare of their families and perhaps even for strangers, then do people have a *right* to become living donors of organs even if transplant surgeons object?

When expressed in terms of a "right" we are referring presumably to free choices made by competent individuals, not to decisions by family to procure organs from incompetent members. Suppose that a parent of a child severely ill with kidney or liver failure is aware that he or she could be the one last hope for saving the child's life. If that person chooses to donate organs, does the transplant surgeon have a moral duty to cooperate and perform the transplant even if the surgeon has reservations (such as believing the risk to the donor is too great or the chance of success too small)?

I raise this as a moral issue, not a legal one. I assume that, at least for now, no surgeon will be forced by law to perform this surgery against his or her will. But under what conditions may a potential organ donor make a moral demand that his or her organs be procured?

This question closely parallels the debate in the United States and elsewhere over so-called futile care.[39] People are increasingly demanding the right to life-prolonging treatment even in cases in which the clinician believes the procedures will do no good. The interesting cases are those in which the intervention (with ventilator or medication) may temporarily prolong the life of a permanently comatose, vegetative, or inevitably dying patient. Increasingly, clinicians are refusing to perform these procedures. Patients or their surrogates are going to court to obtain an order to be treated.

The American courts have uniformly recognized that when certain conditions are met, a right of access to care will be supported that generates an obligation on hospitals and individual clinicians.[40] I am speaking only of interventions that can be expected to prolong life and that are not burdensome, at least in the case of an incompetent recipient. The physician must be competent to provide the care, and an ongoing patient–physician relationship must exist. When all of these conditions are met, the court has always ordered treatment.

This creates interesting questions for transplant. If we are inclined to recognize the right of people with minority views to preserve their own lives or the lives of loved ones by court-ordered continuation of life support, would a willing potential donor of organs have a similar right to have his or her organ procured and transplanted even if the clinician objected?

For now the working presumption is that there is no such right. But the moral logic that supports a right to lifesaving treatment in one case would seem to support it in the other. Granting a right to have one's organs procured would violate the Hippocratic ethic that the physician intervention must be for the benefit of the individual who is treated, but it could be supported by secular liberal ethics as well as Jewish and Christian moral theology, as discussed in Chapter 1. Of course, there would have to be limits on the risk to the donor and the recipient; there would have to be some minimal probability of success. But is there any HLA match that is so poor that live donor kidney transplant should be ruled out when willing and properly screened donors are available? I think not.

It would also violate the Hippocratic ethic that specifies it is the physician's judgment about benefit that is decisive. Recent shifts in American law and ethics have now largely abandoned the idea that it is the physician's judgment of benefit and harm that is decisive. The *Quinlan* opinion[41] clearly rejects the professional standard in favor of judgments by the patient or the valid surrogate.

I suspect that sooner or later surgeons will be confronted with patients who bring with them willing familial donors who have met psychological and physical criteria for transplant. If live donation and transplant is acceptable in general and the normal clinical criteria are met, I see no reason why there is not a moral obligation on the part of the surgeon to cooperate.

Conclusion

The ethics of procuring organs from living donors poses no moral questions that are truly new. In one way or another, we have faced them before for transplant, medical research, and other areas of medical ethics.

We now know that the old Hippocratic Oath is inadequate for twenty-first-century medicine. It violates the autonomy of the patient, prohibits most medical research, and makes all living donor organ transplant extremely difficult.

If we turn to the more appropriate ethic of rights and responsibilities rather than merely benefits and harms, an ethic that recognizes social responsibilities within moral communities while guarding against simple utilitarianism, then procurement of organs from living people becomes more defensible.

ENDNOTES

1. Rihito Kimura, "Japan's Dilemma with the Definition of Death," *Kennedy Institute of Ethics Journal* 1 (1991): 23–31; Yuri Kageyama, "Japan Redefines Death to Assist in Transplants," *Washington Post*, June 18, 1997, p. A20.

2. The best recent review of the technical aspects of living organ donation accessible to the lay person is Richard D. M. Allen, Stephen V. Lynch, and Russell W. Strong, "The Living Organ Donor," in *Organ and Tissue Donation for Transplantation*, ed. Jeremy R. Chapman, Mark Deierhoi, and Celia Wight (New York: Oxford University Press, 1997), pp. 162–99.

3. Richard D. M. Allen, Stephen V. Lynch, and Russell W. Strong, "The Living Organ Donor," p. 163.

4. UNOS Web site: <http://www.unos.org/Frame_default.asp?Category=Newsdata> (March 3, 2000). In the past there have also been living donors of hearts, as many as 12 per year in 1990, but as of this writing only 2 had been performed in the past five years. The living donation of a heart can occur in a patient who has a healthy heart but needs a lung transplant. Some surgeons, believing it easier to implant a heart–lung block rather than lungs alone, have removed the lung recipient's heart as well and implanted a cadaver heart–lung combination, leaving that person's heart available for transplant to another person who needs only a heart.

5. Arthur Caplan, "Must I Be My Brother's Keeper? Ethical Issues in the Use of Living Donors as Sources of Liver and Other Solid Organs," *Transplantation Proceedings* 25 (1993): 1997–2000; James F. Childress, "The Gift of Life: Ethical Problems and Policies in Obtaining and Distributing Organs for Transplantation," *Critical Care Clinics* 2 (1986): 133–48; "Ethics of Organ Transplantation from Living Donors," *Transplantation Proceedings* 24 (1992): 2236–37; Peter A. Singer, Peter F. Whitington, John D. Lantos, Jean C. Emond, J. Richard Thistlethwaite, and Christoph E. Broelsch, "Occasional Notes: Ethics of Liver Transplantation with Living Donors," *New England Journal of Medicine* 321 (1989): 620–22; Mordechai R. Kramer and Charles L. Sprung, "Living Related Donation in Lung Transplantation: Ethical Considerations," *Archives of Internal Medicine* 155 (1995): 1734–38; Aaron Spital, "Living Kidney Donation: Still Worth the Risk," *Transplantation Proceedings* 20 (1988): 1051–58; Carl Elliott, "Doing Harm: Living Organ Donors, Clinical Research, and the Tenth Man," *Journal of Medical Ethics* 21 (1995): 91–96; A. S. Daar, "Living-Organ Donation: Time for a Donor Charter," in *Transplants 1994*, ed. Paul I. Terasaki and J. M. Cecka (Los Angeles: UCLA Tissue Typing Laboratory, 1995), pp. 376–79.

6. Robert M. Arnold and Stuart J. Youngner, "The Dead Donor Rule: Should We Stretch It, Bend It, or Abandon It?" *Kennedy Institute of Ethics Journal* 3 (2, 1993): 263–78; *see also* John A. Robertson, "The Dead Donor Rule." *The Hastings Center Report* 29 (Nov.–Dec. 1999): 6–14.

7. Robert M. Veatch, "The Whole-Brain-Oriented Concept of Death: An Outmoded Philosophical Formulation," *Journal of Thanatology* 3 (1975): 13–30.

8. Robert D. Truog, "Is It Time to Abandon Brain Death?" *Hastings Center Report* 27 (1997): 29–37.

9. Robert M. Arnold, Stuart J. Youngner, Renie Schapiro, and Carol Mason Spicer, eds. *Procuring Organs for Transplant: The Debate Over Non-Heart-Beating Cadaver Protocols* (Baltimore, MD: The Johns Hopkins University Press, 1995).

10. Michael A. De Vita and James V. Snyder, "Development of the University of Pittsburgh Medical Center Policy for the Care of Terminally Ill Patients Who May Become Organ Donors after Death Following the Removal of Life Support," *Kennedy Institute of Ethics Journal* 3 (1993): 131–43.

11. Ronald B. Cranford and Harmon L. Smith, "Some Critical Distinctions between Brain Death and the Persistent Vegetative State," *Ethics in Science and Medicine* 6 (1979): 199–209.

12. Of course, the adequately informed consent of the donor is still required. There is considerable hand wringing about whether family members or others contemplating donation of life-saving organs can really make a rational choice to give their consent. Some people report that, when learning of a loved one's need of an organ, the decision is immediate—without the benefit of an adequate information

session on which to make the choice. Sometimes such decisions are thought to lack freedom. (See Rachel Ankeny Majeske, Lisa S. Parker, and Joel E. Frader, "In Search of an Ethical Framework for Consideration of Decisions Regarding Live Donation," in *Organ and Tissue Donation: Ethical, Legal, and Policy Issues*, ed. Bethany Spielman [Carbondale: Southern Illinois University Press, 1996], pp. 89–101, for an example.) In fact, some offers in such cases may be irresistibly attractive. This may lead to instantaneous decision, but that need not imply that the decisions is not "adequately" informed. Some offers are so obviously compatible with one's basic commitments and life plan that very little if any information is needed. Such poorly informed decisions may nonetheless be autonomous and consistent with one's life plan. These donors, of course, should be worked up psychologically, but the ethics of consent seems rather straightforward. We will discuss these issues later in the chapter.

The risk of morality from a kidney donation is small but real. It is estimated to be about 0.03% (Richard D. M. Allen, Stephen V. Lynch, and Russell W. Strong, "The Living Organ Donor," p. 165. There is also concern about long-term risks of the donor developing renal failure, leading to a need for the second kidney. Although this risk is not fully studied, it is believed that the donor's risk is no greater than in the normal population. Of course, if the recipient's kidney disease is genetically related and the donor is genetically related to the recipient, the donor's risk of developing kidney disease may be much greater.

13. Peter A. Singer, Mark Siegler, Peter F. Whitington, John D. Lantos, Jean C. Emond, J. Richard Thistlethwaite, and Christoph E. Broelsch, "Ethics of Liver Transplantation with Living Donors," *New England Journal of Medicine* 321 (1989): 620–22; Linda R. Shaw, John D. Miller, Arthur S. Slutsky, Janet R. Maurer, John D. Puskas, G. Alexander Patterson, and Peter A. Singer, "Ethics of Lung Transplantation with Live Donors," *Lancet* 338 (1991): 678–81.

14. Mordechi R. Kramer and Charles L. Sprung, "Living Related Donation in Lung Transplantation: Ethical Considerations," 1734–38.

15. S. Grundfest-Broniatowski and A. Novick, "Pancreas Transplantation—1985," *Transplantation Proceedings* 18 (1986): 31–39.

16. Jack Kevorkian, *Prescription Medicide: The Goodness of Planned Death* (Buffalo, NY: Prometheus Books, 1991), p. 33 and passim.

17. The correspondence is published in "A Condemned Man's Last Wish: Organ Donation & a 'Meaningful' Death," *Hastings Center Report* 9 (1979): 16–17.

18. We are not considering unrelated organ sources who are paid. That topic was discussed in Chapters 9 and 10. Some commentators, confusing a paid vendor with a "donor," put forward arguments against markets in organs from living vendors while talking as if they were criticizing living unrelated donation. See M. K. Mani, "The Argument against the Unrelated Live Donor," in *Ethical Problems in*

Dialysis and Transplantation, ed. Carl M. Kjellstrand and John B. Dossetor (Boston: Kluwer Academic, 1992), pp. 163–68.

19. Thomas H. Murray, "Gifts of the Body and the Needs of Strangers," *Hastings Center Report* 17 (April 1987): 30–38; Andrew S. Levey, Susan Hou, and Harry L. Bush, Jr., "Sounding Board: Kidney Transplantation from Unrelated Living Donors," *New England Journal of Medicine* 314 (1986): 914–16; Martyn Evans, "Organ Donations Should Not Be Restricted to Relatives," *Journal of Medical Ethics* 15 (1989): 17–20.

20. Martyn Evans, "Organ Donations Should Not Be Restricted to Relatives"; Andrew S. Levey, Susan Hou, and Harry L. Bush, Jr., "Kidney Transplantation from Unrelated Living Donors"; Aaron Spital, "Unrelated Living Kidney Donors: An Update of Attitudes and Use among U.S. Transplant Centers," *Transplantation* 57 (1994): 1722–26; Carlton J. Young, Anthony M. D'Alessandro, Hans W. Sollinger, and Folkert O. Belzer, "Living-Related and Unrelated Renal Donation: The University of Wisconsin Perspective," in *Clinical Transplants 1994*, ed. Paul I. Terasaki and J. M. Cecka (Los Angeles: UCLA Tissue Typing Laboratory, 1995), pp. 362–63.

21. Lainie F. Ross, David T. Rubin, Mark Siegler, Michelle A. Josephson, and J. Richard Thistlewaite, Jr., "Ethics of a Paired-Kidney-Exchange Program," *New England Journal of Medicine* 336 (1997): 1752–55; F. T. Rapaport, "Living Donor Kidney Transplantation," *Transplantation Proceedings* 19 (1987): 169; Rapaport, "The Case for a Living Emotionally Related International Kidney Donor Exchange Registry," *Transplantation Proceedings* 18 (Suppl. 2, 1986): 5–9.

22. Some of these arrangement are discussed by John Harris, "The Survival Lottery," *Philosophy* 50 (191, Jan., 1975): 571–85; and Francis M. Kamm, *Morality, Mortality: Volume I: Death and Whom to Save from It* (New York: Oxford University Press, 1993), pp. 226–28.

23. For a recent, more critical account of these live donor swaps see Jerry Menikoff, "Organ Swapping," *The Hastings Center Report* 29 (6, Nov.–Dec. 1999): 28–33.

24. James R. Burdick, Jeremiah G. Turcotte, and Robert M. Veatch (Eds.), "Principles of Organ and Tissue Allocation and Donation by Living Donors," *Transplantation Proceedings* 24 (1992): 2226–37.

25. Paul I. Terasaki, J. Michael Cecka, David W. Gjertson, and Steven Takemoto, "High Survival Rates of Kidney Transplants from Spousal and Living Unrelated Donors," *New England Journal of Medicine* 333 (1995): 333–36.

26. Aaron Spital, "Living Kidney Donation."

27. James R. Burdick, Jeremiah G. Turcotte, and Robert M. Veatch (Eds.), "Principles of Organ and Tissue Allocation and Donation by Living Donors," *Transplantation Proceedings* 24 (1992): 2226–37.

28. Robert M. Veatch, *A Theory of Medical Ethics* (New York: Basic Books, 1981).

29. Deborah Josefson, "Prisoner Wants to Donate His Second Kidney," *BMJ* 318 (January 2, 1999): 7.

30. Ruth Faden and Tom L. Beauchamp, in collaboration with Nancy N. P. King, *A History and Theory of Informed Consent* (New York: Oxford University Press, 1986), pp. 337–73.

31. S. Krugman, R. Ward, J. P. Giles, O. Bodansky, and A. M. Jacobs, "Infectious Hepatitis: Detection of Virus during the Incubation Period and in Clinically Inapparent Infection," *New England Journal of Medicine* 261 (1959): 729–34.

32. National Commission for the Protection of Human Subjects of Biomedical and Behavioral Research, *Research Involving Children: Report and Recommendations* (Washington, DC: U.S. Government Printing Office, 1977).

33. *Strunk v. Strunk*, 445 S.W.2d 145 (Ky., 1969).

34. Ibid. at 146.

35. *In Re Richardson*, 284 So.2d 185 (La. App., 1973).

36. Ibid. at 187.

37. U.S. Department of Health and Human Services, "Additional Protections for Children Involved as Subjects in Research: Final Rule: 45 CFR 46," *Federal Register: Rules and Regulations* 48 (46, March 8, 1983): 9814–20.

38. Linda R. Shaw, John D. Miller, Arthur S. Slutsky, Janet R. Maurer, John D. Puskas, G. Alexander Patterson, and Peter A. Singer, "Ethics of Lung Transplantation with Live Donors," 678–81; Mordechai R. Kramer and Charles L. Sprung, "Living Related Donation in Lung Transplantation: Ethical Considerations," 1734–38.

39. Robert M. Veatch and Carol M. Spicer, "Medically Futile Care: The Role of the Physician in Setting Limits," *American Journal of Law & Medicine* 18 (1992): 15–36.

40. *In the Matter of Baby K*, 832 F. Supp. 1022 (E.D. Va. 1993); *Velez v. Bethune et al.* 466 S.E.2d 627 (Ga. App. 1995); *Rideout, Administrator of Estate of Rideout et al. v. Hershey Medical Center*, Dauphin County Report, 1995, pp. 472–98; *In re Doe* 418 S.E.2d 3 (Ga 1992); Cf. Kolata, Gina. "Withholding Care from Patients: Boston Case Asks Who Decides," *New York Times*, April 3, 1995, pp. A1, B8.

41. *In re Quinlan*, 70 N.J. 10, 355 A.2d 647 (1976), *cert. denied* sub nom.; *Garger v. New Jersey*, 429 U.S. 922 (1976), overruled in part. *In re Conroy*, 98 NJ 321, 486 A.2d 1209 (1985).

THIRTEEN

NON-HEART-BEATING CADAVER DONORS

THE TRANSPLANT COMMUNITY has been so committed to procuring organs from people pronounced dead based on brain criteria that it has almost forgotten that, in the earliest days of transplantation, organs—especially kidneys—were obtained from people who were pronounced dead the old-fashioned way: based on heart criteria. Recently, as we have gotten more and more desperate for organs, some people have raised the question of whether we might still be able to obtain some medically suitable organs from the large group of people who are still pronounced dead based on heart stoppage without any tests being performed on their brains. These people have been given the troublesome name *non–heart-beating cadaver donors* (NHBCDs).[1]

Two groups of patients are considered feasible sources of organs following cardiac arrest. The first group are heart attack and accident victims who are brought to hospitals for emergency treatment. They suffer cardiac arrest before or after their arrival and the attempted resuscitations fail. These people are eventually pronounced dead based on irreversible loss of heart function. These have come to be referred to as "unplanned" cases.

The second group involves patients under care for critical illnesses who decide to exercise their right to refuse further life support. When that support is withdrawn they will die. Some patients offer to become organ donors before the withdrawal of treatment. It is clearly illegal to take organs before death; no organ procurement organization in the United States would do so. However, the University of Pittsburgh Medical Center and, more recently, several other centers, have developed protocols by which such volunteers could be taken to the operating room before withdrawal of life support with the intention that as soon as the heart stops and death is pronounced, organs will be procured.[2] These have come to be called "planned" cases, because the death and organ procurement are planned in advance. Although the two groups raise somewhat different moral and policy issues, they are often considered together, as they will be in this chapter.

It is striking that the death of the brain has become so ingrained as the "real" definition of death for organ procurement purposes that some people, especially in Germany, have come to doubt that people who suffer irreversible cardiac arrest are really dead. Nevertheless, American law states that death can be based on irreversible cessation of *either* heart or brain function.

In spite of the doubters, there is a substantial consensus among those who approve of any allograft organ transplantation that, once proper permissions are obtained, there is nothing ethically controversial about procuring organs from cadavers and that it makes no difference in principle whether the death is measured by brain criteria or heart criteria. Individuals are just as dead either way. (Hence I plead once again that we not refer to individuals as "brain dead" or "heart dead." They should be thought of simply as "dead.") That consensus supporting organ procurement extends to the conclusion that no one—not the source of the organ or the health care team involved in the procurement—should participate in the procurement against his or her will and that the organs must, according to law and ethics, be donated.

The procurement of organs from asystolic patients who are dead, whether they are dead as a result of trauma, myocardial infarction, or a decision to forgo life support, appears at first not to present overwhelming problems. Nevertheless, three issues potentially add complexity to the apparently easy-won consensus: respecting the integrity of members of the procurement team, determining that the source of the organs is really dead, and establishing whether there has been a valid consent not only for donation but also for the steps necessary to prepare the body for donation. In particular, once the heart stops beating, the need to cool the body by perfusion is crucial. We shall see that consent for that step has become a critical matter of controversy, particularly when the death is unplanned.

The Rights and Welfare of the Caregivers

Some members of the health care team may be deeply troubled by procuring organs from recently deceased non–heart-beating cadavers.[3] They may be traumatized by discontinuance of resuscitation efforts or termination of life support, the perfusion of the body, and the removal of organs from a still-warm body in which, in some cases, a heart has beat only minutes previously.

The emergency and operating room staff will normally play only a preliminary role—assisting the patient and family in deciding to cease life support, participating in perfusion in the case of trauma and cardiac arrest patients, and preparing the body to be taken to the operating room in the case of patients with advance directives to forgo treatment. Even if there is a careful separation of the procurement team from other caregivers, the problems for professional staffs are potentially serious. Health care teams are normally militantly committed to attempting to prolong life but will be aware that, in the case of unplanned arrests, others are standing by with the interests of other patients in mind. They are aware that, in the case of planned arrests, purposeful cessation of treatment followed by organ procurement is being contemplated. Procurement team members will need to understand that they are dealing with a truly dead body for which proper organ donation has occurred. This will be particularly true in the moments before perfusion when patients will feel warm and manifest some signs often taken to be signs of life.

Compassion for nurses and other professionals on the team requires careful preparation and ample opportunity for those who have reservations to withdraw from the profusion and procurement processes. This may be particularly troublesome for emergency room staff who may not be intimately involved in organ procurement on a daily basis. With care and compassion, these problems can probably be avoided.

The Organ Source Must Really Be Dead

A more difficult problem raised by procuring organs from non–heart-beating cadavers may turn out to be establishing exactly when they are dead. Common wisdom used to suggest that, although it was more difficult to measure death based on brain criteria, measuring death based on heart criteria was straightforward. Now it appears that exactly the opposite may be the case.[4]

The asystolic heart can surely be used as a measure of the death of the individual after prolonged asystole, but there are important reasons why death should be pronounced (and organs procured) as quickly as possible. The Pittsburgh protocol in its original form called for death pronouncement after two minutes of asystole.[5] It was claimed that at this point autoresuscitation was impossible, but it cannot be denied that cardioversion could be accomplished mechanically. It is debatable whether a heart stoppage should be considered "irreversible" if it could be restarted but will not be because a decision has been made not to do so.

Death requires irreversible stoppage, yet it is unclear whether that means the heart *could* not be started again or merely *will* not be. Even more perplexing is whether an individual should be considered dead during the period when a heart could be restarted by people with expert skills and sophisticated equipment if those people and equipment are not available. The concept of irreversibility has become much more complex. Moreover, depending on the exact meaning of irreversibility, the brain tissue is not necessarily dead at the point when the heart is determined to be stopped irreversibly. This raises the problem that in Pittsburgh a patient could be called dead while his or her brain continues to be living, a problem to be addressed later in the chapter.

The significance of these subtle distinctions is not necessarily great in cases in which the patient or surrogate has made an advanced decision not to resuscitate, but in patients suffering unexpected cardiac arrest this could raise serious problems. The initial working presumption of the trauma team must be that resuscitation should be pursued. Longer periods of asystole would be necessary to establish irreversibility, and, therefore, there may be longer periods of warm ischemic time. This means that ethically there must be a sharp separation of responsibility between the organ procurement team and the resuscitation team. This could mean a longer period of asystole will be necessary to establish that the heart has really ceased function irreversibly. If the resuscitation team has been trying unsuccessfully for a long time to resuscitate, the heart may be asystolic for much more than two minutes. Having organ procurement on the agenda creates an incentive to cut resuscitation time because more lengthy attempts could diminish the value of organs. Regardless, according to current law, if the heart is really dead (however *dead* is defined), the dead donor rule will be satisfied. Because the organs can survive as much as thirty minutes of warm ischemia, shifting to a longer period of asystole, say five minutes, probably need not pose an insurmountable problem for transplantation.

A more serious question lurks beneath the surface, however. Although there is a clear recognition in statutory definitions of death that death may be pronounced based on the irreversible loss of either cardiac or brain activity, the possibility of organ procurement based on death pronouncement following short periods of asystole poses a new challenge. Especially if periods as brief as two minutes of asystole are used for pronouncing death (based on irreversible loss of cardiac function), it seems likely that the brain tissue is really not dead at this moment. In fact, much of literature advocating such death pronouncements really does not even present firm evidence that the patient is unconscious. The vision of pronouncing a patient dead after only two minutes of asystole (while brain tissue still lives) starkly poses the question of whether someone really ought to be considered dead if the brain tissue is still alive. The asystolic organ source may force the participants in the definition of death debate to reconsider whether someone can really be pronounced dead based on the loss of cardiac function alone.

It had previously been assumed that if irreversible cardiac arrest had occurred, then all brain functions would necessarily have ceased. That turns out to be not quite true. If brains can function even briefly after irreversible cardiac arrest can be determined to have occurred, then society must reassess whether it should continue to accept a policy by which death can occur when either cardiac or brain function is lost. This challenges the society to reexamine whether it really wants to treat people as dead when brain function exists. Of course, in routine cases of prolonged cardiac arrest we could continue to pronounce death without measuring brain function. Surely all brain function has been destroyed with prolonged heart stoppage. But in planned arrest we may want to insist that enough time pass following cardiac arrest not only to foreclose resuscitation but also to ensure that there has been irreversible loss of brain function.

The reasonable conclusion seems to be that, quite to our surprise, the emergence of non–heart-beating cadaver donors and organ sources has challenged the established definition of death that states simply that death may be pronounced when there is irreversible loss of either brain or cardiac function. This position should be amended to make clear that if cardiac function loss is used as an indicator of death, it must be only because it is a measure—an accurate predictor—that the brain function has been irreversibly lost, not because the loss of heart function per se is significant. It is becoming more and more clear, at least to those who advocate brain-based death pronouncement, that it is the brain's function that is critical, not the beating heart. Thus if we can interpret irreversibility to mean "will not start again" rather than "cannot be started again," we still must use irreversible cardiac function loss to pronounce death only when the loss accurately measures the irreversible loss of brain function. Two minutes of asystole does not do this. Some longer time does. The neurologists need to tell us exactly how long the heart function must be stopped to say safely that the brain will never function again. Five minutes of asystole appears to be a much safer time period than two minutes. Perhaps even a longer time is necessary.

The Organs Must Really Be Donated

The truly difficult problem in procuring organs from the asystolic trauma or heart attack victim is what can be done, legally and ethically, with the deceased before obtaining appropriate permission of the next of kin. Proposed protocols for such procurement call for minimizing warm ischemia time. This means femoral cannulation and perfusion as soon as possible after death is pronounced. The procuring surgeon often will want to perfuse before the time relatives have been contacted or at least before the time they have given permission for organ procurement. The most critical legal and ethical question thus becomes whether perfusion can precede permission for procurement. Generally, it is feasible to obtain the permission before actual organ procurement but often not before perfusion. Two potential policy concerns deserve attention.

Human Research Regulations

First, at least during the early phase, such efforts at organ procurement following cannulation and perfusion might be conceptualized as research on human subjects. The Regional Organ Bank of Illinois (ROBI), which made an early attempt to test procurement from non–heart-beating cadavers, conceptualized its work as an experiment subject to institutional review board (IRB) approval.[6] Federal regulations require that all institutions having multiuse assurances for conducting research on human subjects based on local IRB approval get the informed consent of the subjects or the subjects' surrogates.[7] Normally that consent must be obtained before initiating the investigational interventions. That would appear to require consent before perfusion, not simply before procuring organs.

It is true that federal regulations provide for limited exceptions to the consent requirement. However, exceptions are permitted only when getting the consent would make the investigation impossible. It might be argued that, if procuring organs from asystolic cadavers is investigational, the perfusion should be exempt from the consent requirement on this basis. To qualify for an exemption under federal regulation, however, four conditions must be met: the risk must be no more than minimal, the patient (or surrogate) must be debriefed afterward, the rights and welfare of subjects must be preserved, and the situation must be such that the research could not practically be carried out any other way.[8]

However, one of the rights of human subjects of research is the right to give an informed consent before participating. Thus we are left with the odd situation that one can waive consent only when rights are protected, but one right is the right to consent. If giving consent is a right, then no waiver of the federal consent requirement would ever be acceptable for any research. Therefore, I believe that the waiver provision in the regulations is fundamentally flawed and could not be used in any research.

Even if this argument does not succeed, a waiver would appear not to be acceptable in the case of research on organ procurement from non–heart-beating cadavers. Waivers are permitted only when the study could not otherwise be conducted. In fact, a consent requirement would not make it impossible to procure organs from non–heart-beating cadavers, although it would make it more difficult and might delay the project. It is the nature of an investigation that only a modest number of consents would have to be obtained successfully. Even if most heart attack and trauma victims would not have surrogates reachable in time, some would arrive with valid organ donation cards and others would arrive with relatives who have legal authority to consent to the perfusion and organ procurement. The experience at ROBI shows that with perseverance, some families can be reached and that some of those reached will give permission.

Having argued that the waiver provision in the federal human subjects regulations does not provide an out for the advocate of non–heart-beating cadaver-organ procurement, there is, at the level of law, another response. The federal regulations technically do not apply to body parts or materials from deceased individuals.[9] That would appear to provide a legal out. However, it does not seem to provide an ethical one. Ethically, the consent requirement is designed to show respect for the individual. The duty to show that respect does not cease at death—as is seen by our expectation that economic wills should be respected as well as the traditional requirement in organ procurement that organs not be taken from known objectors. Thus, even if the technical requirements of the human participants research regulations may not restrict perfusion before consent, the underlying ethical concerns might.

The Uniform Anatomical Gift Act

The second locus of potential problems is the legal and ethical requirements specifically addressing organ procurement. Under the Uniform Anatomical Gift Act, all U.S. states require that consent be obtained—from the patient or next of kin—before procuring organs.[10] Various people have offered a number of arguments for not violating the dead body, arguments I examined in Chapter 9. For example, some people argue that even after death the integrity of the human body must be respected. Some say the body does not belong to the society but to the individual who has the authority, while still alive, to refrain from cooperating.

After death, responsibility for the body reverts to the next of kin. There are important social reasons why we should continue to show respect for the individual by honoring his or her wishes about the body's treatment after death occurs. For religious or secular reasons individuals may object to the state assuming control over the body to serve state purposes. Even more plausible is objection to procurement personnel—who are after all merely individual private citizens—claiming the right to perfuse the body for the potential benefit of strangers.

We know that approximately half the people asked say they object to donating organs.[11] Most of the individuals who say they are against organ donation probably object to perfusion as well. Some religious traditions, such as Judaism, have a strong prohibition on mutilation of the corpse, at least if it is not done to preserve another identifiable life. Therefore, the perfusion itself will offend some people. With a deceased patient possessing a valid donor card, there is no problem. With next of kin permission there is not a problem either (assuming the deceased has not registered an objection). But absent such consent or permission, there is a potential problem.

Some people might mistakenly claim that inserting a catheter before consent preserves the family's option to donate until informed consent can be exercised, and, therefore, is more respectful of patient autonomy or informed consent. This claim, however, shows a misunderstanding of the notions of autonomy and consent.

Autonomy generates a liberty right—a right to be left alone. It is on the basis of that liberty right that patients as well as potential organ donors must be asked before their bodies are violated with medical interventions. Autonomy in no way gives one the right to be a subject of a medical procedure, an experiment, or organ procurement. In fact, even if organs are donated, the procurement organization has the legal and ethical right to refuse to procure them. The only relevance of autonomy to perfusion is that any perfusion before consent violates the individual's autonomy rights. This is true not only for the half of the population that would refuse to consent to donation if asked but also of the group who would consent if asked but who would object to invasion of the body without being asked.

Ways around Absence of Explicit Consent

There are three possible ways around absence of explicit consent.

Deferred Consent

First, some have suggested turning to a "deferred consent," getting the consent for the perfusion as well as the organ procurement from the next of kin after the perfusion has taken place. Bruce Miller[12] and others have shown, however, that deferred consent is no consent at all. Even if one agrees to proceed, there is no way one can claim justification for the perfusion based on such deferred consent. Debriefing and even getting approval after the perfusion process does not constitute a consent for the perfusion. Some people, apparently as many as 50 percent based on surveys of willingness to donate organs, will refuse to give an approval after the fact. Even if it is obtained, such approval does not equal consent. Consent must exist at the time of the intervention if it is to serve as the basis of justifying the perfusion.

Presumed Consent

Second, one may attempt to justify perfusing on the grounds of a concept we have encountered in previous chapters: presumed consent. We saw in Chapter 10 that there is terrible confusion over the meaning of *presumed consent*. Many people mistakenly confuse presumed consent with policies authorizing organ procurement without any consent. Thus people mistakenly say that many European countries have presumed consent laws when in fact none does. What they have are laws authorizing procurement without consent, a policy that is consistently rejected by a more autonomy-loving, individualistic American society. Even if the law contains an opting-out provision whereby one can execute a document recording objection to procurement, it is not possible to presume that everyone who has not executed such an opting-out provision in fact would want to have their organs used. Many people do not respond either because they are not aware of the legal provisions or simply do not express their refusals in writing. There is no basis for presuming the consent of those who have not opted out, and, in fact, the European laws do not claim to base their laws on a presumption of consent.

There would be nothing wrong with presuming consent provided there were an empirical basis for supporting the presumption. Thus, as we suggested in Chapter 10, it raises no problems to presume consent for emergency treatment of the trauma victim in the emergency room—because it is clear that almost everyone would, in fact, consent not only to treatment but also to a policy that presumes the consent.[13]

There is presently no basis for such a presumption of consent to the perfusion. We need data, probably hospital-specific data, showing a willingness of an adequate percentage of patients to agree to the presumption of consent for perfusion.[14] Probably data showing with 95 percent certainty that such a presumption is correct should be considered adequate. There is no definitive argument for a specific percentage, but we would, in effect, be predicting that the specific patient would have consented (or would have agreed to perfusion without consent). If we are wrong in that prediction, we would be illegally proceeding without consent. We would be violating the rights of the deceased. Short of such a basis for presuming consent, it is hard to see how presumed consent can provide a basis for perfusing.

Even if one could establish that, say, 60 percent of a particular hospital's asystolic patients would have favored perfusion without consent, that would not be sufficient to justify perfusing the other 40 percent in the absence of a formal, publicly debated policy authorizing invasion of the dead body without consent. The two groups—those who would approve of perfusion without explicit consent and those who would not—are not symmetrical regarding their rights. Each of the group who would object to perfusion can be said to have a right violated— the right not to have one's body invaded without consent. On the other hand, none of the group who would approve perfusion would have any right violated if the perfusion were omitted.

Rights normally have reciprocal obligations. In fact, generally, one is not a bearer of a right if no one has a reciprocal obligation. Yet no one is obligated to perfuse and procure organs. That is true even if explicit consent has been given; it is true even more obviously if no consent has been given. Anyone who feels strongly that it would be a good thing to have his or her body perfused and organs procured has the right to make an explicit donation. In that case, perfusion can take place without any additional consent. But absent a documented prior consent, no one has the right to violate the body; surely no one has a duty to do so.

Conscription without Consent

There is only one other way to justify perfusion before explicit consent. This third way is to change public policy to accept perfusion without consent. Efforts have been made to change U.S. policy for procuring organs to one of routine salvaging without consent, such as many European countries have adopted. They represent very different cultures, however. Although the United States has consistently rejected routine salvaging laws—even those with opting-out clauses—we have not yet had a public debate on perfusion without consent. As long as a significant number object to organ procurement, there is reason to assume they would also object to laws permitting perfusion without consent, but a proposal to the state legislatures to authorize perfusion before consent could be attempted. One jurisdiction, the District of Columbia, has actually passed such an exemption.[15]

It is conceivable that in other jurisdictions enough people who object to procurement without consent would have less objection to profusion before consent provided there was a statutory authorization. Plausibly, that might be the view of some members of the group who would donate but who have never documented their willingness to do so. Still, with about half the population objecting to organ procurement under the best of circumstances, and others objecting in principle to bodily invasions without consent, it seems unlikely that such a law would be adopted in most jurisdictions. Although I have no objection to attempting to pass such legislation, I believe it would not be wise to violate a person's autonomy by perfusing without consent and without statutory authorization.

There are limited examples of legal authorizations to invade a human body without consent even in cases in which we have reason to believe the individual would have objected. Military conscription is one example. Such conscription is usually presumed to authorize invasions, even medical invasions, without consent.[16] The policy decision that troops in Desert Storm could be given experimental vaccines without their consent also illustrates a national policy of legal authorization to treat without consent.[17]

Also, laws providing limited authorization for autopsy without consent provide an analogy.[18] Controversy exists over whether the law permits taking corneas and tissues at autopsy. To the extent that the law permits such removal without consent, this would be another precedent for public policies providing legal authorization for procurement without consent. What is critical is that whenever persons are conscripted into service to others without their consent, specific statutory or judicial law must provide the justification.

My conclusion is that there is no problem with perfusing and procuring organs from asystolic patients who have in the past authorized donation—even without next of kin permission. The advanced consent for medical use of the body for transplant includes consent to the procedures necessary to procure the organs, including the perfusion. There is also no problem with procurement based on next of kin permission before perfusion. That is the easiest, least controversial way to procure such organs, especially on a limited scale experimental basis, but absent such explicit consent or permission, one must either presume consent—a presumption that has not yet been validated—or adopt a public policy authorizing perfusion without consent.

Determining If Planned Donation Hastens Death Unethically

The type of organ procurement that follows a withdrawal of life support and a planned death raises an additional ethical question. Certain drugs, anticoagulants such as heparin and vasodilators such as pheltolamine, can be given in the hours before the withdrawal of life support for the purpose of improving the preservation of the organs.[19] Some of these drugs may actually shorten the life of the dying organ donor. This has led to considerable controversy, particularly in Cleveland, where a case led to an exposé on the television program, "60 Minutes." Critics of a Cleveland Clinic protocol for procuring non–heart-beating cadaver organs claimed that administration of medication actively shortened the donor's life and was therefore unethical and illegal. Some have doubted that the drugs involved actually do shorten the patient's life, but, even if the life is not shortened, the administration is not for the donor's benefit and has therefore been criticized.

Of course, if drugs are administered to the donor before death for the purpose of preserving organs for transplant, the donor would have to be informed of this intervention and consent to it. But assuming that such consent is obtained, would the practice be objectionable? Physicians who subscribe to the pure, unmodified form of the Hippocratic Oath believe that they are justified in their actions only on the basis that they are for the benefit of the patient. That ultraindividualistic ethic is, however, widely rejected among contemporary physicians, many of whom support research for the benefit of society, responsible cost containment, and public health efforts—all of which are undertaken for the benefit of other parties. Whether physicians accept such procedures for the benefit of others, certainly most lay people do. In fact, the entire organ procurement enterprise is precisely for the benefit of others, never for the benefit of the donor (unless the live donor cases are considered beneficial to the donor—an argument we questioned in the previous chapter). Hence the mere fact that the drugs are given for the benefit of the potential recipient does not make the administration unethical provided donor consent is obtained.

The real controversy is over the possibility that these drugs would shorten the donor's life. Of course, there are some who object to all cases of withdrawal of life support. Many right-to-life advocates do. So do some Orthodox Jews. They will, one assumes, also disapprove of giving drugs that hasten death to preserve organs. The real issue is whether, among those who have come to accept the legitimacy of the withdrawing of life support and the procuring of organs from such planned demise, administering a drug that hastens death is also acceptable.

This may look to the untrained observer like a case of converting a forgoing of life support into an active killing. Because active killings are generally considered unethical and are illegal—the implication is that administering the drug that might shorten life potentially converts the non–heart-beating cadaver protocol into a homicide—an auspicious development for the physician who administers the drug. In fact, the Institute of Medicine panel that studied NHBCD protocols seems divided and quite confused about the use of such medication.[20] The report authors seem to believe that if the drug administration actively causes death, then such administration is automatically unethical and illegal.

More careful examination, however, makes clear that the moral and legal analysis is more complex. This may be yet another case that can be analyzed under the "doctrine of double effect." This doctrine, which has its roots in Catholic moral theology, is now widely accepted by lay and medical professional groups. It is accepted by the American Medical Association[21] and by U.S. law.

The doctrine of double effect deals with situations in which an action undertaken for the purpose of producing good consequences also has effects that are bad. It is applied in such classic cases as military engagements in which attacking military targets may be known in advance to risk injury to innocent civilians. It is applied in many medical settings (including abortion and the administration of narcotics to relieve pain).

The general formulation of the doctrine is that such harmful side effects are morally tolerable provided four conditions are met: (1) The intention behind the action must be to produce the good effect and not the evil one; (2) the evil must not be the means to achieving the good effect; (3) the action itself cannot be intrinsically evil; and (4) the good effect must be proportional to the evil.[22] One key to the doctrine is that its adherents believe an unintended evil can be tolerable even if one can foresee that it will occur.

Not everyone accepts the doctrine. Some consider it too conservative, claiming, for example, that if the good consequences exceed the evil ones, that should be sufficient to justify the action. Those who hold this more liberal view[23] might even believe that direct, active killing of the terminally ill with their consent to obtain organs would be justified. This liberal interpretation has been widely rejected, however.

Likewise, some people reject the doctrine of double effect, claiming it is too liberal. They say that if intentional producing of a death is morally wrong, then one that is foreseen should also be wrong even if it is not the actor's intention to produce the death. They claim that the mere lack of intention in the mind of the actor cannot make the action moral provided the evil is foreseen. Nevertheless, this doctrine is widely accepted as a middle position, one that tolerates some foreseen deaths while simultaneously affirming that it is always wrong to intend death.

This doctrine has led some opponents of abortion to the conclusion that it would be acceptable to remove a cancerous uterus even if the patient happened to be pregnant (and therefore a fetal death would result). If the patient and the surgeon can honestly say their intentions are to remove the cancer and not to cause the fetal death, then the death can be tolerated. Likewise, the doctrine has led to the conclusion that it could be acceptable to administer pain-relieving drugs if necessary to relieve a patient's pain, even if the known side effect was respiratory depression that could contribute to hastening the patient's death. These views are now widely accepted even by Catholic moral theologians who consider all directly intended hastening of death unethical.[24]

The application of the doctrine in the narcotic pain-relieving cases is important for the question of administering drugs to potential NHBCD patients. If the intention is not to hasten the death of the donor but to preserve the organs to provide benefit to a recipient, then the doctrine of double effect can potentially apply. It seems obvious that if the drug is given, the purpose is not to hasten the patient's death. It is not the quicker death that preserves the organs. If the physicians injected potassium for the purpose of producing a quick cardiac arrest, that would be a different story. That would be a directly intended causing of death. We can assume, however, that the purpose of administering the heparin or phentolamine is not to get the donor dead more quickly. Hence the practice seems to meet the criterion that the hastening of the death is not directly intended. Moreover, it is not the hastening of death that is the means to the good intended end. The drug has a mechanism of action that is independent of the death of the donor. Thus the second criterion of the doctrine is satisfied.

Surely the administration of the drug is not intrinsically evil. The third criterion is easily satisfied. That leaves the question of whether the good achieved—providing higher-quality organs for transplant, potentially for several patients, and perhaps saving one or more lives—is proportional to the harm done. One might argue that hastening a death is a tragedy (although the hastening is only a matter of minutes), but we must realize that the case only arises for a patient who has decided that his or her prognosis is so bleak that it is appropriate to withdraw life support even though doing so will inevitably lead to a rapid death. If we can accept the negative of the inevitable death of the patient, surely, the fact that this death will occur a few minutes earlier is a minimal harm—if it is considered a harm at all.

The result seems to be clear. The harm to the donor is minimal, and the benefit to several other critically ill human beings could be enormous. As long as the death is not intended, any holder of the doctrine of double effect should have no moral objection to the practice of administering medications to preserve organs even if the unintended side effect may be the hastening of the donor's death.

If this is our conclusion in the case in which the drug was administered to preserve organs in the planned non–heart-beating cadaver case, then it is obvious that administering any drugs that have less dramatic impact on the demise of the donor will also be acceptable. The act of choosing to become a donor is a noble one. Many such donors will realize that, as long as the decision to withdraw life support is reached independently from the organ donation decision, there is nothing morally objectionable. In fact, many individuals would conclude that the benefit to others is a legitimate part of the patient's decision to withdraw support. If such a donor has reached the decision to withdraw life support on his or her own and is adequately informed about the use of drugs to help preserve organs, it seems that many individuals in that position would also consent to the use of the drugs. If they do and if the burdens sustained are minimal or nonexistent, then the practice of administering the drugs with the consent of the recipient seems morally defensible, in fact, morally the right choice.

ENDNOTES

1. Robert M. Arnold and Stuart J. Youngner (Eds.), "Ethical, Psychological, and Public Policy Implications of Procuring Organs from Non-Heart-Beating Cadavers," *Kennedy Institute of Ethics Journal* 3 (Special Issue, June 1993): 103–278; Robert M. Arnold, Stuart J. Youngner, Renie Schapiro, and Carol Mason Spicer (Eds.), *Procuring Organs for Transplant: The Debate over Non-Heart-Beating Cadaver Protocols* (Baltimore: Johns Hopkins University Press, 1995).

2. Michael A. De Vita and James V. Snyder, "Development of the University of Pittsburgh Medical Center Policy for the Care of Terminally Ill Patients Who May Become Organ Donors after Death Following the Removal of Life Support," *Kennedy Institute of Ethics Journal* 3 (2, 1993): 131–43; "University of Pittsburgh Medical Center Policy and Procedure Manual," *Kennedy Institute of Ethics Journal* 3 (2, 1993): A-1–A-15.

3. Robert M. Arnold and Stuart J. Youngner (Eds.), "Ethical, Psychological, and Public Policy Implications of Procuring Organs from Non-Heart-Beating Cadavers."

4. Stuart J. Youngner, Robert M. Arnold, and Michael A. DeVita, "When Is 'Dead'?" *The Hastings Center Report* 219 (6, Nov.–Dec. 1999): 14–21.

5. For comment, see Robert M. Arnold and Stuart J. Youngner (Eds.), "Ethical, Psychological, and Public Policy Implications of Procuring Organs from Non-Heart-Beating Cadavers."

6. "Non-Heartbeating Donor Procurement Attempted," *UNOS Update* 8 (6, 1992): 15.

7. U.S. Department of Health and Human Services, "Federal Policy for the Protection of Human Subjects; Notices and Rules," *Federal Register* 46 (June 18, 1991): 28001–32.

8. Ibid. at 28017.

9. Ibid. at 20813.

10. For both the text of the act and comment, see Alfred M. Sadler, Blair L. Sadler, and E. Blythe Stason, "The Uniform Anatomical Gift Act: A Model for Reform," *Journal of the American Medical Association* 206 (1968): 2501–06.

11. Gallup Organization, "The American Public's Attitudes toward Organ Donation and Transplantation," conducted for the Partnership for Organ Donation, Boston, Feb. 1993.

12. Bruce L. Miller, "Philosophical, Ethical, and Legal Aspects of Resuscitation Medicine. I. Deferred Consent and Justification of Resuscitation Research," *Critical Care Medicine* 16 (1988): 1059–62.

13. David W. Meyers, *The Human Body and the Law*, 2nd ed. (Stanford, CA: Stanford University Press, 1990), pp. 128–29; *Canterbury v. Spence*, 488 F.2d 772, 778 (1972); *Stafford v. Louisiana State University* 448 So.2d. 852 (La. App. 1984).

14. Examples using this methodology are Ruth R. Faden, Catherine Becker, Carol Lewis, and Alan I. Faden "Disclosure of Information to Patients in Medical Care," *Medical Care* 19 (1981): 718–33; and Richard Winer, Robert M. Veatch, Victor W. Sidel, and Morton Spivack, "Informed Consent: The Use of Lay Surrogates to Determine How Much Information Should Be Transmitted," in *The Patient as Partner: A Theory of Human-Experimentation Ethics*, ed. Robert M. Veatch (Bloomington: Indiana University Press, 1987), pp. 153–68.

15. Anatomical Gifts, D.C. Code § 2-1509.1 (1998), D.C. ANN. tit. 2, ch. 15.

16. Stephen E. Deardorff, "Informed Consent, Termination of Medical Treatment, and the Federal Tort Claims Act—A New Proposal for the Military Health Care System," *Military Law Review* 115 (Winter 1987): 68, 74.

17. U.S. Department of Health and Human Services, Food and Drug Administration, "Informed Consent for Human Drugs and Biologics; Determination That Informed

Consent Is Not Feasible; Interim Rule and Opportunity for Public Comment," *Federal Register* 55 (December 21, 1991): 52814–17.

18. Neil L. Chayet, "Consent for Autopsy," *New England Journal of Medicine* 274 (1966): 268–69.

19. Roger Herdman and John T. Potts, *Non-Heart-Beating Organ Transplantation: Medical and Ethical Issues in Procurement* (Washington, DC: National Academy Press, 1997), pp. 39–40, 52.

20. Ibid., p. 52.

21. American Medical Association, Council on Ethical and Judicial Affairs, *Code of Medical Ethics: Current Opinions with Annotations, 1998–1999 Edition* (Chicago: American Medical Association, 1998), p. 46. Here the AMA endorses administration of pain-relieving drugs to dying patients even though such medications may actively hasten death. The standard justification for this exception to the prohibition on active killing is that the death is not intended—that is, the doctrine of double effect. Although the AMA endorses procurement of organs from NHBCDs and supports perfusion of the deceased donor (with appropriate consent), it does not explicitly address the administration of organ-preserving drugs that might hasten death.

22. Charles E. Curran, "Roman Catholicism," in *Encyclopedia of Bioethics*, 2nd ed., ed. Warren T. Reich (New York: Free Press, 1995), pp. 2321–31; Donald B. Marquis, "Four Versions of Double Effect," *Journal of Medicine and Philosophy* 16 (1991): 515–44; Richard A. McCormick and Paul Ramsey (Eds.), *Doing Evil to Achieve Good: Moral Choice in Conflict Situations* (Chicago: Loyola University Press, 1978); Edmund D. Pellegrino, "Intending to Kill and the Principle of Double Effect," in *Ethical Issues in Death and Dying*, 2nd ed., ed. Tom L. Beauchamp and Robert M. Veatch (Englewood Cliffs, NJ: Prentice-Hall, 1995), pp. 240–42.

23. For example, Jack Kevorkian, *Prescription Medicide: The Goodness of Planned Death* (Buffalo, NY: Prometheus Books, 1991).

24. United States Bishops Committee on Doctrine, "Ethical and Religious Directives for Catholic Health Care Services," *Origins* 24 (27, 1994): 449, 451–62.

REPORT OF THE ANENCEPHALY TASK FORCE OF THE WASHINGTON REGIONAL TRANSPLANT CONSORTIUM*

WHILE TRANSPLANTATION HAS come of age in the 1980s, relatively little progress has been made in the transplantation of tissues and organs in neonates. Part of the difficulty rests in the fact that relatively few organs have been available of suitable size. Infants normally do not die from conditions that leave organs intact suitable for transplantation. They do not die from conditions that lead to irreversible loss of brain function while other organs remain viable. At the same time a number of infants are born each year with the severe brain pathology known as anencephaly. It has been suggested that if these organs could be made available for transplantation, much good would be done. The interests of infants suffering serious and potentially fatal heart, liver, and kidney damage and their parents might be served if organs from anencephalic infants were made available. Moreover, there are numerous reports of couples who have conceived fetuses suffering from anencephaly who are seriously committed to salvaging some good from their tragedy and are willing to carry their fetus to term and donate organs from their anencephalic child in order that other infants may have a chance to live.

At the same time there have been serious obstacles to procurement of organs from anencephalic infants. The organs of some anencephalic infants are not salvageable for technical reasons. Transplantation of tiny organs has posed an obstacle as well. Anencephalic infants also have a higher incidence of congenital

---

*The issues of organ procurement from anencephalic infants were addressed by a special task force of the Washington Regional Transplant Consortium. I served as the chair of the task force. Presented here is the report of that task force, March 29, 1990. It is reprinted here by permission of the Washington Regional Transplant Consortium.

anomalies. However, other important limits on the transplantation of organs from anencephalic infants are moral and legal. It is widely presumed, both morally and legally, that, with very special exceptions, organs should only be procured from human beings after they are deceased. This position has generally been held even for humans who are inevitably near death and who are irreversibly unconscious or in a persistent vegetative state. This commitment to procure organs only from the dead is sometimes referred to as the "dead donor rule." The term is not always precisely correct since some of these individuals who are potential sources of organs have never been in a position to consent to make a donation. For this reason we will refer to anencephalic infants as possible sources of organs rather than "donors."

Anencephalic infants who are potential sources of organs for transplant are not yet dead. Although they are sometimes referred to as "brain absent" and thus might be thought to be dead (or more accurately to never have lived) according to the well-established concept of death based on irreversible absence of brain function, they, in fact, have brain tissue. In many cases that tissue is alive and functioning at least at lower-brain levels so that certain clinically manifest functions including spontaneous respiration may be present. Thus, these infants are alive by current legal standards.

These problems have left such doubts that many clinicians and transplant organizations have chosen simply to avoid the issues by refusing to become involved in anencephalic organ procurement. Important moral, legal, and policy questions need to be addressed if the good envisioned in anencephalic organ procurement is to be served. While it would be unacceptable to modify our current practices solely to obtain additional organs, if it turns out that current practices can be modified for good, independent reasons, it would be irresponsible to fail to clarify our policy. It is the purpose of this report to propose a policy regarding such organ procurement for the Washington Regional Transplant Consortium.

The Need for and Availability of Organs and Tissues

There is considerable dispute over the question of how much need exists for organs and tissues from neonates and whether that need could be met by procuring organs and tissues from anencephalic infants. One source indicates there are presently 47 children less than one year of age awaiting transplant. These numbers are misleading, however, because it is common practice for clinicians to tell parents of seriously afflicted newborns (such as those with hypoplastic left heart syndrome) that no feasible treatment is available. If infant heart transplant were feasible and sufficient transplantable organs were available, the number of infants awaiting transplant could increase significantly. It seems reasonable that the limiting factor will not be the number of children who could be recipients of organs, but the number of organs available.

One source estimates that 1125 anencephalic infants potentially are born each year in the United States based on an incidence rate of 0.3 per 1000 live births and a national number of births of 3.75 million.[1] Many adjustments need to be made in this estimate, however. More than two-thirds of anencephalics are reportedly stillborn. Some of those born alive are too small to provide transplantable organs. Some organs will be medically unsuitable because of organ malformations. Additional problems of size- and tissue-matching will further reduce the number of organs suitable for transplant. Prenatal diagnosis will also have some impact on the number of available organs. Some expect that the parents of anencephalics who are diagnosed prenatally will choose to abort rather than carry the fetus to term. On the other hand, there are persistent reports of parents who claim to be willing to carry pregnancies to term if other children may benefit. In at least one case the anencephalic fetus was one of twins who was carried to term at least partly to avoid interfering with the development of the unaffected twin.

Thus, it is extremely difficult to predict exactly how many infants will actually benefit from organs procured from anencephalic infants. One conservative group of critics of anencephalic organ procurement estimates that ten years from now there could be as few as 25 kidneys, 12 hearts, and 7 livers transplanted from anencephalic infants.[2] That estimate is based in part on the fact that clinicians presently are choosing to dialyze infants in kidney failure waiting until the infants reach an older age when transplantation is more feasible. The staff for the task force estimated that somewhat more organs would be transplanted: 69 hearts and 61 livers. If, however, a substantial supply of organs were available, technical improvements in surgery and immunosuppression emerged, and infants with critical disease were to become more routine candidates for transplant, the numbers could potentially be much larger.

The task force is convinced that it would be a mistake to imply that, at present, there are large numbers of infants who may benefit from transplant from anencephalic infants. On the other hand, we believe that if even the conservative estimates of approximately 40 to 130 lives a year could be saved, it is well worth the effort to clarify our standards for morally and legally acceptable organ procurement.

We conclude that given the need for organs suitable for transplantation as well as education, research, and other therapeutic uses, organ procurement from infants, including anencephalic infants, should be considered acceptable provided the requirements associated with anatomical gift statutes are met. These must include the appropriate pronouncement of death of the infant and the consent of the next of kin prior to organ procurement. At the same time health care providers and families of anencephalic infants should be advised realistically of the probability of obtaining usable organs and tissues for transplant purposes or for education, research, and other therapies.

Present Requirements that Organ Sources Be Dead

It is critical to understand that it is almost universally agreed that any human who serves as a source of organs and tissues must be dead prior to organ procurement. The exceptions normally are limited to cases of a competent adult willing to donate renewable tissue or a paired organ (a kidney) to a relative after giving adequately informed consent. In rare cases, minors and persons who are mentally incompetent have also served as the source of kidneys. It is universally agreed, however, that no unpaired organs (such as hearts or whole livers) should be procured from humans if they are not dead. To the task force's knowledge there is no precise law other than homicide law requiring that the individual who is the source of the organs be dead. We examined the possibility that some group of humans including anencephalics might have organs procured prior to death but concluded that the dangers of abuse are so great that no policy authorizing any organ procurement prior to the death of anencephalic infants should be adopted, at least not without major public discussion and specific statutory authorization.

It may appear that requiring that the infant who is the source of the organs be dead prior to procuring organs imposes only a technical requirement and that the decision to pronounce death should be left to the clinicians caring for the infant. However, we have found that there are complex technical, conceptual, philosophical, and policy questions raised that require that the consortium articulate precisely when it will consider an anencephalic infant dead for purposes of consortium involvement in organ and tissue procurement.

First, we note that in the District of Columbia individuals may be pronounced dead based on the criteria of irreversible cessation of heart and lung function. While infants found to be dead on this basis will generally not be suitable sources of solid organs, they may be suitable providers of tissues including bone marrow, skin, and bone.

In adults, it has generally been found that individuals pronounced dead based on criteria measuring irreversible loss of all functions of the entire brain provide most of the organs suitable for transplant. The law in all jurisdictions in which the Consortium is involved defines death as a condition in which there is irreversible loss of all functions of the entire brain including the brain stem. We see no problem in principle in pronouncing death in anencephalics on that basis. If organs or tissues can then be procured that are suitable for transplantation or other authorized medical uses, we endorse that procedure.

There are serious problems, however, in determining what it means for an infant to have lost all functions of the entire brain and establishing criteria that accurately predict that state. Questions have arisen over what precisely is meant by loss of *all* functions. Does that include functions at the cellular level? Does it include electrical functions or only clinically manifest functions? How can one predict the irreversibility of these losses and how certain does one have to be in predicting?

In 1981, the Uniform Determination of Death Act proposed by the president's commission would define an individual as dead who has sustained either (1) irreversible cessation of circulatory and respiratory functions or (2) irreversible cessation of all functions of the entire brain, including the brain stem.[3] In talking about "whole-brain" definition of death, the commission relied on two arguments—the integrated-functions and the primary-organ views.[4] The first focuses on the integrated functioning of the body's major organ systems, while recognizing the centrality of the whole brain, since it is neither revivable nor replaceable. The other identifies the functioning of the whole brain as the hallmark of life because the brain is the regulator of the body's integration.[5]

Going further on the integrated functions, the commission commented, "death is that moment at which the body's physiologic system ceases to exist to constitute an integrated whole. Even if life continues in individual cells or organs, life of the organism as a whole requires complex integration and without the latter, a person cannot properly be regarded as alive."[6]

More recently, a set of guidelines has been endorsed by the American Academies of Neurology, Pediatrics (Section on Neurology), American Neurologic Association, and the Child Neurology Society. This statement does not provide for a definitive diagnosis of brain death in infants less than 7 days of age based on a few cases who questionably fit clinical brain death criteria and who survived, most of them severely neurologically damaged. For infants greater than 7 days they recommended but did not require EEGs 48 hours apart because of neurologic immaturity.[7]

These groups did not try to deal with the problem of the anencephalic infant who, when properly diagnosed has virtually no cerebrum and a brain stem that will function for varying short periods of time and who basically is an infant with no ability to have integrative functioning of the brain and no chance of recoverability. Therefore none of these guidelines can be used for the infant with anencephaly, at least prior to 7 days after birth.

Investigators at Loma Linda Medical School have tried to see whether anencephalic infants could be supported long enough to fit brain death criteria as traditionally described for infants with brains.[8] They had great difficulty and no organs were procured. This therefore does not seem to be a viable alternative for using the organs of these infants.

Thus it would seem that there are only three possibilities:

1. To use no anencephalic infants as organ sources until the present legal definition of death is satisfied.
2. To create exceptions that would permit the use of living anencephalic infants as organ sources.
3. To clarify or modify the definition of death, which may have the effect of making clear that additional anencephalic infants are dead.

For the present, we recommend that, for the purposes of the Washington Regional Transplant Consortium, organs and tissues be procured only from those infants who have been pronounced dead based on either traditional criteria measuring irreversible heart and lung function loss or based on criteria that measure irreversible loss of all functions of the entire brain. It is our recommendation that, for consortium purposes, we consider infants, including anencephalic infants, as dead based on irreversible loss of all functions of the entire brain only when the criteria of the Task Force for the Determination of Brain Death in Children have been satisfied. At the present time we have been able to find no empirical evidence or consensus of relevant expertise that would support any claim that any group of anencephalic infants who do not meet these criteria can be definitively diagnosed as having irreversibly lost of all functions of the entire brain. At the same time we recognize that these criteria were not developed for anencephalic infants. We encourage those with the appropriate neurological expertise to attempt to develop such criteria.

Possible Changes in Public Policy

The task force acknowledges that under the present law it will be extremely difficult to procure solid organs for transplant from anencephalic infants. The mere fact that the current definition of death makes it difficult to procure usable organs, however, should not rule out changing the law. There may be reasons to insist that all humans who are sources of organs be dead before organs are procured and that death has not occurred if any functions of the brain remain possible. However, there may be good independent reasons why current policy should be changed.

Exceptions to the Dead Donor Rule

We have noted that in our society it is generally accepted that, except for certain narrowly defined exceptions, no organs should be procured from humans prior to death. Some have proposed providing additional exceptions. For example, some have suggested that there should be a specific exception for anencephalics. A rule could be established specifically permitting procurement from living anencephalic infants on the basis of a diagnosis of anencephaly.

We think that would be a mistake. If exceptions are to be made, we believe the criteria for permitting procurement from these special classes of living individuals should be articulated carefully. For example, some have proposed that the reason why we might procure from living anencephalics is that they are very near death. Others have proposed that it is because they are unconscious and will never again recover consciousness. Other criteria might be identified. Whatever those criteria are, they would appear to apply—at least in theory—to other individuals who are permanently unconscious or who are dying imminently who do not have anencephaly. If an exception is to be made, it should not be based on a specific diagnosis but should apply to all who fit the relevant criteria.

We are convinced that it would be implausible and dangerous to permit an exception to the rule that those who are to be sources of organs be dead. While there may be legitimate reasons for the exceptions related to the consent of the competent living adult to donate a paired organ to a relative and to the procuring of a paired organ from an incompetent when it is deemed in the interest of the incompetent to do so, procurement from anencephalics can never be said to be with the consent of the individual or in his or her interest.

We are convinced that those who are attempting to identify criteria for procuring organs from living anencephalic infants are really articulating criteria for diagnosing death. To be dead for social and policy purposes is to have lost the status in which it is intrinsically necessary to protect individual rights and bodily integrity. We believe that if there are some situations where it would be acceptable to procure organs from individuals now considered alive, it is because such persons really ought to be treated as dead. We thus suggest a change in the definition of death.

An Amendment to the Definition of Death

Some have proposed a specific and ad hoc change in the definition of death to include anencephalics by diagnosis. Such a law might read, in part, that an individual shall be considered dead when there is an irreversible loss of all brain functions except for anencephalics who shall also be considered dead even if some brain function remains. That proposal seems irresponsibly idiosyncratic, however. It seems to be a gerrymandering of the definition of death to include anencephalics. Rather we should consider whether there are some cases where humans may reasonably be treated as dead for all public policy purposes (including organ and tissue retrieval) even though some rudimentary brain function remains.

We believe the most plausible modification in the definition of death is one that would authorize death pronouncement when there is an irreversible absence of either cerebral function or cerebral substance. We urge the Transplant Consortium to endorse and work for an amendment in the definition of death in all relevant jurisdictions that would permit death to be pronounced when there is irreversible absence of either all cerebral function or all cerebral substance.

Criteria for the Humane Treatment of Living Anencephalic Infants

Some parents and clinicians may want to intervene medically during the course of the final days of the infant's life to assure that organs are maintained in a viable condition. Such interventions are sometimes attempted in adults and other potential donors and we do not, in principle, object in the case of anencephalic infants provided some strict criteria are met.

One problem is in determining whether anencephalic infants are capable of perceiving pain or other sensation. Of course they demonstrate withdrawal reflexes and crying, but it is not clear whether these are evidence of actual pain perception rather than reflex responses. It is widely held that since anencephalic infants lack all or a substantial part of the cerebrum they are incapable of experiencing anything including pain. If that is true, then it is a confusion to worry about inflicting physical or mental suffering on such an infant. In fact, certain medical procedures for example, administering analgesic medication, that would be appropriate in a normal infant to relieve pain may be inappropriate in an anencephalic infant.

There is some opinion that anencephalic infants may be able to perceive pain either in rudimentary portions of cerebral tissue that may be present or in midbrain structures that may have such capacity. We word our criteria for the humane treatment of the living anencephalic infant with the goals of avoiding suffering should the particular infant be capable of it and also of avoiding trauma or burden on parents, caregivers, and others who may be distressed with the appearance of pain. With that in mind, we propose the following criteria for the humane treatment of the living anencephalic infant who may be the object of medical interventions for the purpose of preserving viable organs.

1. The living anencephalic infant should be treated with the same respect and dignity as other living patients.
2. The deceased anencephalic infant should be treated with the same respect and dignity as other deceased patients.
3. Efforts should be made to avoid all trauma to the parents and caregivers and all appearance of pain to the infant.

4. Educational efforts should be made to assure that parents and caregivers understand the nature of the interventions and the reasons for them.

5. To the extent that the anencephalic infant can be said to have an interest in avoiding risks, the procedures designed to preserve organs in a condition making them viable for transplantation or other uses should involve only minimal risk to the infant.

6. Prior to initiating any medical intervention for living anencephalic infants for the purpose of preserving organs and tissues for procurement after death, a specific decision should be made with the consent of the parents of the infant pertaining to which interventions should be made and what the duration of those interventions should be.

Conclusion

The anencephalic infant presents a complex set of legal, ethical, conceptual, and policy problems to those involved in transplantation. We insist that all infants, including the anencephalic infant, be shown respect and be protected from any significant risk of harm. We conclude that organs should never be procured from infants who are still alive even if they are dying imminently and have no capacity to perceive sensation. For this reason we recommend that the Transplant Consortium do the following:

1. Adopt a policy of procuring organs only after the individual is declared dead based on standard heart criteria or based on brain criteria established in the Guidelines of the Task Force for the Determination of Brain Death in Children.

2. Make every effort to amend the statutes defining death in the District of Columbia, Maryland, and Virginia to permit individuals to be treated as dead who have irreversible absence of either all cerebral function or all cerebral substance.

3. Adopt the criteria for the humane treatment of anencephalic infants and others being maintained with interventions for the purpose of preserving organs in a condition viable for transplantation and other medical uses.

ENDNOTES

1. Alan D. Shewmon, Alexander M. Capron, Warwick J. Peacock, and Barbara L. Schulman, "The Use of Anencephalic Infants as Organ Sources," *Journal of the*

American Medical Association 261 (1989): 1773–81; Shewmon, "Anencephaly: Selected Medical Aspects," *Hastings Center Report* 13 (Oct./Nov. 1988): 11–18.

2. Alan D. Shewmon, Alexander M. Capron, Warwick J. Peacock, and Barbara L. Schulman, "The Use of Anencephalic Infants as Organ Sources," at 1775.

3. President's Commission for the Study of Ethical Problems in Medicine and Biomedical and Behavioral Research, *Defining Death: Medical, Legal and Ethical Issues in the Definition of Death* (Washington, DC: U.S. Government Printing Office, 1981), p. 2.

4. Ibid., p. 32.

5. Ibid.

6. Ibid.

7. Task Force for the Determination of Brain Death in Children, "Guidelines for the Determination of Brain Death in Children," *Neurology* 37 (1987): 1077–78.

8. Joyce L. Peabody, Janet R. Emery, and Stephen Ashwal, "Experience with Anencephalic Infants as Prospective Organ Donors," *New England Journal of Medicine* 321 (1989): 344–50; Marsha Goldsmith, "Anencephalic Organ Donor Program Suspended; Loma Linda Report Expected to Detail Findings," *Journal of the American Medical Association* 260 (12, 1988): 1671–72.

Addendum: Events Related to Anencephalic Organ Procurement since the Writing of the WRTC Report

Since the writing of the Anencephaly Task Force Report in 1990,[9] two important developments have occurred that have helped clarify public policy regarding anencephalic organ procurement.

First, an infant named Baby Teresa was born with anencephaly in the state of Florida.[10] Her parents sought unsuccessfully to gain legal authority to donate her organs while she lived. One strategy to deal with the legal prohibition on anencephalic organ procurement while these infants are still living has been to attempt to make an exception to the dead donor rule and procure organs so that the procurement need not wait for the death to occur. Because anencephalic infants are permanently unconscious, they would feel nothing. Because death of anencephalics who are not given aggressive life support is inevitable and rapid, such an exception to the dead donor rule would end up painlessly advancing the procurement somewhat while shortening the period of agony for the parents and providing organs that have not been exposed to the trauma of waiting for the death to occur.

The second event of importance relates to a significant endorsement of this approach. In 1995 the American Medical Association Council on Ethical and Judicial Affairs endorsed such an approach, although it remains illegal in the

United States and all other jurisdictions.[11] Within 24 hours of the publication of the AMA report, the national ethics committee of the United Network for Organ Sharing (UNOS) rejected the AMA position, claiming that such procurement from living anencephalic infants is unethical and illegal.[12] They were unanimous that organs could not be procured while the anencephalic infants are considered living. Some of the committee members would have been open to further change in the definition of death law so that these anencephalic infants would be classified as dead. These people essentially concurred with the WRTC task force recommendation to adopt a cerebral (i.e., a higher-brain) definition of death proposed in Chapter 5 of this book. However, such a position was never formally adopted by the UNOS Ethics Committee. I remain convinced that the higher-brain view I originally proposed in 1972 is the best policy. It would permit pronouncing anencephalic infants dead and, with parental permission, procuring their organs.

The AMA almost certainly made a conceptual mistake. Many philosophers of medicine would argue that being dead *means* being in a state in which the individual is not provided usual moral and legal protections granted members of the moral community, including protection from having organs procured. Organs may be procured from the anencephalic infant, such as Baby Teresa, but only if she is not fully a part of the moral community. Thus the project is to figure out whether anencephalic infants are members with full standing in the moral community, in which case we would label them as "alive," or alternatively they lack some essential feature of full moral standing, in which case they would be considered "dead" or, perhaps more appropriately, "never having lived."

Thus anencephalic infants such as Baby Teresa may be "dead" even though they continue to have heartbeats and respiration. For those who accept what in Part One of this book was called a higher-brain definition of death, they may lack full moral standing and therefore not exist within the community of the "living" even though certain lower-brain functions remain. Thus someone who holds a moral position like that of the AMA Council would more appropriately advocate changing the law so that anencephalic infants did not meet the criteria necessary for full moral standing. Anencephalic infants would then be considered "dead." The policy would be to hold to the dead donor rule, simply making clear that one is advocating organ procurement from anencephalic infants with beating hearts because they do not meet the criteria for full standing rather than advocating an exception to the dead donor rule so that organs could be procured from living infants with anencephaly. Such a law would need to authorize pronouncing death when there was irreversible loss of cerebral functions or whatever is deemed to be the "higher" functions. The anencephalic infant would be an instance in which procurement would then be legal. (Others who were classified as dead by higher-brain criteria—such as the permanently vegetative—would also thereby be candidates for organ procurement.)

Although the court opinion in the case of Baby Teresa rejected procurement of organs in a way that would cause death, it made a very strange and controversial move. It permitted procurement of non–life-prolonging organs and tissue from Baby Teresa even while she was alive, organs such as one kidney, or perhaps pancreatic tissue, as well as corneas. The judge apparently took the view that one could not shorten the living infant's life but that nonharmful contributions to others would be acceptable. There is no record of organs being procured. The idea was repulsive to many people, even those deeply committed to organ procurement.

The key moral arguments supporting such procurement are as follows: (1) If the patient is alive, she is a member of the moral community. (2) One cannot do anything to a patient that will cause serious harm or death, at least without the patient's consent. (3) Infants and children can never consent. (4) Nevertheless, one can do certain "minimal risk" procedures to children for the good of others even though they cannot consent. For example, some argue one can do low-risk research on infants solely for the purpose of advancing science.[13] Arguably one can take a small sample of blood; possibly one can take bone marrow from a healthy sibling although that is pushing the moral limits. In the case of a terminally afflicted anencephalic infant who cannot feel pain, it is hard to determine what constitutes minimal risk. Arguably procuring a kidney would be of no risk or only minimal risk as long as the infant can feel no pain and will not have his or her life shortened by the procedure. Hence someone like the judge could develop an argument to support such organ and tissue procurement.

If a kidney can be procured on this basis, eyes, skin, and bone could be as well. Most of us, however, believe that only if anencephalic infants are reclassified as dead—that is, as not full members of the moral community—could organs be procured, even if those organs are traditionally classified as "life prolonging." This seems to be the position finally adopted by the AMA when it reversed its endorsement of organ procurement from anencephalic infants.[14]

ENDNOTES FOR ADDENDUM

9. The reader will note two minor inconsistencies in substance between the report of the WRTC Task Force and earlier chapters in this book. The report endorses pursuit of a revised definition of death that would classify anencephalic infants as dead—a position consistent with the views expressed in Part One of this book—but in the task force report the revised definition of death was described as one involving irreversible loss of "cerebral" function, whereas in Chapter 5 I used the language of "higher-brain function." This is because it seems clear that if the

"higher" function involved relates to consciousness, it is theoretically possible that one could have irreversibly lost consciousness without having lost all cerebral functions. Although "cerebral" function is an approximation of "higher" function, I generally prefer the more vague, but more accurate, use. Second, the task force report refers to procuring a paired organ (such as the kidney) from an incompetent patient "when it is deemed in the interests of the incompetent to do so." In earlier chapters, I have suggested that often the claim is hard to sustain that it serves the interests of an incompetent to have a kidney removed. I went on to suggest that, nevertheless, incompetents may have very limited duties to serve the interests of other family members and that this limited duty could provide a moral basis for procuring blood and possibly procuring bone marrow or even a kidney. Neither of these differences between the task force report and earlier chapters were considered substantial. They resulted primarily from the cumbersomeness of the committee process in which not every sentence of a document will be expressed precisely the way every member would want it expressed.

10. *In Re TACP*, 609 So 2d 588 (Fla. 1992).

11. American Medical Association, Council on Ethical and Judicial Affairs, "The Use of Anencephalic Neonates as Organ Donors," *Journal of the American Medical Association* 273 (1995): 1614–18.

12. Committee Reports: Ethics, *UNOS Update* 11 (1995): 22.

13. United States National Commission for the Protection of Human Subjects of Biomedical and Behavioral Research, *Research Involving Children: Appendix to Report and Recommendations* (Washington, DC: U.S. Government Printing Office, 1977).

14. American Medical Association, Council on Ethical and Judicial Affairs, *Code of Medical Ethics: Current Opinions with Annotations, 1996–1997 Edition* (Chicago: American Medical Association, 1996), p. 33.

FIFTEEN

THE ROLE OF AGE IN PROCUREMENT: MINORS AND THE ELDERLY AS ORGAN SOURCES

THE ROLE OF age in organ transplant has become an increasingly controversial issue as transplant becomes more successful and the shortage of organs increases. Age poses problems both for organ donation and for organ allocation. The allocation issues—whether elderly persons deserve an equal shot at an organ even though they may have less capacity to undergo the rigors of surgery and a shorter time to enjoy the benefits of the transplant—will be the topic of Chapter 22. The procurement issues—whether it is acceptable to take organs from youngsters who cannot consent and whether organs can be procured from older people whose organs may be of poorer medical quality and may not survive as long—are the issues of this chapter.

"Donation" from Minors

On the procurement side of transplant, the first group to consider for whom age is important is infants and children. I have previously stressed that infants and young children can never be "donors." They cannot give consent to have their organs used for transplant. The younger ones cannot even comprehend the idea of transplantation. For this reason, I will continue (as I have done throughout this book) to avoid calling any minors donors. As with mentally incompetent adults, I will use the more noncommittal term "organ source."

The Analogy to Human Subjects Research

The problems of organ procurement are in many ways like those of conducting research on human subjects, an analogy first suggested in Chapter 12 when we were dealing with organ procurement from living, incompetent persons. It is an analogy we can now extend to the question of procuring organs from deceased persons who were not mentally competent at the time of their deaths. In both human subjects research and organ procurement human beings (alive or deceased) are being "used" for the benefit of other humans. If we accept the model of gift giving, we commit to the position that humans must offer their bodies or organs rather than having them taken for public purposes. That was the position taken earlier in this book and is generally the position of the American transplant program as well as the human subjects research enterprise. However, unless some provision is made for surrogate decisions to authorize the use of bodies or body parts from incompetents, the implication is that they could never be procured from infants, children, or others who have never been competent. Using one human as a means to benefit another, whether in human subjects research or transplantation, requires consent, and incompetent persons cannot give consent.

There is somewhat more ambiguity about the requirement for access to a cadaver in human subjects research. Most interpretations hold that the federal human subjects research regulations apply only to research on living humans.[1] Nevertheless, many hold that the principle of respect for persons requires some form of consent for research on tissues of the deceased. We generally accept a limited authority of parents to give that permission to do research on deceased minors and, under even more rigid conditions, on living minors. Even if the human subjects regulations do not apply to the deceased, the clear meaning of the Uniform Anatomical Gift Act is that consent or permission is required for *all* uses of the dead body, whether for transplant, education, therapy, or research.

We generally recognize that the parent or guardian of a living minor can give permission for research on the minor. Not all medical ethical commentators accept that approach.[2] However, many do,[3] and this is the dominant view as well as the view expressed in both medical ethical codes[4] and federal regulation.[5] Research that is not connected with therapy that promises benefit for a child is permitted with parental permission provided certain conditions are met, including the requirement that the risk to the child is strictly limited. Of course, in the case of a deceased minor, it is hard to imagine what risk there would be in organ procurement. Respect of the body would certainly be required, but, normally, parental permission should be sufficient to permit such research. Likewise, it should be sufficient for organ procurement.

Assent of Older Minors

The human subjects research regulations pertaining to children impose an additional requirement. In the case of older children, they must be asked to "assent" to participation. *Assent* differs from *consent* in that it involves mere approval or disapproval, not the requirement that the person have the capacity to comprehend and make a reasoned choice. In research not involving therapy, in addition to obtaining parental permission, the investigator must ask older children for their assent.[6] If older children decline, they cannot be used. Because the premise that makes research ethical is that the research intervention is not known in advance to be better or worse than the standard treatment, assent poses no risk to the child and could even be extended to so-called therapeutic research.[7]

The same reasoning might be applied to organ procurement from older children. It is unlikely that a child will have formed an opinion in advance about organ procurement, but if the child has expressed revulsion or otherwise has objected, then the child's opinion should be taken as a veto even in the case of parental permission.

Children as Living Organ Sources

What has been said thus far applies to cadaveric organ procurement from infants and children. If one contemplates using children as living organ sources, matters become much more complicated. The risks involved in solid organ procurement from a living organ source are not insignificant. I have explored the justification of procuring organs from living children and other incompetents in detail in Chapter 12. I examined two moral justifications for the acceptance of organ procurement from living incompetents. The first was the claim that in some cases providing an organ to another family member would provide benefit to the organ source. That was the court's rationale in the legal case of *Strunk v. Strunk*,[8] the case in which it was claimed that it was in the interests of a mentally retarded sibling to provide a kidney to his mentally normal brother so that the brother would survive to provide future support. I suggested that this "organ-source-benefit" rationale for procuring organs from incompetents was limited at best and perhaps disingenuous. It may merely be a rationalization for doing what the family wanted to do to serve the recipient brother's interest.

I then suggested a second justification: that as members of the human moral community even incompetents owe certain minimal obligations to serve others. This seems particularly true when the others are members of the same family. It is this restricted obligation to serve others that justifies parents who offer their children as subjects in minimal risk research. It could also be the basis for limited approval of the use of minors and other incompetents as organ sources. It would at least justify modest procurement of blood, probably bone marrow, and maybe even a kidney. Beyond that I claimed society almost certainly could not go if the potential source was not competent to give a valid consent. That would rule out the use of living minors as a source of liver and lung lobes or pancreata and small bowel segments.

Donation from Older Persons

Although infants and children generally cannot give a valid consent to donation, surrogate consent may partially address this problem. In the case of older donors, similar problems may arise. Older persons may be mentally incompetent. If they have never expressed while competent a willingness to donate organs, they may be in a position similar to that of minors. If so, similar reasoning should apply.

If the older adult has given adequate consent or if adequate consent is obtained through a surrogate, a second, quite different, problem may arise. The problem is whether the organs are of sufficient quality medically that they can be given to recipients. If organs from older donors will not survive as long as young recipients into whom they are placed or if older recipients have a life expectancy much shorter than the organs procured from young donors, serious moral and practical questions are raised. The problem is especially acute if the recipient is a young person who might well outlive the physiological life of the organ. For shorthand I will refer to organs from older donors as "older organs."

It is widely believed that older organs do not do as well as those procured from younger donors. The United Network for Organ Sharing (UNOS) 1997 survival rate data support that belief. Controlling for other variables, it appears that failure rates increase when the age of the donor increases above the mean, first gradually and then more precipitously. Thus the mean age of donors in the UNOS 1997 study was 32. Recipients receiving kidneys from 42-year-olds experienced failure 1.096 times more often; kidneys from 52-year-olds, 1.361 times as often.[9] This means that whatever reasoning leads to a policy limiting use of organs from those over, say, age 65, would apply also to somewhat younger donors whose organs predictably will fail more often than those of a 32-year-old.[10] Similar findings were reported for other organs. For livers (for which the data were reported in a somewhat different form), one-year graft failure was 1.131 times as great for 38-year-old donors compared with 28-year-olds and 1.462 times as great for 48-year-old organs than for 38-year-old organs.[11] For hearts graft failure was 1.140 times more likely when organs were obtained from 36-year-olds as compared with 26-year-olds and 1.434 times more likely for 46-year-olds.[12]

A Categorical Maximum Age for Procurement

There was a time when older organs were considered unusable. A categorical cutoff of age 65 was one policy considered plausible. As organs are perceived as more and more valuable as life-saving devices, transplant surgeons are reassessing the wisdom of such a categorical prohibition based on donor age. At least for older recipients, some surgeons would now consider no chronological age of a donor as per se too old to provide useful organs. Only case-by-case medical assessment can rule a donor out, and even then judgment calls will be required.

Clearly, some organ sources will be of ages suggesting that the organ has only a slightly worse than ideal chance of graft survival. The increased risk of using older organs is one that changes gradually as age increases. If a surgeon or organ procurement organization (OPO) is to decide that advanced age rules out certain organs, it must decide how much greater risk is too great. For example, if an organ from a person who was slightly older than the ideal age statistically has only a 1 or 2 percentage greater chance of one-year graft failure, should that be enough to rule out the use of the organ? Would a 10 percent increased risk rule the organ out? Keeping in mind that ruling out an organ means someone will go without a transplant, these judgments about when an organ is too old are both subtle and important. There is no reason to believe that surgeons or OPO personnel have any special moral skills in making the calls. If we wanted to maximize transplant, we would want a system that accepts organs that are known in advance to be somewhat suboptimal. We might even have to develop a policy that targets those organs according to certain principles. For example, we could allocate the suboptimal organs on a purely random basis, giving everyone on the waiting list an equal chance of getting an organ from an ideally young and healthy donor or one from an older, less healthy source. Alternatively, we could target the older organs for recipients with shorter life expectancy. We could target them, for example, for older recipients.

Older Organs for Older Recipients: The Potential Problems

At one OPO in the United States, the current policy is that the organ-procuring surgeons assess the potential usefulness of organs of older donors. No donor is excluded categorically on the grounds of age alone. Once an organ is procured, it is offered to the surgeon of the patient who scores highest in a computer-based algorithm for allocating the organ in question. For kidneys, for example, human lymphocyte antigen (HLA), panel reactive antibodies (PRA), blood type, and time on the waiting list all play a role.

AN INFORMAL, AGE-BASED ALLOCATION

If a surgeon is offered an organ from an older patient to be transplanted into a younger one, that surgeon has the right to decline the organ. If it is declined on behalf of a young potential recipient who happens to have emerged as first on the list, it will then be offered to the next potential recipient on the list. Eventually, an older recipient will emerge at the top of the list. At that point his or her surgeon may consider the risk of the patient outliving the organ less and may accept the older organ.

The first issue this approach raises is whether it should be the potential recipients rather than their surgeons who should be given a chance to accept or refuse the organ. A younger person may be desperate for an organ, conceivably even suicidally depressed from the uncertainty of a prolonged wait. It is possible for such a person that getting the older organ immediately is preferable to a prolonged uncertainty of having to wait for a younger organ.

Surgeons are not always in a position to determine whether it is in the young person's interest to decline an older organ. Consider a patient with a high PRA, unusual HLA antigens, and an O blood type who is quite miserable on dialysis. Such a person can only receive an organ from someone of O blood type, and the donor must not have antigens that will react with the recipient's antibodies. If an older organ is declined, it could be a long time before another suitable one became available. Even if it could be shown that the long-term organ survival was better with a younger organ, it is quite hard to determine whether it is in the patient's interest to wait. It will depend on how much better the young organ survival is, how miserable the patient is on dialysis, and how well the patient can tolerate the emotional strain of the wait. At the very least, it seems the patient should have a right to participate in the decision to decline the older organ in favor of a longer wait.

A case can be made that the decision to decline the older organ should rest with the patient rather than the surgeon. It seems clear that, if the young recipient scores highest in the allocation of an older organ, he or she has a right to the organ. Many rights, however, are alienable—that is, they may be waived. It is sometimes not unreasonable for a young person to waive his or her right to the older organ even if it means waiting for an additional one. Assuming the patient participates in the waiving of this right, such waivers seem reasonable. At the very least it should be a shared decision made after consultation about the likelihood of another younger organ becoming available soon and about the subjective and objective burdens to the patient of having to wait.

Likewise, the older patient who might receive the organ "handed down" after several surgeons had declined it for younger patients might have a right to be informed that he or she has risen to the top of the list only because other surgeons (or even the patient's own surgeon) have declined the organ on behalf of other patients because of the advanced age of the donor. The present policy of leaving these choices entirely in the hands of surgeons needs to be reassessed.

THE BIAS IN FAVOR OF THE ELDERLY

A second issue is raised by this system of having surgeons for younger patients decline organs from older donors. The result is an informal age-based allocation with refusals on behalf of younger recipients leading to older organs tending to go to older recipients.

Although this has the effect of keeping older organs from younger recipients, there are complex policy implications. If an older patient scores highest in the algorithm when the donor was a young person and the surgeon's moral duty is to serve his or her patient's interests, there is no reason why the surgeon would decline the organ. On the other hand, older organs would more reasonably be declined for young patients. The effect would be that older patients get all the organs that naturally are assigned to them plus all those that are first declined by surgeons for their younger patients. This allocation policy seems designed so that older persons get more than their fair share of organs, a strangely counterintuitive arrangement.

DETERMINING IF INDIVIDUAL PATIENTS AND SURGEONS ARE IN THE POSITION TO DECLINE OFFERS OF OLDER ORGANS

To the extent that organ procurement and allocation is a *social* system involving appeals to donors to give organs to a public organ procurement organization, a case can be made that neither the patient nor the surgeon should have the final word. A full analysis will entail judgments about whether a year of life from a graft in a younger person should count the same as one from a graft in an older person, as well as whether the overall goal is to maximize the number of years of aggregate graft survival. These are not questions that either the individual patient or the clinical surgeon is in a good position to answer. Some more formal policy seems appropriate. Although the complex details of allocation will be addressed in Part Three of this book, the integration of donor age into the allocation should be addressed at this point.

A Formal Donor-Related Allocation Formula

If data support the claim that older organs have a shorter life expectancy, it seems reasonable to strive to place them in older recipients, reserving younger organs for younger recipients. One way to facilitate this without making it the sole consideration in allocation might be to create a factor in organ allocation based on the difference in age between donor and recipient. In allocation algorithms that assign points for various factors (as the U.S. allocation system does), some "negative-point" consideration could be assigned for each decade of difference in age between donor and recipient. About one point per decade difference would probably work well. Hence a recipient who was between 50 and 59 years older than the donor would lose five points in the allocation calculation. (A recipient who was that much younger than the donor would also receive negative points, but those organs might be declined by the surgeon or the patient anyway.) This would achieve the goal of matching donors and recipients for age and eliminating the unfair advantage that older people would receive from the informal system of ad hoc refusals of organs offered to young recipients.

This would be far better than a categorical age cutoff for donors over age 65. Under this arrangement only those organs that are medically unsuitable for any patients would be excluded. Any patient who wanted to could decline an organ based on the age of the donor, but a young person would only be offered older organs if there were some telling factors (such as zero-antigen mismatch or a negative cross-match for a high-PRA patient) that offset the age difference between the donor and the recipient. These factors should naturally incline the potential recipient to accept the organ notwithstanding the age difference. On the other hand, the older recipient would receive an offer of a young organ only in special cases in which other considerations offset the age difference, thus justifying the offer. Some version of a factor in the organ allocation formula based on difference in age between donor and recipient seems to be morally necessary if the allocation formula is to be efficient and fair.

An allocation factor based on difference in age is not the only age-based consideration that needs to be addressed. Independent of the consideration of donor age, some critics have argued that younger recipients deserve priority either because of the extra benefit that accrues to young recipients or because older people will get the benefit for a shorter time. These issues of recipient age will be discussed in Part Three.

ENDNOTES

1. U.S. Department of Health and Human Services, "Federal Policy for the Protection of Human Subjects," 45 C.F.R. 46, revised June 18, 1991, reprinted March 15, 1994.

2. Paul Ramsey, "Consent as a Canon of Loyalty with Special Reference to Children in Medical Investigations," in *The Patient as Person*, ed. Paul Ramsey (New Haven, CT: Yale University Press, 1970), pp. 1–58.

3. Richard A. McCormick, "Proxy Consent in the Experimentation Situation," *Perspectives in Biology and Medicine* 18 (1974): 2–20.

4. World Medical Association, "Declaration of Helsinki—1989," in *Encyclopedia of Bioethics*, Vol. 5, rev. ed., ed. Warren T. Reich (New York: Free Press, 1995), pp. 2765–67.

5. U.S. Department of Health and Human Services, "Additional Protections for Children Involved as Subjects in Research: Final Rule: 45 CFR 46," 48 Fed. Reg. 9814 (March 8, 1983).

6. Ibid. at 9819.

7. This is formally known as the *null hypothesis*. In randomized clinical trials the investigator is hypothesizing that there is no difference between the standard treatment and the experimental one. For such research to be ethical, that hypothesis must be plausible. Therefore, there should be no risk to an incompetent if the individual refuses to be randomized and simply receives the standard treatment.

8. *Strunk v. Strunk*, Ky., 445 S.W.2d 145 (1969).

9. Hung-Mo Lin, H. Myron Kauffman, Maureen A. McBride, Darcy B. Davies, John D. Rosendale, Carol M. Smith, Erick B. Edwards, Patrick Daily, James Kirkin, Charles F. Shield, and Lawrence G. Hunsicker, "Center Specific Graft and Patient Survival Rates: 1997 United Network for Organ Sharing (UNOS) Report," *Journal of the American Medical Association* 280 (Oct. 7, 1998): 1155.

10. The story is more complicated still. The study reported what it called *three-year conditional survival*. This refers to survival for three years among those who survived the first year. This is considered an important statistic because it provides an assessment of risk factors independent of those related to the transplant and such factors as prolonged organ preservation and acute infection. Conditional three-year graft failure was 1.143 times as great for organs from 42-year-old donors compared with 32-year-olds and 1.448 as great if the donor was 52 years old.

11. Hung-Mo Lin, H. Myron Kauffman, Maureen A. McBride, Darcy B. Davies, John D. Rosendale, Carol M. Smith, Erick B. Edwards, Patrick Daily, James Kirkin, Charles F. Shield, and Lawrence G. Hunsicker, "Center Specific Graft and Patient Survival Rates: 1997 United Network for Organ Sharing (UNOS) Report," p. 1157.

12. Ibid., p. 1158.

Sixteen

Tainted Organs:
HIV-Positive and Other
Controversial Donors

A transplant coordinator learns a patient has died and meets the initial tests for death based on brain criteria. The patient has succumbed to an overdose of heroin. He is known to have a long history of IV drug abuse. The first question that enters the coordinator's mind is, "Is he HIV positive?"

He has repeatedly tested negative. Still, there is some risk he has not sero-converted. The standard antibody test for HIV will not be positive in the weeks after infection before antibodies have formed. Thus the patient with a dead brain who only days earlier had been a young, apparently healthy man may be carrying the virus for AIDs. The procurement professional faces two problems. Can she refuse to expose herself to the risk of contact and can she let the organs be transplanted into a willing donor?

Age turns out to be only one of the factors that can make organs procured for transplant less suitable in the eyes of transplant surgeons and potential recipients. Some organs are medically marginal. Others may be damaged during the procurement, from warm ischemic time that is too long or by experiencing too long a period between procurement and implantation. Others may come from patients with diseases that could be transmitted to the recipient. Some of these diseases are so troublesome that they clearly rule out the organs for anything but research. Metastatic cancer is an example. Other diseases such as cytomegalovirus are tolerated.

The danger that places the greatest fear into transplant personnel and recipients alike is HIV. HIV-positive donors are rejected by organ procurement organizations (OPOs). This seems reasonable, even though it excludes a significant number of organs potentially available for transplant. Moreover, it overlooks the possibility that some people, including some already HIV-infected, may be at death's door and might consent to an implant from such a donor.

Moreover, many potential organ sources who are not known to be infected but who are known to live high-risk lifestyles—such as some homosexuals and I.V. drug users—are also rejected. Is this because surgeons fear exposure during procurement or perhaps because they are repulsed by giving someone the virus—even though taking such a risk may be rationally in the recipient's interest? More likely it is because transplant professionals cannot tolerate the thought that they would be agents to the transmission of the virus to a patient who may become infected and eventually die from AIDS. Similar concerns may arise with other potential donors whose organs are rejected because of fear that disease will be transmitted or because organs are otherwise unacceptable.

Types of Tainted Organs

I will refer to these as "tainted" organs. In this chapter I will argue that recipients should be informed about the risk and receive tainted organs if they so consent.

Donors Known to Be HIV Positive

Cases of HIV transmission from transplant are known to have occurred.[1]

MANDATORY SCREENING

Currently, all potential organ donors must be tested by use of a screening test licensed by the U.S. Food and Drug administration for human immunodeficiency virus antibody.[2] Because not all people who have acquired the virus will be identified, especially those who have acquired it recently, additional steps must be taken. If the potential donor has received a blood transfusion, it must be determined if a pretransfusion test is available and if all transfusions have been screened. If not, the recipient transplant center must be provided with the screening results and a complete history of all transfusions received for the ten days before organ removal.

HISTORY-TAKING

In addition, the donor history must be obtained to attempt to determine whether the potential donor is in a "high-risk" group. The history must be communicated to any transplanting center. The person consenting to procurement should be informed that a screen will be performed "for medical acceptability for organ donation and that such tests may be the basis for not using the organ in transplantation."[3] There should be a consent to the screening as well as the organ procurement. Such vague language as screening for "medical acceptability" is, however, not sufficient to authorize HIV antibody testing. More explicit consent to HIV screening is necessary.

Problems Arising from Screening without Explicit Consent of
the Next of Kin

In a still-living patient, detecting HIV can create serious problems—for employment, insurance, and personal relationships. Although it is important that people know their HIV status, it is not a good thing for patients to be screened without understanding that the testing is going on. If a positive result occurs when the patient has not explicitly understood that screening for HIV was taking place, the health personnel are left in a very awkward position. They must either impose the unsolicited information on the patient or take it on themselves to withhold this potentially important finding. Neither choice is attractive. Arguably, neither is morally nor legally acceptable.

In the case of a deceased patient, the harm that can result from learning the deceased was HIV positive is somewhat less. Nevertheless, spouses or close relatives learning unexpectedly that their loved one was diagnosed as HIV positive can leave them in a difficult and psychologically stressful position. They may be forced unexpectedly to confront the possibility that they may have been exposed themselves. The transplant coordinator and others on the procurement team are not necessarily trained in counseling for HIV testing. Withholding the HIV findings from any family member consenting to organ procurement is ethically unacceptable as well. The only plausible policy is to explicitly inform the next of kin or any other party with authority to consent to organ procurement that an HIV test is to be performed and to reach an explicit understanding with that person about what will be done with the results. The only possible exception might be screening persons who have already recorded their consent to be organ donors, either through signing a donor card or by agreeing to become a non–heart-beating donor through a planned treatment stoppage, as discussed in Chapter 13.

The Emergency Exception to Screening for HIV Antibody

The United Network for Organ Sharing (UNOS) permits one exception to the screening requirement. In the case of nonrenal organs when there is an "extreme medical emergency" in the eyes of the staff of the procuring OPO and the recipient institution, an organ may be used without screening provided the consent of the recipient or next of kin is obtained.[4]

HIV-Negative Donors with High-Risk Lifestyles

The insistence on obtaining an adequate medical and social history is to rule out patients who do not test positive for HIV but may nevertheless be infected with the virus. This can occur if the exposure is so recent that antibodies have not formed. Although the UNOS regulations do not preclude organ procurement from persons who test negative but have a history of high-risk activity (such as

I.V. drug use or permiscuous lifestyle), the history must be communicated to any institution receiving an organ. It is standard practice to refuse such organs.

Organ Sources without Medical or Social Histories Available

This means that any potential donor or organ source for whom no history can be obtained is, in effect, excluded from the procurement process. This has the effect of making signed donor cards almost useless in authorizing organ procurement. Even if someone has engaged in the socially noble behavior of taking the time to learn about donation and has signed a donor card (including those on drivers' licenses), he or she will be ignored as a donor if relatives cannot be located who will provide such a history. Likewise, relatives who are uncooperative will be able to veto donation even from someone who has a valid, signed donor card simply by refusing to cooperate.

The law is quite clear that the donor card is sufficient, without the next of kin's further consent, to authorize organ procurement. I argued in Chapter 9 that in a society that values individual autonomy, it is the potential organ donor whose consent should be primary. Only in cases in which the potential organ source's wishes cannot be established should we resort to next of kin permission. Thus even though the donor's valid, signed card is legally sufficient and morally superior to the next of kin's permission, the need for a history gives a resisting relative an opportunity to veto the procurement. Relatives should be counseled in these situations to understand that the deceased's wishes are legally and morally primary and ought to prevail. It is possible that some relatives who object for their own reasons can be made to see that it is their duty to cooperate in fulfilling the deceased's wishes by providing the history. They need not and should not be asked to also "consent" to the procurement—merely to provide the history. Although some might seize the opportunity to block the procurement, others may understand that their loved one's desires should prevail and cooperate sufficiently to rule out high-risk lifestyles.

Other Diseases

Other diseases such as HTLV-I, hepatitis, and cancer also raise concerns in organ procurement. Although none automatically rules organs out, they pose ethical and policy problems that must be addressed.

Human T-Lymphotropic Virus Type I (HTLV-I) Antibody

The UNOS policies have provisions for screening and excluding persons infected with the HTLV-I virus. Histories must be obtained, and donor consent is recommended. Exceptions are once again permitted for "extreme medical emergency."[5]

HEPATITIS

Hepatitis B can also be transmitted during an organ transplant.[6] In this case, however, if the donor is known to be infected, someone will have to make a judgment about whether the risk is worth it. Although intentionally risking transmission is very troublesome to clinicians, patients may consider the risk worth it, especially if the alternative is certain, rapid death. Moreover, there is a high prevalence of naturally occurring immunity to hepatitis B, so that immune recipients might be located. In that case, however, immune recipients might claim they are being treated inequitably if they do not have an equal chance of receiving an organ from a negative donor. And although the risk to the immune recipient is greatly reduced, it might not be zero.

There is also evidence that hepatitis C is transmitted via transplant. The risk appears to be about 50 percent that recipients receiving organs transplanted from positive donors will develop non-A, non-B hepatitis.[7] Although this risk has not been considered an absolute contraindication for the use of organs from donors with hepatitis C, some centers restrict their use to life-saving procedures.

CANCER

Potential donors with cancer seem as dangerous as those with HIV. Cancers can metastasize to distant sites so that even an apparently disease-free organ can harbor microscopic cancer cells. Almost no transplant surgeon would be willing to transplant an organ procured from someone with cancer. Once again, however, there are complications. Primary cancers of the brain are believed not to pose a serious threat to other organs and so provide an exception to the cancer exclusion. More critically, we can raise questions about whether it would ever be in the interests of someone on the waiting list for an organ to accept a transplant procured from someone with cancer. Keeping in mind that many people on the waiting list end up dying for want of an organ and that some cancers can be determined to be unlikely to have metastasized, it seems that some potential transplant recipients who are nearing death from their organ failure would rationally be willing to accept an organ from someone with a malignancy that appears not to have spread. We need to ask whether the prohibition on procuring organs from persons with cancer is really based on the interest of the potential recipient or whether it is more to serve the psychological needs of surgeons. Surely, a surgeon should be troubled with the thought that his or her actions might be the cause of a cancer in a transplant recipient. On the other hand, a surgeon should also realize without the transplant of the tainted organ, his or her patient will die needlessly. It is hard to imagine an argument supporting a categorical prohibition on organ transplant from organ donors with cancer.

MORE RARE AND LESS TROUBLESOME DISEASES

Cytomegalovirus (CMV) can be transmitted during transplantation,[8] as can many other viruses such as herpes simplex, Epstein-Barr, rabies, and the virus causing Creutzfeldt-Jakob disease, as well as bacteria, fungi and yeast, toxoplasmosis, and other microorganisms.[9] In each of these cases, if the donor is known to be infected, a decision will have to be made about whether the disease is an absolute contraindication for the transplant or whether it would be tolerable as a side effect of obtaining the usable organ. Such decisions will have to take into account the fact that a graft recipient will be immunosuppressed and thus at greater risk, but it must also take into account the technology that is available at the time that could decrease risk of infection. For example, pulsatile perfusion of the kidney may decrease the infectious load. For some tissues (but not currently for solid organs) techniques are available to attempt to sterilize or render the tissue safe for transplant, but more studies are needed to confirm the effectiveness of these techniques.[10] For at least some organisms "excellent results following inadvertent use of infected organs" have been reported, including one series in which actual one-year survival of contaminated grafts did not differ statistically from that of "sterile" kidneys.[11]

In the case of CMV, excluding positive organs would significantly decrease the supply. One study reports 42% of donors of kidneys are seropositive.[12] Some transplant programs reserve CMV-negative organs for negative recipients. The result has been a decrease in morbidity and mortality and graft loss from primary infection.[13] The policy raises serious questions, however. The result was a greater mismatch in human lymphocyte antigen (HLA) for the seronegative recipients. Also, because fewer recipients were negative than donors and positive recipients do worse receiving positive than negative organs, the policy has the potential of producing inequities. However, this notion of reserving organs for recipients whose infection status matches the donor suggests a model that has provocative implications for HIV.

HIV-Positive Recipients and Transplant

Although HIV-positive donors and even those who test negative but are at high risk or from whom no history can be obtained are excluded from donation, HIV-positive persons in need of organ transplants are not precluded from receiving them. UNOS policy is that to become a candidate for screening to receive a transplant patients must be tested for HIV antibody unless state or federal laws or regulations prohibit it.[14] The UNOS policies note that asymptomatic patients who are HIV-antibody-positive need not be excluded from transplant, but they indicate that such patients should be informed of the increased risk of morbidity and mortality because of the immunosupressive therapy that will be required.

With increasingly effective treatment regimens for HIV, many positive persons have long life expectancy and could potentially benefit from organ grafts if they have such needs.

There are good reasons for testing prospective recipients. Patients need to know if they are carrying the virus. It influences their judgment about possible futures and changes the nature of the risks of transplant. Moreover, operating room personnel have an interest in knowing. The policies support informing health care personnel caring for patients who test positive (without indicating whether patient consent is expected). Even though they are supposed to be using "universal precautions," any person at risk for coming in contact with blood or body fluids of an HIV-positive transplant recipient is bound to want this information and will undoubtedly take extra precautions if they know. Whether informing these personnel could lead to discriminatory treatment is a question of concern. The policies also specify that treatment of HIV-positive patients is not optional or discretionary for health care personnel.

An Assessment

The combination of precluding all HIV-positive donors and those who are at high risk or whose histories cannot be determined while including HIV-positive recipients raises some troublesome questions. Even though it at first seems only common sense to exclude from donation those who are HIV positive, that may not be a wise policy.

HIV-Positive Recipients

HIV-positive patients presently are on the organ transplant waiting lists. In fact, recent reports indicate more interest in transplants by HIV-positive patients and several successful transplants for such persons.[15] Given the serious shortage of organs, some of them will die waiting for their transplants. Does it make sense to discard perhaps hundreds of organs, some of which show no evidence of infection, when positive patients are dying for want of organs?

A strong case can be made that organs from HIV-negative persons who are in high-risk categories and those for whom no history can be obtained should be procured and offered to HIV-positive persons on the waiting list. Of course, potential recipients should be informed that these are "tainted organs"—that is, organs for which we cannot establish a "clean" history. Some HIV-positive patients might decline, but others might accept. In fact, some might be willing to accept organs known to have come from an HIV-positive donor. At least for those who are at the end-stage of their organ-specific disease that makes them a candidate for transplant, they might prefer such a risk to the alternative of certain death. It is striking that an exception is made for emergencies that require transplant before screening, but no exception is made for emergencies to implant an HIV-positive organ into an HIV-positive patient.

There are empirical medical questions as well as moral questions raised by such a proposal. There is very little information available on the risk of transmission of HIV when organs are transplanted either from an HIV-positive donor or from one known to be engaging in high-risk activities. It seems that there would be some increased risks from placing the virus into a person who is already positive. There could be an increased viral load created or a different strain of the virus introduced, giving the recipient a double infection. On the other hand, we know that some people exposed to the virus do not get infected. The only reasonable conclusion seems to be that an HIV-positive person should probably try to avoid an additional exposure, but it is hard to argue that intentionally choosing to receive an organ from an infected person or one engaging in high-risk lifestyle choices would be irrational in all cases (including those when the already HIV-positive recipient is desperate).

The case in which the HIV-positive recipient altruistically decides to leave the untainted organs for recipients who do not have the virus is also an interesting case. Although that kind of altruism seems to be beyond the call of duty, it would be hard to criticize someone who made such a choice. Deciding what course of action is in the recipient's self-interest is a very difficult judgment. No one but the recipient is capable of making that choice.

HIV-Negative Recipients in Desperation

This suggests an even more controversial proposal: If it is reasonable for HIV-positive persons to accept organs for which HIV cannot be ruled out and maybe even organs from persons known to be HIV positive, is there ever a case in which it would be rational for an HIV-negative person to accept one of these high-risk organs? If death is the only alternative for someone who cannot obtain a negative organ, I do not see why someone would decline. There is no firm evidence on the incidence of transmission in such a situation. The risk surely should be presumed to be high. But the risk of dying without transplant may also be very high. Given the fact that people with infection are now living many years symptom free, I can imagine some people preferring that risk to certain, rapid death.

Determining Why Surgeons Reject Tainted Organs

It is worth asking why surgeons and other transplant personnel might resist procuring organs until it can be established that the donor is a low risk.

RISKS TO PATIENTS

By tradition, physicians are committed to benefiting their patients and protecting them from harm. Implanting a vitally contaminated organ sounds terrible. No one would like the possibility that they have performed a successful, life-saving transplant only to see the patient die of an HIV infection.

RISKS TO HEALTH PROFESSIONALS

It probably should not be overlooked that health care professionals also have a self-interest in this controversy. They put themselves in harm's way when they handle HIV-positive tissue and organs. The procuring team is particularly exposed to contaminated blood and fluids. Enthusiastic support of the prohibition on procuring HIV-positive organs and those from high-risk donors may reflect, in part, the awareness on the part of health professionals that the exclusion is in their interest.

PHYSICIAN FEAR OF IATROGENIC DEATH

The self-interest of the professional should not be overemphasized, however. Health professionals are routinely at risk for HIV and other infectious diseases. They understand the necessary precautions. They provide treatment for HIV-positive patients regularly. Many health professionals are remarkably dedicated in their service during epidemics. They have a generally good record of maintaining their presence in the face of infectious disease. They show dedication in caring for infected patients even at significant personal risk.

Why, then, do they resist procuring HIV-positive organs and even antibody-negative organs from high-risk donors? Part of the explanation may be that physicians have a great fear of iatrogenic disease and death. They do not want to be the one who caused the patient's death even if risking exposure was the rational thing for a patient to do. We see this in surgeons who militantly oppose letting so-called do-not-resuscitate orders remain in effect in the operating room.[16] Even though a patient may have very carefully thought out reasons why resuscitation should not be attempted, surgeons may flatly refuse to perform surgery on a patient who will not suspend his or her do-not-resuscitate decision, even though that patient understands that resuscitation in the operating room may be easier and more successful than when it is performed elsewhere.

The real issue seems to be that physicians, especially surgeons, simply do not want to be the direct cause of the patient's death. This may also be behind many physicians' insistence on a distinction between omitting and withdrawing life support. Although almost all theorists, lawyers, and policy makers insist there is no valid distinction between the two, many clinicians still feel powerful emotional resistance to actively withdrawing support, even when the patient insists on it.[17]

I suspect that surgeons and other organ transplant professionals resist implanting HIV-positive organs because of the revulsion at being directly in the causal chain that might lead to the death of the patient. Reason tells us that it is as bad or worse to be in the causal chain by refusing to perform a transplant that has a good chance at extending life. Philosophers recognize both actions and omissions as potentially leading to causal responsibility.

There is a significant philosophical difference between being causally responsible for omitting desired life-saving surgery and being causally responsible for a death that occurs when a patient withdraws consent for a life-sustaining ventilator. In the case of withdrawal of consent for life-supporting treatments, the physician is legally and morally obliged not to touch the patient. There is no longer a valid consent. The physician could enter the causal chain by refusing to withdraw the life support when the patient withdraws consent, but that would be illegal as well as unethical. It is, technically, an assault to treat a patient without consent.

That is quite different from the case in which a physician enters the causal chain by refusing to implant an HIV-positive organ that eventually might lead to the patient's death. In the latter case, at least in the system I envision, the patient will have consented to the risk of the HIV-positive organ. It will have been a rational consent in those cases in which the probability of survival with the infected organ significantly exceeds that of going without. The surgeon who unilaterally refuses to perform a life-saving intervention that the patient wants is responsible for the death of the patient just as he or she would be if the death results from implanting an infected organ. It is quite different from the death resulting from omitting life support because the patient has demanded not to be treated. The surgeon, indeed, enters the causal chain by implanting the organ, but he or she can enter that causal chain by refusing the patient's request for the surgery as well.

Many physicians concerned about medical ethics are quick to point out that a professional is not required to treat a patient simply because the patient demands it. In fact, the right of the physician to refuse to treat is by no means absolute. Several legal cases have recently been brought to the courts in which patients demand so-called futile treatment—that is, treatment that will only extend life temporarily and at a burden that many feel is unacceptable. These cases raise the issue of whether a physician can refuse to deliver temporary life-prolonging treatment on the grounds that the benefits are not worth it. Of the eight court cases that have given rise to some form of written legal opinion, all have been decided in the patient's favor—even though the benefits may be very minimal and very brief.[18]

The dilemma for a surgeon with the opportunity to implant an HIV-positive organ is more like that of an anesthesiologist than it is like a physician who withdraws life support at the patient's request. The anesthesiologist knows that every time anesthesia is administered there is some finite risk of an unintended adverse reaction that could kill the patient. The lethal effect is not expected; surely not intended, but it is foreseen that occasionally such accidents will happen. This does not lead the anesthesiologist to refrain from practicing the art. It would, in fact, be immoral to refuse to anesthetize merely because we foresee that occasionally a bad event, even death, may be actively caused by the action. So, likewise, implanting an HIV-positive organ (or a high-risk one) may be the only rational thing for a surgeon to do. The policy of refusing to procure all organs from this class of donors forecloses the possibility of this life-saving surgery in patients, many of whom may already be HIV positive and quite able to understand and take the risk.

It is hard to predict whether a surgeon would be required by a court to implant an HIV-positive organ in a patient who was dying and demanded the transplant. Certainly, the expected benefit to the patient is greater than the more classical "futile care" cases. But the complexity of the procedure is greater also. Perhaps the eventual conclusion of a court would be on the side of the surgeon refusing to operate.

Although the law may not require a physician to treat in these cases, it is hard to see on what ethical grounds the refusal would rest. The surgeon surely cannot claim that his personal risk is too great. Surgeons perform surgery on HIV-positive patients routinely. He cannot even claim the operation would be futile (in the sense of being doomed to fail to achieve the objective sought). In some cases, the benefit measured in expected days of survival will surely be much greater with the HIV-positive transplant than without. The expected difference in benefit with an organ that is from an HIV-negative, high-risk donor will be even greater. The moral imperative for a licensed health care professional to use his or her professional skill to significantly increase the life expectancy of an ongoing patient is powerful. Even if the law would not require such surgery, ethics surely does.

A Proposal for a Policy Change

Given the seeming inconsistency in U.S. policy of refusing to procure HIV-positive and high-risk organs while accepting the right of HIV-positive patients to be on the waiting list for organs, I suggest that the existing policy can no longer be defended and a new one is needed. The new policy would affect not only organs at risk for carrying HIV but also other diseases that lead to classifying the organs as "tainted."

People are dying today for want of organs. Some of them are already infected with HIV and understand enough about the risks of exacerbating the infection to be able to choose between a good chance at living with an infected organ and dying without one. The current policy of categorical refusal to procure not only forecloses the choice for life that these patients should have, it also forecloses the right of some transplant surgeons to implant such organs.

I propose that all patients be asked when they are placed on the waiting list for an organ whether they would be willing to accept an otherwise medically suitable HIV-positive organ or one from a donor at high risk for HIV. They should be further told that, if such an organ is not in their interest at the present time, they would have the opportunity at any time to add their names to the group of those willing to accept such organs. They would, of course, also be permitted to withdraw their names at any time. Similarly, they should be given the opportunity to consent to receiving organs tainted with the risk of other diseases, as well as organs procured from older persons.

For any patient willing to receive such an organ, a discussion with his or her surgeon should then take place, including information about whether the surgeon is willing to implant such an organ if it were to become available. Although I have argued that surgeons who are committed to doing what is best for their patients should feel themselves under moral pressure to agree to do the surgery, for the time being, I would not force any unwilling surgeon to engage in the surgery against his or her will. If the surgeon declined to agree to the potential of doing the surgery with an infected or high-risk organ, that should be a stimulus for the physician and patient to explore whether they have a mutually acceptable agreement. The patient would, of course, be free to change surgeons, seeking one willing to pursue what is in the patient's interest if the original surgeon declined to do so.

If such information were part of the database for patients on the waiting list for organs, we could then make a rational judgment about the probability of an organ from a positive or high-risk person being used if it were procured. I would then expect all OPOs to facilitate organ procurement of such organs unless they could establish that there was little likelihood of anyone using the organ at the time the procurement decision had to be made.

I realize that it is often impossible to run the program to establish whether there is a suitable, willing recipient before the organs would have to be procured. From the waiting list supplemented by data on patient willingness to accept positive and high-risk organs, however, the probability of the organ being used could be calculated. As long as the probability of being used was similar to that of other organs that are procured, then it ought to be retrieved.

ENDNOTES

1. Svetlozar N. Natov and Brian J. G. Pereira, "Transmission of Disease by Organ Transplantation," in *Organ and Tissue Donation for Transplantation*, ed. Jeremy R. Chapman, Mark Deierhoi, and Celia Wight (New York: Oxford University Press, 1997), pp. 128–29; K. M. Gottesdieneer, "Transplanted Infections: Donor-to-Host Transmission with the Allograft," *Annals of Internal Medicine* 110 (12, June 15, 1989): 1001–16; A. Schwarz, F. Hoffman, J. L'age-Stehr, A. M. Tegzess, and G. Offermann, "Human Immunodeficiency Virus Transmission by Organ Donation. Outcome in Cornea and Kidney Recipient," *Transplantation* 44 (1, July 1987): 21–24; V. Briner, W. Zimmerli, G. Cathomas, J. Landmann, and G. Thiel, "HIV Infection Caused by Kidney Transplant: Case Report and review of 18 Published Cases," *Schwweiz Med Wochenschr* 119 (30, July 29, 1989): 1046–52; M. Quarto et al., "HIV Transmission through Kidney Transplantation from a Living Related Donor," *New England Journal of Medicine* 320 (June 29, 1989): 1754.

2. UNOS Policy 4.1, available on the Internet at <http://www.unos.org/frame_Default .asp?Category=About> (Sept. 22, 1998).

3. Ibid.

4. UNOS Policy 4.1.3, available at <http://www.unos.org/frame_Default.asp?Category =About> (Sept. 22, 1998).

5. See G. Mate, C. Gonzalez, J. M. Bronsoms, M. Valles, P. Torguet, and J. M. Marie, "Transplant and Organ Donor-Associated Transmission of Human T-lymphotropic Virus Type I and II," *Transplant Proceedings* 27 (4, 1995): 2417.

6. K. M. Gottesdieneer, "Transplanted Infections: Donor-to-Host Transmission with the Allograft"; T. Eastlund, "Infectious Disease Transmission through Cell, Tissue, and Organ Transplantation: Reducing the Risk through Donor Selection," *Cell Transplant*, 4 (5, Sept.–Oct. 1995): 455–77; Svetlozar N. Natov and Brian J. G. Pereira, "Transmission of Disease by Organ Transplantation," pp. 129–31.

7. Svetlozar N. Natov and Brian J. G. Pereira, "Transmission of Disease by Organ Transplantation," p. 133.

8. M. Ho, "Epidemiology of Cytomegalovirus Infections," *Review of Infectious Diseases* 12 (Sept.–Oct. 1990, Suppl. 7): S701–10; M. E. Falagas et al., "Primary Cytomegalovirus Infection in Liver Transplant Recipients: Comparison of Infections Transmitted Via Donor Organs and Via Transfusions," *Clinical Infectious Diseases* 23 (Aug. 1996): 292–97.

9. Svetlozar N. Natov and Brian J. G. Pereira, "Transmission of Disease by Organ Transplantation"; K. M. Gottesdieneer, "Transplanted Infections: Donor-to-Host Transmission with the Allograft"; A. Schwarz, F. Hoffman, J. L'age-Stehr, A. M.

Tegzess, and G. Offermann, "Human Immunodeficiency Virus Transmission by Organ Donation. Outcome in Cornea and Kidney Recipient," 21–24; T. Eastlund, "Infectious Disease Transmission through Cell, Tissue, and Organ Transplantation: Reducing the Risk through Donor Selection."

10. Svetlozar N. Natov and Brian J. G. Pereira, "Transmission of Disease by Organ Transplantation," p. 129.

11. Ibid., p. 121–22.

12. M. L. Smiley, C. G. Wlodaver, R. A. Grossman, cited in ibid., p. 125. Similar problems arise with hepatitis B where in some cultures up to 10 percent of the population is positive.

13. J. R. Ackerman, W. M. LeFor, S. Weinstein, cited in ibid., p. 125.

14. UNOS Policy 4.2, available at <http://www.unos.org/frame_Default.asp?Category= About> (Sept. 22, 1998).

15. Christopher Snowbeck, "Longer-Living HIV Patients Raise a New Transplant Question," *Online Post-Gazette*, September 7, 1999. <http://www.post-gazette.com/ healthsceince/19990907transplant3.asp> (Sept. 7, 1999).

16. Peter J. Cohen and Cynthia B. Cohen, "Do-Not-Resuscitate Orders in the Operating Room," *New England Journal of Medicine* 325 (26, Dec. 26, 1991): 1879–82; Allan L. Smith, "DNR in the OR," *Clinical Ethics Report* 8 (4, Winter 1994): 1–8; Jean M. Reeder, "Do-Not-Resuscitate Orders in the Operating Room," *AORN Journal* 57 (4, 1993 April): 947–51; Guy Micco and Neal H. Cohen, "Do Not Resuscitate Orders in the Operating Room: The Birth of a Policy. [Article and Commentary]," *Cambridge Quarterly of Healthcare Ethics* 4 (1, Winter 1995): 103–10; American College of Surgeons, "Statement on Advance Directives by Patients: 'Do Not Resuscitate' in the Operating Room," *Bulletin of the American College of Surgeons* 79 (9, Sept. 1994): 29.

17. President's Commission for the Study of Ethical Problems in Medicine and Biomedical and Behavioral Research, *Deciding to Forego Life-Sustaining Treatment: Ethical, Medical, and Legal Issues in Treatment Decisions* (Washington, DC: U.S. Government Printing Office, 1983).

18. Robert M. Veatch and Carol Mason Spicer, "Medically Futile Care: The Role of the Physician in Setting Limits," *American Journal of Law & Medicine* 18 (1 & 2, 1992): 15–36; for the most famous court case see *In the Matter of Baby K*, 832 F. Supp. 1022 (E.D. Va. 1993). Other cases include *In Re the Conservatorship of Helga Wanglie*; State of Minnesota, District Court, Probate Court Division, County of Hennepin, Fourth Judicial District, June 28, 1991; *Rideout, Administrator of Estate of Rideout et al. v. Hershey Medical Center*, (1995); *Velez v. Bethune et al.*, 466 S.E.2d 627 (Ga. App. 1995); Gina Kolata, "Withholding Care from Patients: Boston Case Asks Who Decides," *New York Times*, April 3, 1995, pp. A1, B8.

SEVENTEEN

THE ETHICS OF XENOGRAFTS

Baby Fae was born October 12, 1984. She was born with a fatal condition, hypoplastic left heart syndrome, a condition in which the left atrium and ventricle are seriously underdeveloped.

The baby was transferred from a community hospital to Loma Linda University Medical Center in California, a medical facility associated with the Seventh Day Adventist Church and its medical school. The mother was told that the baby's condition is usually fatal within the first week of life. A Norwood procedure, a palliative two-stage surgical procedure, was explained to them. They were told that the procedure was "generally unsuccessful." The mother left the hospital with the baby.

Four days later the pediatrician called the mother informing them of the possibility of a xenograft cardiac transplant—that is, a transplant of an organ taken from a nonhuman animal. The mother, accompanied by the grandmother and a friend, met with Leonard Bailey, a surgeon at Loma Linda who had been developing a proposal for experimental xenografts, for approximately seven hours. He reviewed the Norwood procedure and explained to them that a human heart transplant was unlikely because size-matched and histocompatible infant human hearts only rarely become available.

The mother consented to the xenograft transplant, signing a form that summarized the procedure.

Although the initial transplant appeared to be successful, the baby died November 15. There was considerable dispute over the cause of death. There were initial reports that the tissues did not show evidence of cellular graft rejection. A report that the death was related to a blood-type mismatch was disputed.

Following the death and enormous publicity, there was widespread criticism. The problems raised included claims that animal-to-human transplant is intrinsically unethical and a violation of divine orders of creation, concern that the family was inadequately informed, the suggestion that this was an abuse of a baby in a procedure that was more for the purpose of advancing knowledge than serving the baby's interests, and the claim that it was an unethical use of scarce resources.

A National Institutes of Health team visited the site and prepared a report reviewing these charges. The report praised the candidness of Loma Linda personnel and acknowledged that internal reviews of the protocol had taken place by an ad hoc committee in the department of surgery as well as a neonatal cardiac transplantation committee, the hospital ethics committee, the executive committee of the medical staff, and the advisory committee to the Loma Linda vice president for medical affairs in addition to the institutional review board required to review all research on human subjects. The review team was critical of some shortcomings in the consent procedure: The expected benefits were thought to be overstated, it failed to discuss the possibility of searching for a human heart, and it failed to explain the institution's compensation policy. The controversy surrounding the case and lingering moral doubts about the wisdom of xenografts have led to a moratorium on such procedures since that time.[1]

Transplanting of organs from one species to another congers up images filled with ethical controversy. When the source or recipient species is a human, that controversy is particularly acute. Because xenografts into humans are medical procedures, the ordinary, traditional ethical requirements must of course be met. There must be adequately informed consent and protection of confidentiality. There must be adequate review, especially of any procedures that are experimental. Any discussion of the ethics of xenografts must be premised on the expectation that all of these standard requirements of medical ethics will be fulfilled.

Assuming adequately informed consent is obtained and the surrogate choice is not clearly contrary to the patient's interests, what are the special ethical problems of transplantation between humans and other species? Although many more xenografts have been performed from human to animal species than the other way around, I shall focus primarily on cases in which the nonhuman species is the source of the organ. (With the same reasoning I have used to suggest in the case of infants, children, and mentally retarded individuals, it is not acceptable to refer to the nonhuman as a "donor." Clearly, the animal did not decide to engage in an act of gift-giving the way some humans do when they are appropriately called donors.) I shall address five special ethical problems raised by xenografts. I shall refer to them as (1) the natural law problem, (2) the animal rights problem, (3) the nontherapeutic interventions problem, (4) the scarce resources problem, and (5) the virus issue.

The Natural Law Problem

The first problem that is unique to xenografts is whether the intermixing of biological material from different species somehow violates fundamental morality in and of itself. We saw this question arise in Baby Fae's case. Especially when we transplant vitally important and emotionally significant organs such as hearts, are we tampering with nature in a way that goes beyond what humans are supposed to do? Are we, to use the religious language, violating God's plan for creation? The question was raised initially when concern was expressed about transplantation of organs from one human to another. There is an initial feeling of shock if not repulsion by many people when they think of baboon organs replacing those of humans.

Some have maintained that the human is unique, not in any way in continuity with other species. Anyone who holds that view might be uncomfortable with xenografts involving humans. It is therefore important to realize that there are no principled objections from the major religious traditions to the transferring of material from one species to another, even if it involves humans. Catholic theologian Richard McCormick, a member of the National Institutes of Health (NIH) panel reviewing the Loma Linda cardiac xenograft transplant, raises the issue and refers to the "special concern" about cross-species grafts.[2] He focuses primarily on more practical psychological problems of xenografts: how people will be viewed by others and themselves, not on any violation of the natural law that would be involved. Although it is a special problem it is not insuperable.

Orthodox Jews go even further in affirming the fundamental morality of cross-species transplants. Fred Rosner, one of this country's leading authorities on medical ethics in Judaism (who happens also to be a physician), examines the problem of cross-species transfer. He concludes that "the preservation of human life is of infinite and supreme value."[3] Provided the rules for respectful treatment of animals are followed, the standards governing human experimentation are met, and a human being stands a chance of benefiting from the procedure, then it is permissible in Jewish thought to use an animal organ to save a human life.

Although the movement of essential organs from one species to another at first appears shocking, it involves no more of a violation of any natural law than does the movement of an organ from one human to another, as long as the animal is treated respectfully.

The Animal Rights Problem

The qualifier that the animal must be treated respectfully suggests a second possible problem with xenografts. Assuming that therapeutic use of xenografts occurs primarily to humans from other species, some may argue that this is an abuse of animals. In fact, this issue also arose in Baby Fae's case.

The animal rights movement is increasingly powerful and has raised objections to xenografts. Anyone who has fundamental objection to the use of animals for any human ends would logically object to interspecies transplants for the purpose of benefiting humans.

Tom Regan, a professor of philosophy committed to the animal rights perspective, refers to the baboon as "the other victim."[4] Charging anthropocentrism, he argues that animals are experiencing subjects who command respect. They cannot be viewed solely as means for the support of other living beings.

His is a view that is being taken increasingly seriously. It at least has been a force sufficient to overcome patterns of abusive brutality and unnecessary slaughter of animals for research purposes. The broader question of animal rights clearly cannot be resolved within the explicit context of xenografts. It does seem clear, however, that if there is ever a case for using an animal for the benefit of humans, it would be when the sacrifice of one animal will offer the possibility of saving an identifiable human life. The case for xenograft use of animals is, for example, much stronger than the case in any general use of animals in the research labs, for food, or for sport. Jews, for example, will object to animal experimentation solely to satisfy human curiosity.[5] They and many others, however, find at least some uses of animals acceptable. Animals are thus viewed as morally distinct from humans with their own moral claims.[6]

There is another dimension to the animal rights concern. It is apparently still a minority of the population that objects in principle to animal research. Yet the reduction of animals to instruments of human welfare could take on an added perspective if xenografts became acceptable. Clearly, one of the major problems of human to human transplantation is inadequate tissue compatibility. If it is established that animals such as primates can be the source of badly needed organs for human transplantation and that their immune systems are similar to humans, then there would be a greatly increased incentive to breed large numbers of primates so that eventually there could be a "grocery store" approach, with primates available on the shelf to provide virtually all of the thousands of tissue-type combinations that might be needed by humans. Revulsion with this image of thousands of primates bred specifically for their organs may increase the possibility that people will join the camp of those who object to using animals, especially sensate animals, for human ends.

The Nontherapeutic Interventions Problem

The third major objection to xenografts that has emerged, especially in conjunction with the Baby Fae procedure, is the concern that Baby Fae was, in effect, the unconsenting subject of an experiment on a human being that had no therapeutic justification. It is now common to distinguish between interventions justified for their therapeutic intent (even if they are novel or experimental procedures) and interventions solely for research purposes. The distinction was once referred to as the difference between therapeutic and nontherapeutic research. That language has been criticized,[7] but the underlying distinction between interventions justified by consideration of the potential welfare of the patient and those justified by the potential value of the knowledge to be gained remains valid.

A number of critics have questioned the Baby Fae xenograft on the grounds that it constituted a nontherapeutic intervention—that it was really done just to see what could be learned with no hope of benefit for the baby.[8] If that were true, it would be a valid criticism. It is well recognized that novel procedures, especially nontherapeutic ones, should first be tested on consenting adults when possible. They are justified on nonconsenting subjects only when the risks are very minor.

There is room for controversy, however, over whether Baby Fae had a realistic chance to benefit. Some have argued that Baby Fae could not consent to the experiment. The parental permission to operate has also been questioned. There is some public doubt that the parents had adequate information about the alternatives. The review of the Office for the Protection from Research Risks, which is part of the National Institutes of Health, casts some doubt on the adequacy in this case. At any rate, I assume that adequate consent based on the duty to communicate what the parents would reasonably want to know would be a minimal necessary condition for ethically acceptable xenograft surgery.

Some have gone on to argue that even if the parents did have adequate information, they did not have the right to volunteer their child for a procedure so experimental that it could be said that it was undertaken for the knowledge rather than for the benefit of the patient. We are increasingly coming to the conclusion that parents, in making medical decisions for their wards, must attempt to approximate the ward's interests. A parental decision that the xenograft best served their child's interests does not strike me as totally unreasonable. We are increasingly coming to the conclusion that society should not insist that the parents have made the most reasonable choice. Their choice should be tolerated according to this view, provided it is a choice within the realm of reason.[9] Although the most reasonable parental decision might have been against the surgery on the grounds that it did not serve the baby's interests, I am not persuaded that the parental decision was so unreasonable that it should have been overridden.

Considering the alternatives available to Baby Fae, it is hard to fault parents who opt for a chance of success no matter how slim. A principle is emerging in contemporary debate about parental and guardian decision making that helps justify a parental choice for a xenograft—assuming the parent is adequately informed and not pressured into a decision, beyond the natural pressures caused by the critical illness of their daughter.

Today it is increasingly recognized that the decision about whether a child will benefit from a novel procedure should first be made by the parents. Parents will differ in such judgments, but if the parents conclude that the xenograft is more in their daughter's interest than any available alternative, normally their judgment should not be challenged. It should be reviewed and overturned only in those cases in which the parental judgment was so unreasonable that it would constitute child abuse. It would have to be beyond the limits of reason.[10] I do not see how anyone could conclude that the parents who opted for a xenograft heart transplant for their dying daughter when their options were so constrained were beyond reason when they judged it to be not only potentially beneficial but the best option available to them. Assuming their consent was adequately informed and voluntary, such parental choice strikes me as well within reason. Thus even if we agree that it would be wrong to conduct xenograft experiments on nonconsenting patients who do not stand to benefit, it would not follow that they should never be tried on those patients who could benefit, according to their own judgment, if they are competent, or the reasonable judgments of their guardians, if they are not.

The Resource Allocation Problem

This brings us to a fourth controversy surrounding the ethics of xenografts. It has been argued that even if xenografts do not violate any law of nature and do not violate any rights of animals and do not necessarily constitute nontherapeutic interventions on nonconsenting subjects, they still consume significant resources that are better spent elsewhere. Xenografts surely, according to this argument, constitute exotic technological innovation with low probability of short-term payoffs. The critics ask whether our resources would not better be spent on more basic interventions in preventive care and more simple treatments.

A number of people have suggested that even if the animal rights issues and consent problems are solved, it is unethical to spend hundreds of thousands of dollars on exotic, high-technology care when others in our society are doing without the basics of preventive care, maternal and child health services, and other basic medical needs. This argument is usually offered against experimental transplant surgery such as Fae's. It is that argument that deserves further attention.

Such an argument rests fundamentally on a cost–benefit reasoning that is insensitive to basic questions of social justice and, therefore, incompatible with the Judeo–Christian tradition. The observation that appears to drive the critics of expensive, high-technology medical interventions is that more good could be done if the resources currently invested in the Baby Faes of the world were spent on primary care. Assuming that is true, however, it does not follow that care should be so diverted. The hidden moral premise is that net utility in aggregate should be maximized as a matter of social policy even when aggregating utility masks any consideration of the distribution of benefits and harms. Although that may be good-act utilitarianism, it violates the moral insights of the Judeo–Christian tradition.

The argument takes us into the center of the ethics of distributive justice. It hinges in large part on how one ought to be evaluating benefits. Two basic strategies are available for assessing how resources ought to be distributed. One, the approach dominating much contemporary health planning and public health, emphasizes the maximization of the aggregate net welfare that will come from an investment in health care. It is the strategy that leads to the methods of cost–benefit and cost-effectiveness analysis, two devices that are really nothing more than sophisticated strategies for adding up the benefits and harms of alternative courses of action. The underlying philosophical premise is that of utilitarianism—doing the greatest good for the greatest number.

Under such an ethic of distribution, quite frankly, xenografts are going to be difficult to justify. It is the approach that leads to invitations to imagine how many immunizations against measles could be provided for the cost of one organ transplant. Conceivably even on these grounds xenografts would come out ahead in the calculation. The short-term benefits are admittedly not very likely, but if there were a success, the reward would be great. Moreover, in the long-term countless lives might be saved, not only from hearts but from other organ transplants as well. It is nevertheless quite difficult to imagine that spending equal resources on xenografts and preventive medicine would lead to greater net benefits in aggregate from the xenografts.

There is a second way of assessing the ethics of distribution, however. This second alternative will be emphasized in Part Three of this book when we deal with allocation of organs. Some people argue that it is a mistake to look only at the net aggregate benefit from alternative courses of action. They say that, instead, one needs to focus on the special needs of special groups. The least well-off among us, according to this second strategy, have special priorities. According to philosopher John Rawls the basic institutions of the society should be arranged so that the least well-off groups have their interests served.[11] This suggests that policies should be arranged to devote significant resources to the least well-off even if they do not efficiently maximize the payoff for the society as a whole.

Others, those who consider themselves egalitarians, reach a similar conclusion, arguing that resources should be arranged to provide for greater equality. I[12] and, if I understand it correctly, much of the Judeo–Christian tradition, hold to this theory of distribution, a theme I will develop further in Chapter 25. The important thing is that resources get skewed toward the least well-off rather than toward approaches that simply produce great aggregate societal benefit.

Although the application of this to health care is complex, a case can be made that the egalitarian principle of justice requires that, whenever possible, an individual be given an opportunity for health equal to that of any other individual. That probably means that there are enough resources for both primary prevention and high technology. If a choice must be made, however, the resources should go to the least well-off. According to egalitarian justice, primary care would get priority only if those who did not get it would be worse off than those needing, but not receiving, the high-technology interventions.

What does all this mean for xenografts? Where do those who might receive xenograft transplants stand in relation to others in the society? Are they among the least well-off? At first, it would appear that anyone who is sick enough that a xenograft is likely to benefit is in very bad shape, plausibly among the least well-off in the society. I am convinced that is true for some but not all possible xenograft recipients.

The critical question is whether we evaluate how well-off people are at a moment in time or over their lifetimes. Some older persons are admittedly very sick at the moment, but they may have had long, productive, enjoyable lives. If this over-a-lifetime perspective is adopted, then some persons who have completed their life cycles could be said to have very low claims on societal medical resources even though they will not live long without treatment. On the other hand, the very young who are critically ill would appear from the over-a-lifetime to be very poorly off indeed. They are dying without having had the benefits of many years of life. This perspective would place Baby Fae near the top of the list in terms of how poorly off she was. She and similarly ill infants could easily be considered the worst off of the society. (These issues will be explored further in Chapter 22.)

This suggests that even if xenografts are not terribly efficient in improving societal health statistics—mortality and morbidity rates—there are claims of justice from certain among our number for significant investments in resources. If a xenograft is, according to the parental judgment, likely to offer some chance of benefit for an infant who is surely among the least well-off of our society, and if we are a society who responds to the needs of the neediest, then a xenograft for that infant is going to have a high-priority claim of justice. It will have such a claim even if the payoff is not very great and even if other critically ill patients—

those who have had long, happy lives—do not have such a priority claim. Thus even if the consenting adult ought to be first from the standpoint of a theory of informed consent, it may be that infants whose needs are great deserve even higher priority.

The Virus Problem

One final issue has emerged with xenografts that may become the most difficult to surmount. Over the past several years increasing concern has been expressed about the transmission of viruses from animals to humans during the process of xenograft transplantation.[13]

The Science of Cross-Species Virus Transmission

Some of the concerns about the use of primates as organ sources have been mitigated by the development of the transgenic pig as a potential source.[14] Pigs are easily bred, already mass-bred for human consumption, and offer anatomical and physiological fit encouraging for human transplant. Transgenic pigs, with human genes introduced that code for complement regulatory proteins, can be protected from hyperacute rejection.[15] Concern now exists, however, about the small but real risk that viruses could be transmitted from the pig to humans receiving organs and then from the human organ recipient to other humans. With the history of the HIV virus moving from nonhuman animals to humans vivid in our consciousness, even a small risk raises great concern. There is the possibility that porcine endogenous retroviruses (PERVs) would be transmitted to humans. Particularly in the immunosuppressed patient, viral recombination could pose a potential threat.[16] Although recent observations are encouraging to those who are eager to develop xenograft transplantation using the pig,[17] the science is evolving very rapidly. It would be a mistake to make any final judgments at the time of this writing about the eventual outcome of this debate.

As of early 1999, Britain had developed a set of national guidelines for controlled clinical trials and the United States had draft guidelines, but the Council of Europe had adopted a moratorium on clinical trials and several European countries were in the process of imposing moratoria.[18] By April 1999 the U.S. officials had reversed course. The FDA, citing risks to third parties, announced a de facto ban on xenotransplant trials. It informed anyone wanting to apply for approval of protocols that it would not be possible to satisfy the FDA that the procedures are safe.[19] The issue to be addressed is what the ethics of proceeding with xenograft development is assuming that there can be no guarantee for the near future that the risk of viral transmission will be completely eliminated.

The Ethics of Third-Party Risks

The possibility of viral transmission poses the one truly new issue of xeno-transplant. In the case of human to human transplant the risks to the transplant recipient—risks of being exposed to HIV, cytomegalovirus, cancer, and other diseases as well as rejection risks and graft-versus-host disease—were risks that could be evaluated and accepted or rejected by the recipient. The same is true for any theoretical risk that the transplant recipient will be exposed to endogenous viruses from other species. However, in the case of these viruses, there is also a possibility that other human beings will be exposed (just as they are with the HIV virus). This means that when the recipient of a xenograft consents to the risk, he or she is, in effect, consenting to some risks to other parties.

That, of course, poses serious ethical problems. It would seem fair that those other parties who are put at risk should have to agree in some way to that risk. Close relatives, such as spouses, may be among those most at risk, and they are theoretically capable of being educated about the risk and consenting to it or not. However, some of those at risk will inevitably be children and others incapable of making autonomous choices and incapable of consenting. Also, direct consent to the risk is not feasible for distant relatives, friends, and strangers. The real question, then, is whether potential transplant recipients who are willing to take their own personal risks of viral infection to get an organ have a right to take these risks without any explicit approval of the other exposed parties. This is essentially a problem of what economists would call "externalities" of such decisions—risks that the decision maker may not take into account in making his or her choice.

Part of this problem will be addressed by requiring governmental and other public agencies (the U.S. Department of Health and Human Services or the United Network for Organ Sharing [UNOS], for example) to approve of the regulations or guidelines. That simply shifts the moral question, however, to one of the basis on which these agencies ought to approve of these risks to third parties without their direct and explicit consent.

The most restrictive standard would be that no third party be put at any risk without his or her explicit consent. That would, of course, make xenotransplant impossible. It would also make impossible most other socially worthwhile programs—for example, constructing roads, building schools, and developing a police force. A policy requiring explicit, individual consent is not plausible.

Another approach that could be used is to endorse xenografts only if it can be shown that the benefits from the xenograft can be expected to exceed the harms—including the harms to third parties. This would be the utilitarian justification. There are two problems with that criterion, however. First, the quantification of expected benefits as well as expected harms is almost impossible. The problem is not just the usual one of having to quantify uncertainties and subjective goods and harms; it is also that the potential benefits and harms are both almost unlimited. On the one hand, if xenografts from a commonly available animal such as a pig become successful, thousands—eventually millions—of life years could be the result. On the other, if the worst fears were realized, another HIV epidemic or worse could result.

The real issue is whether assessment of benefits and risks to the society is the real basis for making this choice. Another approach would be to rest the decision on the principle of justice, focusing on the needs or interests of the worst-off persons. As we have seen previously, the principle of justice supports arranging social practices to benefit these worst-off people or to give them opportunities to be as well-off as others insofar as that is possible. It would support such practices even if the effect were a net decrease in the amount of good in the society—provided that was necessary to improve the lot of the worst off.

The implications of the principle of justice, although also not easy to determine in the case of viral transmission risk via xenotransplant, may turn out to be easier to estimate than if the principle of utility were the criterion. People so ill that they are candidates for transplant are surely not well-off. Those on waiting lists who are so ill that they are willing to volunteer to be pioneers in an experiment to transplant organs from pigs or other nonhuman animals are probably particularly poorly off. They would be members of the kind of group that would have a special claim grounded in the principle of justice, a claim for society to adopt social practices that are designed to benefit them, even if the interests of others in the society are to the contrary.

But even very sick people in organ failure are not helped if they should contract a serious viral disease from a pig. That risk, however, is one that people desperate for an organ might rationally be willing to take. Thus assuming they are reasonably well informed and rational about their decision to take the chance on the xenograft, their choice to undergo the procedure would be understandable and, for egalitarians, justified.

Still, someone approaching this issue from the perspective of the principle of justice would have to ask whether the others in society have interests that must be taken into account. Surely they do, and potential xenograft experimenters would be decent to take those interests into account. But how ought society to take them into account in deciding policy about whether to permit volunteers to receive experimental xenografts when we do not know the risk of virus transmission?

The justice theorist, at least one who interprets justice as requiring arranging practices to serve the interests of the worst off among us, will ask whether it is possible that the others at risk from introducing the virus into the human species could plausibly end up even worse off than the transplant candidate. Any such even-worse-off bystanders would have a legitimate claim to block the xenograft experiment.

Although it cannot be denied that someone who became infected via human to human transmission of the hypothetical virus from a xenograft recipient could be even worse off, it is important to note how unlikely that would be. First, the xenograft recipient would be in double jeopardy. He or she would be very poorly off from organ failure—a failure so severe that the individual is willing to risk experimental xenograft. Second, if it should turn out that some virus was indeed a danger to humans, that recipient would also be a victim of the virus. If we are trying to identify who is the worst off, the person with severe organ failure combined with the serious viral infection is surely worse off than the one contending only with the virus. There is more to consider. The dose of the virus received by the transplant recipient is quite likely to be larger than one passed on to other humans through blood, body fluids, or other modes of transmission. If the seriousness of the risk is dose-dependent, the transplant recipient is statistically in a worse position.

Finally, there is a technical problem in how we calculate how poorly off people are. If a large group of people each have a small chance of being exposed to a deadly disease, do we view each person statistically as being relatively well-off because his or her harm is considered to be the harm of getting the disease multiplied by the probability of getting it or do we describe the group as being made up of many people who are well-off because they will not get the disease plus a small number who are in a very bad position because they will get it? If the former approach is used, then no one can be identified who is very poorly off (because each person is viewed as having only a small chance of getting the disease). If the latter approach is appropriate, then a few people are very poorly off. However, even if the latter approach is the right one, the unfortunate ones who get the viral disease are still better off than those who receive the transplant and get the virus as well.

Of course, there may be some people in society who are even worse off than people with the worst imaginable outcome of a virus exposure—people with amyotrophic lateral sclerosis (ALS) or extreme poverty or pain, for example. According to the principle of justice, they would have prior claims. But if the virus-risk issue is one of whether the risk to others in society is justified to benefit those needing transplants, the correct question is what can be done to benefit them (even if others who are better off are put at risk). For those who have been reasonably well-informed about the risks and the alternatives and still choose to volunteer to receive the xenograft, they have a strong claim of justice to getting the organ. The interests of those in society who are better off do not have the moral weight that they would in a more straightforward utilitarian analysis.

Thus an ethic that focuses on justice would probably be more supportive of xenografts in the face of possible viral risks than a utilitarian one would. In Chapter 2 I suggested that the only considerations that legitimately compete with a principle such as justice are the other non–consequence-maximizing principles (veracity, fidelity, autonomy, and avoidance of killing). By contrast beneficence and nonmaleficence—maximizing the aggregate good and minimizing the aggregate evil—should come into play only when the other principles are satisfied or when they offset each other so that beneficence and nonmaleficence are tie-breakers.

If this is the proper approach, then the viral-transmission issue would be a problem only if some people getting the virus from transplant recipients were even worse off or if one of the other principles militated against permitting the exposure. For example, fidelity or promise-keeping is one of these principles. If members of the public had somehow been promised that no xenografts would take place as long as there was a risk of virus transmission, the duty to keep that promise would count against the justice argument I have presented. This seems quite unlikely, however. If the mere fear of harm to others who are actually better off than the transplant candidate is not a legitimate moral concern, then it seems that ethical support for xenografts would exist. Of course, utilitarians might reach a different conclusion, but they would have to show that the risks to the population exceeded the benefits to the transplant recipients (including all future recipients who could eventually benefit from establishing that animal organs were adequately safe and effective). This would be very hard for a utilitarian to show. In that case, respect for the autonomy of consenting transplant recipients would seem to support those who want to volunteer for xenografts. Thus even a utilitarian might end up supporting policies that take prudent risks to conduct studies to see if the viral transmission problem was real.

Conclusion

Where does that leave us? If xenografts do not violate any natural law, if they are found not necessarily to violate the rights of animals, if they do not constitute research without hope of benefit on unconsenting patients, if the patient is among the least well-off in the society, and if the virus issue can be settled—if all of those conditions are met and if the more traditional requirements of medical ethics having to do with confidentiality and consent and respect for the rights of patients are met—then xenografts will have passed the test of ethics. It is a stiff test, but one that some xenografts surely will be able to meet.

If so, someday the inherent shortage of human organs may be overcome. In the meantime, if our transplants are constrained by the natural limits of the supply from brain-dead and non–heart-beating deceased humans, we must face the other major challenge in the ethics of organ transplant: Who will receive this precious, but scarce resource. It is the allocation of organs that is the topic of Part Three.

ENDNOTES

1. This summary is based on "Report of the National Institutes of Health" [the report of the NIH team investigating the Baby Fae transplant], *Spectrum* 16 (1, April 1985): 19–26. See also Leonard L. Bailey, Sandra L. Nehlsen-Cannarella, Waldo Concepcion, and Weldon B. Jolley, "Baboon-to-Human Cardiac Xenotransplantation in a Neonate," *Journal of the American Medical Association* 254 (23, Dec. 20, 1985): 3321–29.

2. Richard McCormick, "Was There Any Real Hope for Baby Fae?" *Hastings Center Report* 15 (1, Feb. 1985): 12.

3. Fred Rosner, "Artificial and Baboon Heart Implantation: The Jewish View," *Archives of Internal Medicine* 145 (July 1985): 1330.

4. Tom Regan, "The Other Victim," *Hastings Center Report* 15 (1, Feb. 1985): 9.

5. Fred Rosner, "Artificial and Baboon Heart Implantation: The Jewish View."

6. Samuel Gorovitz, "Will We Still Be 'Human' If We Have Engineered Genes and Animal Organs?" *Washington Post*, Dec. 9, 1984, p. C4.

7. Robert J. Levine, *Ethics and Regulation of Clinical Research* (Baltimore: Urban & Schwarzenberg, 1981).

8. Alexander Morgan Capron, "When Well-Meaning Science Goes Too Far," *Hastings Center Report* 15 (1, Feb. 1985): 8–9; George Annas, "Baby Fae: The 'Anything Goes' School of Human Experimentation," *Hastings Center Report* 15 (1, Feb. 1985): 15–17; Richard McCormick, "Was There Any Real Hope for Baby Fae?"

9. President's Commission for the Study of Ethical Problems in Medicine and Biomedical and Behavioral Research, *Deciding to Forego Life-Sustaining Treatment: Ethical, Medical, and Legal Issues in Treatment Decisions* (Washington, DC: U.S. Government Printing Office, 1983), p. 212; Robert M. Veatch, "Limits of Guardian Treatment Refusal: A Reasonableness Standard," *American Journal of Law and Medicine* 9 (4, Winter 1984): 427–68.

10. Robert M. Veatch, "Limits of Guardian Treatment Refusal: A Reasonableness Standard."

11. John Rawls, *A Theory of Justice* (Cambridge, MA: Harvard University Press, 1971).

12. Robert M. Veatch, *The Foundations of Justice: Why the Retarded and the Rest of Us Have Claims to Equality* (New York: Oxford University Press, 1986).

13. M. G. Michaels, "Xenotransplant-Associated Infections," *Laboratory Animal Science* 48 (1998): 228–33.

14. F. N. Bhatti, M. Schmoeckel, A. Zaidi, E. Cozzi, G. Chavez, M. Goddard, J. J. Dunning, J. Wallwork, and D. J. White, "Three-Month Survival of HDAFF Transgenic Pig Hearts Transplanted into Primates," *Transplantation Proceedings* 31 (1–2, 1999): 958; T. Kozlowski, A. Shimizu, D. Lambrigts, K. Yamada, Y. Fuchimoto, R. Glaser, R. Monroy, Y. Xu, M. Awwad, R. B. Colvin, A. B. Cosimi, S. C. Robson, J. Fishman, T. R. Spitzer, D. K. Cooper, and D. H. Sachs, "Porcine Kidney and Heart Transplantation in Baboons Undergoing a Tolerance Induction Regimen and Antibody Adsorption," *Transplantation* 67 (1, 1999): 18–30.

15. M. Schmoeckel, F. N. Bhatti, A. Zaidi, E. Cozzi, P. D. Waterworth, M. J. Tolan, G. Pino-Chavez, M. Goddard, R. G. Warner, G. A. Langford, J. J. Dunning, J. Wallwork, and D. J. White, "Orthoptic Heart Transplantation in a Transgenic Pig-to-Primate Model," *Transplantation* 65 (1998): 1570–77.

16. J. Brown, A. L. Matthews, P. A. Sandstrom, L. E. Chapman, "Xenotransplantation and the Risk of Retroviral Zoonosis," *Trends in Microbiology* 6 (10, Oct. 1998): 411–15.

17. Ehsan Masood, "Xenotransplant Experts Face Good and Bad News," *Nature* 394 (1998): 513; W. Heneine, A. Tibell, W. M. Switzer, P. Sandstrom, G. V. Rosales, A. Mathews, O. Korsgren, L. E. Chapman, T. M. Folks, and C. G. Groth, "No Evidence of Infection with Porcine Endogenous Retrovirus in Recipients of Porcine Islet-Cell Xenografts," *Lancet* 352 (1998): 695–98; C. Patience, G. S. Patton, Y. Takeuchi, R. A. Weiss, M. O. McClure, L. Rydberg, and M. E. Breimer, "No Evidence of Pig DNA or Retroviral Infection in Patients with Short-Term Extracorporeal Connection to Pig Kidneys," *Lancet* 352 (1998): 699–701; Leibniz Research Laboratories for Biotechnology and Artificial Organs, "Porcine Endogenous Retrovirus (PERV) Was Not Transmitted from Transplanted Porcine Endothelial Cells to Baboons in Vivo," *Transplant International* 11 (4, 1998): 247–51.

18. Nigel Williams, "Paving the Way for British Xenotransplant," *Science* 281 (Aug. 7, 1998): 767; U.S. Department of Health and Human Services, "Draft Public Health Service (PHS) Guideline on Infectious Disease Issues in Xenotransplantation (Aug. 1996)," 61 Fed. Reg. (Sept. 23, 1996): 49920–32; Declan Butler, "Europe Is Urged to Hold Back on Xenotransplant Clinical Trials," *Nature* 397 (1999): 281–82; U.S. Department of Health and Human Services, Food and Drug Administration, "Guidelines for Industry: Public Health Issues Posed by the Use of Nonhuman Private Xenografts in Humans," 64 Fed. Reg. (April 6, 1999): 16743–44.

19. Declan Butler, "FDA Warns on Primate Xenotransplants," *Nature* 398 (1999): 549.

PART THREE

ALLOCATING ORGANS

Who Empowers Medical Doctors to Make Allocative Decisions for Dialysis and Organ Transplantation?

The title for this chapter was assigned to me as a title for a lecture to a large international group of transplant surgeons meeting in Germany. To this day I do not know if the person assigning the title knew what he was asking for. There is a short answer to the question, "Who empowers medical doctors to make allocative decisions for dialysis and renal transplantation?" and that answer is "No one." Rather than simply stopping at this point, I would like to develop the argument why, in my opinion, it is a serious mistake for the public to expect clinicians to take on the responsibility for allocating any health resource, including dialysis and transplantation.

The Reality of Allocation

The reality, at least in the United States, of the health care system with which I am most capable of speaking, is that no physician in his or her role as clinician is ever expected to allocate either a dialysis machine or an organ for transplantation. The normal limiting factor for dialysis is the availability of machines and the funding to operate them. The U.S. Congress has, through an amendment to the Medicare laws, categorically covered all appropriate dialysis patients. Of course, clinicians will continue to be expected to determine which patients will benefit medically from dialysis, but in the normal sense of rationing—as we were forced to allocate scarce hemodialysis machines in the 1960s—allocation need not take place. In other countries, there may be fewer machines available, but even then, I shall argue, physicians ought not be the ones who allocate.

For transplantation the story is quite different. Organs are inherently scarce. It is not just a matter of money but also of the availability of the organs themselves.

The problem has recently become more acute because, although the need for organs continues to grow, the supply of organs has not. Even if organ availability were maximized through freedom-infringing routine salvaging of cadaver organs, we probably would not have enough—or would not have enough if technical problems were solved. Someone must allocate.

Still it does not follow that clinicians are expected to do the allocating. By law, in the United States all organs are made available through organ procurement organizations in cooperation with the national United Network for Organ Sharing (UNOS). Its board, under legislative guidelines, sets the principles for allocation of scarce organs and creates a formula for allocating them. Local practices must conform to UNOS policies or to authorized variances, and UNOS policies must, in turn, conform to nationally set public principles. No clinician can gain access to an organ for transplant unless he or she conforms to the decisions of the local procurement organization, UNOS, and the U.S. Congress.

To take kidney allocation as an example, whenever a kidney becomes available in a local procurement organization, a nationally approved formula determines a priority list of possible recipients. The formula takes into account histocompatability, panel-reactive antibody levels, logistics, waiting time, whether the recipient has previously been a living organ donor, and, under special circumstances, medical urgency. Whenever a kidney becomes available, a computer generates a priority list among all eligible patients awaiting kidney transplant. The organ procurement organization is required to offer the organ to the person scoring highest according to the allocation formula. This has the advantage of eliminating any charge of special ad hoc considerations or prejudices influencing the allocation. It also has the effect of completely removing the clinician from the allocation decision at the local level. To be sure, physicians are well represented in both the local and national boards that establish and operate the allocation formulas. Physicians, primarily transplant surgeons, make up about half of the UNOS board. When other health professionals—nurses and transplant coordinators—are included, this group makes up a dominant majority of the board. I will show throughout the chapters that follow that this dominance of the moral perspective of transplant professionals skews the allocation principles in ways that are not fully supported by the general public. Nevertheless, individual clinicians at the bedside do no direct allocating involving their own patients. I am convinced that this is the only morally defensible arrangement. My only quarrel is with the way points have been assigned in the formula. It is the public's responsibility to make sure that the UNOS allocation formulas fairly reflect the proper moral principles. That probably means eventually readjusting the UNOS board so that it is not as heavily dominated by transplant surgeons and other health professionals. For example, the president of UNOS has always been a physician, even though a significant minority of the board has always included transplant recipients, donor-family representatives, philosophers, attorneys, and representatives of community perspectives. I would like to summarize the argument that leads to this conclusion that clinicians should not be making allocation decisions at the bedside and should play a less dominant role in the policy-making process.

Allocation as a Moral Rather Than a Technical Matter

To understand why bedside clinicians should have no role in allocating dialysis machines or transplantable organs, we need to understand why someone might be inclined to assign this life-and-death task to them. I think the working assumption of those who would expect clinicians to be allocators is either that allocations can be made on the basis of factual medical information about patients or that allocations should be made on the basis of the values of physicians. My thesis is that key features of allocations are not factual in the medical sense; they are necessarily evaluative, but should not be made on the basis of the personal values of physicians.

The Role of Medical Facts in Allocation

Surely medical data are relevant in deciding how to allocate scarce medical services. We should continue to expect clinicians to determine the probable effects of transplant in patients who are potential candidates for these services. It is certainly sound to hold that no patient should be a candidate for these procedures whose medical condition will not be affected by them. But the patient who would not be affected is not likely to want the procedures anyway. The real debate is over how to allocate in cases in which more patients wanting care have medical conditions that will be affected than there are organs to respond to those needs. The issue is particularly controversial when we can expect different patients to benefit in different degrees, yet all of the potential recipients will benefit to some degree.

If we could assume that the scarce resource should automatically go to the person who would benefit most, it might appear that clinicians would be in a good position to play a role in deciding who should get the organs. As we shall see, however, it is very implausible to allocate organs on the basis of who will get the most benefit and, even if that were the correct principle, determining what counts as a benefit is inherently controversial and independent of medical facts. One patient may have the greatest chance of survival of acute illness; another may have the greatest predicted years of survival; still another may receive the greatest relief from suffering or morbidity; and another get the most satisfaction. Medical facts alone cannot tell us which of these patients will benefit the most from transplant.

More critically, even if we knew which patient would benefit the most medically from the procedure, we cannot automatically conclude that that patient should receive the medical procedure. Social utilitarians would insist that we take into account social and other nonmedical consequences to all parties of assigning the scarce resource to a particular person—a determination about which physicians surely are not expert. Utilitarians would, for example, ask not only about the benefits to the recipient of an organ but also about how much good for others providing the organ would do. Saving some lives could be thought to do more total good than others. People who are in responsible positions—public officials, business leaders, brilliant scientists, and so forth—will contribute more aggregate good than more ordinary citizens. In fact some transplant candidates may actually provide net disutility if they receive organs. Even if they gain benefit, it could be offset with the expected harms to others. There is, for example, a controversy over whether convicted criminals, particularly those convicted of serious, repeat offenses, should receive organs. Critics argue that even if one takes into account the benefits to the recipient and those family and friends who still care about the recipient, the net effect of saving the life may be negative when one considers the consequences to others.

On the other hand, trying to quantify the net consequences of saving one life rather than another is an enormously difficult task. In the early days of dialysis, the committees responsible for allocating dialysis machines had to face these questions. The committees charged with allocating machines might someday have had to decide whether a head of a large corporation, a poet, or a mother of three small children would contribute most benefit to society. These early committees also began to discover that the people chosen looked strangely like the members of the committee. There were even disutilities of the process of deciding which candidates would contribute most to society—paralyzing controversies over which people were most valuable. This is a controversy I will revisit in Chapter 23 when I discuss the role of status in organ allocation.

The end result of this debate was a widespread social consensus that social consequences—benefits to third parties—should be excluded from the allocation process. Some people reach that conclusion because they believe it is intrinsically wrong to give organs on this basis. They challenge the basic approach of social utilitarianism. They believe that people deserve to be treated more equally regardless of their ability to make social contributions. Others may accept social utilitarianism in principle but reach the pragmatic conclusion that allocating organs and other medical technologies on the basis of such vague and complex considerations causes more harm than good. The time spent in deciding what the long-term social consequences are of giving an organ to one person from a long list of candidates might not be worth it when one realizes how complex the calculations would be and how much discord could be generated from the feuds over the calculations.

Critics of social utilitarianism may insist that the allocation be made solely on the basis of patient-centered reasons. They would exclude all third-party effects. This is the moral principle of the Hippocratic Oath and seems to support the notion that physicians might be the proper allocators after all. However, limiting allocation considerations to the effects on the potential recipient does not imply that the organ should go to the one who would benefit the most medically. Among those in the Hippocratic camp, some people would emphasize considering total good in all spheres of a potential recipient's life—economic, social, educational, aesthetic, spiritual, and other benefits, as well as those measured in medical terms. That is one interpretation of the Hippocratic mandate. Making these assessments of total individual benefit would still require skills well beyond those of the bedside clinician. Others, however, would constrict the relevant considerations still further, limiting them to medical benefits—in other words, changes in morbidity and mortality expected to result from the organ graft. Deciding whether to consider medical benefits to the individual or total benefits to that recipient is, once again, a question that physicians are not in a good position to answer. In fact, we should expect that physicians might be more inclined than others to give special consideration to medical benefit. It is plausible that those who have found medicine so important that they have chosen to give their lives to the field might give special emphasis to the medical component (just as professional specialists in other areas might be biased in favor of their areas—artists emphasizing the aesthetic, clergy the spiritual, etc.). It is reasonable that specialists in any area would overemphasize their area of concern when compared with the values of the general public.

Even if we could agree that the allocation decision should be limited to expected medical benefits, that does not mean that clinicians can be considered to be authoritative. Certainly, they will be expert in deciding what the effects are likely to be of a transplant, but deciding what is a medical benefit is a deceptively complicated issue. Medical benefits involve many different considerations. Some might emphasize years of added life expected, using added survival as the criterion of a medical benefit. Others might use predicted graft survival, recognizing that the person with the best predicted graft survival (based on, say, human lymphocyte antigen [HLA] matching considerations) might not be the same person who has the longest predicted survival. In estimating length of predicted survival, we would take into account probability of graft survival, but also how long the person is expected to live if the graft is successful. An 80-year-old with a zero-mismatched kidney may have a shorter predicted survival than a 20-year-old receiving a significantly mismatched organ.

Survival is not the only medical benefit worth considering. Some people would see curing of disease a legitimate goal of medicine. Some transplant recipients may still have underlying pathology, either pathology that caused the organ failure in the first place or concomitant disease unrelated to the organ involved. The kidney recipient may also have heart disease unrelated to the kidney problem. That heart problem may have an impact that shows up in predicted years of life following transplant, but it may also affect morbidity. Should a life expectancy of 20 years following transplant be considered the same whether or not the survivor has incapacitating heart disease? Many would attempt to adjust the expected years of survival for the quality of life, taking into account the presence of comorbidities. Deciding whether to adjust years for expected quality is a controversial topic. The point is that if bedside clinicians were to do the allocating, they would have to decide whether to adjust life expectancy for quality, and they would have to determine how to make the adjustment. That is a skill that physicians do not have. There is a value choice to be made in deciding whether and how to make the adjustment, and physicians have no special skill in making those value choices. In fact, as I have suggested, they may have unique, profession-specific inclinations so that clinicians (or any other professional group) can be expected to make the choices atypically.

Deciding how much medical benefit will accrue from a graft is even more complex. Some people will include improved subjective sense of well-being as part of medical benefit; others will not. If two people could receive a graft with equal predicted life expectancy and equal expected medical morbidity but one will be more "nervous" about recurring disease than the other and therefore have less of a sense of medical well being, can we say that one person is expected to receive more medical well being than the other, or is his or her expected medical benefit objectively equal? Which of these criteria would be appropriate in allocating organs? Deciding overall medical well being will involve trade-offs among mortality, curing of disease, relief of suffering, and prevention of future disease. Being an expert in medicine does not make one an expert in making such trade-offs.

All of this discussion assumes that the goal of the decision is to use the medical resources with maximal efficiency, doing what will provide the most benefit. I have argued that physicians are not really expert in making the choices needed to determine which benefits count. But even if we were somehow to establish that physicians at the bedside were uniquely good at determining what allocation would do the most good, we need to recognize that most ethical theories deny that maximizing benefit is the proper ethic for resource allocation. Major theories of ethics insist that other considerations are morally relevant. Most important, adherents to such theories insist that fairness or justice be taken into account as well as medical or social utility in deciding what is an ethical allocation of organs.

For example, some might argue that justice requires that each candidate receive an equal chance of getting a scarce, social, life-saving resource such as a kidney even if not all have an equal chance of benefiting. They may insist that those who have waited longest or those who are sickest get priority, recognizing that these patients may not be the ones who would predictably benefit the most.

We need not solve the complex ethical problem of what is the correct basis for allocating scarce resources. The point is merely that, in principle, even perfect knowledge of the medical facts about the patients who are candidates cannot determine which patient should receive an organ or a dialysis machine. If the presumption of a clinician role in allocation is based on their expert medical knowledge of the patient, that cannot provide an adequate basis for defending a role for clinicians in the allocation decision. This perhaps suggests an important role for the clinician in providing medical data about the medical condition of the patient—histocompatability, prognosis without treatment, and likely outcomes with treatment—but these alone cannot determine the appropriate allocation. On this basis the clinician should provide data for those who create and run the allocation system; they should not make the allocation itself.

The Role of Clinician Values in Allocation

Sophisticated clinicians, especially those with knowledge of contemporary medical ethical literature, will readily concede that all medical judgments require ethical and other value judgments and that this includes decisions about dialysis and transplant. They argue at this point that there are values inherent in the medical profession that provide the clinician with a basis for deciding.[1] They point to the traditional values of preserving life, relieving suffering, and maintaining health.

There are serious problems, however, with permitting allocations to be made on the basis of the clinician's interpretation of these traditional medical professional values. First, as we have seen, the medical values in the interesting cases, i.e., those that are not simplistic, lead to contradictions among themselves. The allocation that most preserves life may not be the one that best relieves suffering or promotes health. Clinicians will differ among themselves over how these conflicts should be resolved. Even if they could agree completely, it would not follow that lay people—the ones whose lives are at stake and the ones who created the pool of resources to be allocated—would concur in the ranking.

The problem is even more severe when one realizes that it is not at all obvious that the goal is to maximize medical values. If clinicians can disagree among themselves and can disagree collectively with the general public over the ranking of medical values, they can disagree much more dramatically over the question of how medical values would relate to social, nonmedical goods and over how pursuing the maximum good should be related ethically to other moral norms such as promoting a just allocation.[2] Because these choices have nothing to do with medical knowledge, there is no reason why clinicians should be the ones making them. It is the general lay public that creates the money pool to support dialysis and creates the pool of cadaver organs to be allocated. They should be the ones making the moral choices relating medical to nonmedical goods and relating the pursuit of maximum benefit to maximum justice or fairness in allocation. Clinicians should remain free to give undivided loyalty to their patients. That is incompatible with asking them to be resource allocators.

The U.S. Kidney Allocation Formula: An Example

To make the nature of the problem concrete, imagine two patients under the care of different nephrologists in the same community, both of whom are awaiting kidney transplants when a single kidney becomes available. Patient A, 30 years old, has a 2 AB, 2 DR match, that is, the patient matches on 2 AB antigens and 2 DR antigens (four of the six that are possible), with a potential donor and has been waiting three months for a kidney. Patient B is 58 years old, and has only a 1 AB, 1 DR match with the donor. He has 80 percent panel reactive antibodies (PRA) but is a negative cross-match with the donor. In part because of the high PRA, he has been waiting for 18 months for a transplant. His medical condition has deteriorated during the wait so that his condition is now described as urgent. Nevertheless, considering the deteriorating medical condition and cross-match history and his age, his probability of successful graft survival is considered less than Patient A. What contribution could the physicians for each of these patients make to the allocation decision?

Each historically has an ethical duty to serve the interests of his or her own patient. Presumably, each would make the argument that served those interests. Patient A's physician would emphasize the greater likelihood of success and, based on age, the longer expected life of his candidate; Patient B's physician would emphasize the equity issues related to long waiting time, high PRA, and the more serious medical condition of her patient. Even if either really believed in the moral case the other made, it is doubtful he or she should be swayed by that belief to abandon his or her own patient. Even if both physicians came to the conclusion, for instance, that medical benefit took precedence over equity, that might simply reflect the unique value perspective of medical professionals as a group. It cannot be taken to imply that the general public would support the priority of medical benefit over equity. The formula used for kidney allocation in the United States in the early 1990s assigned two-thirds of its points to medical benefit. It has not always been that way. An earlier formula used in the United

States gave much more emphasis to matters of fairness to patients who had special needs.[3] In rough terms three-fourths of the weight was given to equity, only one-fourth to predictors of good medical outcome. The current formula seems to swing back in the direction of emphasizing equity. Points assigned for HLA match are included as predictors of medical benefit. There remains a mandatory absolute priority for zero-HLA mismatched organs and up to seven points for other good matches. Those who have previously served as live donors of organs receive four points, a provision that is probably included to encourage donation (and therefore more benefits from the program) but also could be thought of as promoting fairness by rewarding behavior thought to be virtuous. Likewise, the points assigned to minors (to be discussed in Chapter 22) promote greater medical benefit but also can be defended on justice or fairness grounds. The four points included for having a high PRA are primarily to make the system more fair to a group who otherwise may have a difficult time finding a suitable organ. Finally, the points for time on the waiting list are clearly there to make the system fair to those who are hard to match with suitable organs. The present formula is thus about evenly balanced between consideration of medical benefit and justice or fairness.

Conclusion

For the moment, we need not determine what the correct balance of points is. For our purposes the question is whether individual clinicians or clinicians as a group should be empowered by the general community to choose the principles on which allocations will be made. In the case of a formula for organ allocation, the critical question is what should be the relative number of points given to medical benefit and to need or equity. Later in the book I will propose that as a compromise equal weight be given to each of the two considerations. Regardless of the answer, there seems to be no reason why clinicians should be empowered to make the choices. They are not related to the relevant medical expertise of the clinician; on the contrary the clinician ought to be committed to the welfare of his or her patient and therefore ought to come up with the wrong allocation decision. When we realize that any specialized professional group is likely to have ingrained commitments that lead it to unique answers to the key ethical question, I cannot see any reason why we should empower the medical professional to make allocative decisions.

ENDNOTES

1. Allen R. Dyer, "Virtue and Medicine: A Physician's Analysis," in *Virtue and Medicine: Exploration in the Character of Medicine*, ed. Earl E. Shelp (Dordrecht, Holland: D. Reidel, 1985), pp. 223–35; Leon R. Kass, *Toward a More Natural Science* (New

York: Free Press, 1985); Edmund D. Pellegrino and David C. Thomasma, *For the Patient's Good: The Restoration of Beneficence in Health Care* (New York: Oxford University Press, 1988).

2. Frances Kamm has also observed that clinicians have a unique set of moral commitments that lead them to strive to do what is maximally beneficial for their patients. See F. M. Kamm, *Morality, Mortality: Volume I: Death and Whom to Save from It* (New York: Oxford University Press, 1993), pp. 272, 293.

3. Thomas E. Starzl, Thomas R. Hakala, Andreas Tzakis, Robert Gordon, Anderi Steiber, Leonard Makowka, Joeta Klimoski, and Henry T. Bahnson, "A Multifactorial System for Equitable Selection of Cadaver Kidney Recipients," *Journal of the American Medical Association* 257 (1987): 3073–75.

Nineteen

A General Theory of Allocation

Once organs are procured, they must be allocated among the hundreds or thousands of potential recipients. In the United States there is a legal federal mandate that the allocation system must take into account both efficiency and equity.[1] In Chapter 2 I set out a general ethical theory and suggested that efficiency and equity are code words for two major principles in ethical theory: maximizing utility and distributing consequences justly. In some cases efficiency and equity are both served at the same time by the same allocation. They come together and the implications for an allocation decision are clear. But often the concepts are ambiguous and, once the meanings are clarified, efficiency and equity can come into conflict. Moreover, there are additional ethical considerations that are not accounted for by the principles of utility maximizing and justice in distribution. Western society is committed to respect for persons, including respect for their autonomy, for keeping commitments made to them, and dealing honestly with them. Overwhelmingly, we are committed to avoiding killing of humans, even in cases in which people are willing, indeed eager, to end their lives. These notions I refer to as the principles of *autonomy*, *fidelity*, *veracity*, and *avoiding killing*. Together with *utility* and *justice* they make up the core ethical principles.

An ethically acceptable allocation must conform to the requirements of these principles. Because any resulting policy will have to take many moral and practical concerns into account, we need a formula that integrates these multiple concerns in a concrete way. The point systems used to allocate organs in the United States should reflect these moral principles. Each point can be seen as being incorporated into the formula because it is a marker for one or more moral concerns. For example, we include points for human lymphocyte antigen (HLA) tissue typing in the kidney allocation formula because we believe that HLA match is an empirical predictor of the likelihood of graft survival. Tissue typing is included because it predicts good outcomes. By contrast points for time on the waiting list are included because we believe that treating people equally requires that we do something to respond to the needs of those who have waited the longest. There is no reason to assume that those who have waited the longest will do better or get more benefit from the available organs. In some situations that may be the case, but time on the waiting list is a factor in allocation because of our concern for justice. Assuming that most will consider both utility and justice—in other words, efficiency and equity—relevant, we need to examine the factors that might come into play in any allocation formula.[2]

Utility

It is obvious that we are interested in organ transplant because we are convinced that it can be beneficial to those in need of organs. There is utility in transplant. The utility is not limited, however, to the medical benefits to the recipients. There is also a broader social utility. Saving people's lives leaves them potentially able to return to society as productive citizens, which can produce social utility.

Social Utility

A pure social utilitarian would take all envisioned benefits of alternative uses of organs into account in deciding how to allocate organs. If giving the organ to the president of a company (or a nation) would do much more good than giving it to a homeless, unemployed person, this is the kind of information a utilitarian would find morally relevant. A straightforward utilitarian allocation policy would rank potential recipients on the basis of the amount of good that would result from receiving organs.

As we saw in the previous chapter, that ranking of recipients could get very controversial, however. It would require generating some interpersonal agreement on the amount of good that can be expected to be produced by each use of an organ. It was the original policy approach to the allocation of hemodialysis machines in the 1960s when they were still scarce resources. Shana Alexander has provided a detailed account of the chaos that resulted at the University of Washington when the dialysis selection committee tried to pick patients based on their social worth.[3] As we discussed in the previous chapter, it generates significant controversy to try to determine who is the most socially valuable in picking among a business executive, a poet, and a parent of three small children.

For various reasons there is widespread agreement that the social worth of recipients should be excluded from the organ allocation process. Utilitarians might argue that the very process of ranking recipients would be so controversial that there would be net disutility in opening the door to such considerations. One can envision investigators doing background checks on those on the organ waiting list. Even on utilitarian grounds, it may not make sense to consider social utility in organ allocation.

Of course, those who focus more on justice would have their own reasons for excluding social worth from the allocation. If they believe in the equal moral worth of all people regardless of their social contribution, they would reject such considerations in principle, even if it were easy to determine something called "social worth."

Medical Utility

Even if social utility is ruled out of bounds, the utilitarians are not finished using their approach in making allocation decisions. Considering *medical utility* has a much better press. Clearly, the goal of transplant is to save life, or at least make it more tolerable. If a transplant can be predicted to be very likely to do a great deal of medical good for one recipient but has almost no chance of helping another, that medical fact seems relevant. Just as there is a consensus against using social utility, there is also a consensus that medical benefit is morally relevant. Calculating the expected medical benefit of a transplant, however, can be a very difficult task. Several different factors have seemed relevant.

Patient Survival

The most obvious medical benefit from transplant is saving life. Of course, not all transplants are life-saving. Kidney transplant is more likely simply to improve life quality by sparing the patient from dialysis, but in some cases, such as those in which veins become inaccessible for dialysis, it can truly be life-saving.

Even if we agree that patient survival is an enormous benefit, it can present serious problems for utilitarians calculating the benefit of a transplant. Not only is there the complicated scientific question of predicting graft survival, there is the more theoretical problem of whether each life saved should count as an equal benefit. This is not the "social worth" question revisiting us—although that could become an issue. The first problem is whether it is the fact of a life saved that counts or whether we should, instead, count years of life added from transplants. Does saving a 50-year-old from imminent heart failure, leaving the beneficiary with a 20-year life expectancy count the same or half as saving a 30-year-old, leaving that person with a 40-year life expectancy? There is no factually correct answer to the question of whether it is lives saved or years of life added that should be counted. Both seem important, but deciding which is more important and how much to weight each in a formula is a serious problem for utilitarians.

Graft Survival

The story is made more complicated by the fact that people do not die just because organs fail, and not all organ failures lead to death. We measure graft survival as well as patient survival. Particularly in kidney transplant a graft failure merely puts one back on dialysis and back on the waiting line for another organ. Even in the case of life-prolonging solid organs, a graft failure could lead to a second transplant, although the case would certainly be a more urgent one.

It is clear that a graft failing is a bad thing even if the patient survives. At best, it will mean another transplant and the consumption of another scarce organ from the donor pool.

The problem for a theory of allocation is how much weight one should give graft survival as compared with patient survival. Should the calculation of medical utility of a transplant take into account both? If so, should the attention focus on the straight measure of expected years of graft survival or should it also take into account the expected impact of retransplant on those on the waiting list, on the insurance system, and on the patient and his or her family? Insofar as we are concerned about medical utility, it seems that the proper criterion, at least to begin the analysis, is the predicted number of years of life. For each organ available we should consider each potential recipient and determine life expectancy without transplant and life expectancy with transplant. The difference, taking into account the probability of a successful graft, would be the expected number of years added for each candidate. We shall start the consideration of medical utility with the assumption that the goal, insofar as medical utility is concerned, is to give the organ to the person expected to gain the greatest number of years of life from the organ.

PSYCHOLOGICAL STATE OF THE PATIENT AND QUALITY OF LIFE

Saving lives and minimizing graft failure are not the only medical good resulting from a successful transplant. Patients normally see a dramatic improvement in their psychological well-being and quality of life. A serious utility calculation would have to take these into account as well. Measuring such benefits is difficult. To use these benefits in allocation, we would have to determine differential psychological benefit to different people on the waiting list.

The more serious problem, however, is deciding how much weight to give changes in psychological well being compared with saving life. A strategy for dealing with comparing the quality of well being with the saving of life that is used in health planning is calculating what has been called a quality-adjusted life year (QALY).[4] It discounts the number of expected years of life by their quality by asking people to compare years of life in a particular compromised state (such as being on dialysis) with a shorter number of years in good health. Using responses, tables can be created that, for example, might view ten years on dialysis as the equivalent of eight healthy years. A year on dialysis then equals 0.8 QALYs. This ingenious strategy permits the integration of data measuring years of life with estimates of the quality of that life. Some utilitarians believe that the best health policy is the one that maximizes QALYs. Thus for each candidate for an organ we would estimate the number of additional years of life added (taking into account probabilities) and then adjust the estimate for the quality of the added years as well as the changes in quality of the years that the patient would have lived without the transplant. Differential QALYs is, then, the criterion for determining the expected medical utility that would result from giving the organ to each candidate. Because both quality and quantity of added life expected will vary as a function of the status of the donor (the donor's HLA antigens, blood type, and so forth), these estimates have to be made anew for each organ that becomes available.

The calculation of QALYs as a health planning tool has been criticized because it discriminates against hard-to-treat patients. These critics consider the approach to violate the principle of justice.[5] A more basic problem for organ allocation, however, is that no one has ever claimed that such strategies can be applied at the micro level in which, say, individual patients on a waiting list can be compared. At best these statistics could be used to compare organ transplants for different diagnoses or different candidate groups. The result would be, at best, an approximation of the amount of good done by transplanting a typical or average patient in a particular diagnostic category. To simplify the allocation decision, defenders of the criterion of maximizing expected medical utility favor basing the allocation on certain empirical factors that are known to correlate with medical outcome. These empirical factors become crude surrogates for predicting the number of QALYs each candidate can expect from an available organ. The factors need to be considered individually.

IMMUNOLOGIC FACTORS

For kidney transplants, the degree of HLA match is a predictor of graft survival. Although the science is not completely understood, it is known that each person has at least three pairs of HLA antigens (called A, B, and DR). Because there are many possible antigens of each type, there are literally thousands of possible combinations. With six antigens for donor and recipient there is a maximum match or mismatch of six antigens. It is common to report HLA by degree of mismatch rather than degree of match, thus making zero-mismatch the best status. This is done in part because not all six antigens can be identified in all patients. If not all six antigens are identified, either an antigen is present but unidentifiable or there is a homozygous pair (two copies existing of the same antigen). By reporting degree of mismatch, it is as if we assume missing antigens are present in duplicate. If, in fact, an unusual antigen is present but not identified, reporting mismatches provides a slight advantage to those with unidentifiable antigens, whereas reporting the number of matches would provide a disadvantage. Hence racial minority groups, who are more likely to have antigens that cannot be identified, would be disadvantaged if priority were based on degree of match but are advantaged if priority is based on degree of mismatch. Table 19.1 shows overall graft survival rates based on degree of antigen mismatch.

Thus the degree of match (or mismatch) is a predictor of graft survival. If the goal is to get as many life years as possible per graft, giving priority to recipients with the smallest number of mismatches with the particular donor makes sense. Points are therefore awarded based on number of mismatches. Logically, the points should be assigned in proportion to the influence of the particular mismatch on graft survival. If there are no mismatches, there is, as a matter of current policy, a mandatory priority, even if this involves sharing the organ with some other organ-procuring organization (OPO) or even some other region of the country. Beyond these mandatory shares, points are awarded as follows: seven points if there are no D or DR mismatches, five points if there is 1 B or DR mismatched, and two points if there is a total of two mismatches at the B and DR loci.[7]

There is much more to be learned about the science of tissue matching. At some point we are likely to know much more. Therefore the formula and the points assigned are likely to change. From the view of the theory of allocation, this raises questions about the legitimacy of using factors that we know are only crude approximations. Moreover, what HLA is predicting is graft survival, something already in our working list of factors that would interest a utilitarian. In the end what a utilitarian would want is a complex formula that assigns consideration based on the percentage of variance explained by each factor known to predict graft survival (or, more accurately, the number of QALYs expected to be added). We are only part way toward being able to construct such an algorithm.

TABLE 19.1 Kidney Graft Survival by Level of Human Lymphocyte Antigen (HLA) Mismatch (percentage)[6]

HLA mismatch	1-year survival	3-year survival	5-year survival
0	89.9	82.4	72.4
1	86.5	74.9	66.6
2	87.8	74.7	64.1
3	87.4	73.1	62.8
4	85.4	70.5	61.0
5	85.4	69.3	58.6
6	84.6	68.4	57.4

AGE

Age is another factor that predicts graft survival. Younger patients are believed to have more resiliency when facing major surgery. A good utilitarian would want to take that into account, giving more priority to younger patients on the waiting list. Chronological age, however, is not a perfect predictor of physiological age, what utilitarians would really be interested in. This, of course, poses problems of deciding how to incorporate age into a utilitarian calculus for predicting overall benefit from a transplant.

There are further complications. If we are using predicted years of patient survival as our criterion of medical utility, younger patients will not only have better results from their surgery, they will also have more years of future expected life. In a world in which antirejection medication were completely effective, many organs might survive until the patient's death. The older one is, the shorter the patient survival and therefore the shorter the predicted years of benefit from the graft. This is another reason why a consistent utilitarian would give greater weight to younger patients.

Finally, in the case of kidney transplant, age plays another role. Small children cannot only be expected to have their organs survive longer, they may get greater benefit from the transplant.[8] Small children in kidney failure experience growth problems and neurological damage that is not completely controlled by dialysis. Thus a utilitarian would want to give small children extra consideration over and above the belief that the surgery will go better and the expectation that they will get more years of graft use from their organ. That is one reason why the kidney allocation awards extra points to children (currently four additional points for children under age 11 and three for those older than 11 but less than 18).

AVAILABILITY OF ALTERNATIVE TREATMENTS

Another factor that a utilitarian would want to consider is the availability of alternative treatments. Other things being equal, we would want organs to go to those who had no alternative. The net good of such a policy would be greater because more lives would be saved. Hence most patients in end-stage renal failure have dialysis available. The few for whom veins are not accessible for dialysis would get priority not only because they are in greater need (that would be of concern to those committed to justice in allocation) but also because more net good is done.

Structuring a Utilitarian Allocation Formula

The project for a utilitarian who wanted to allocate organs according to the strategy of maximizing the net good from the transplant program regardless of the distribution of the good would be to construct a formula that adequately took into account all of these factors in their proper proportion. We have seen that a consistent utilitarian would have to factor in the social good that could come to society from each life saved (unless one could successfully argue that the disutilities of making these comparisons outweighed any benefits). When considering medical goods, one would first have to establish the overall outcome goal. Would it be short-term patient survival of the transplant (avoidance of acute rejection), expected years of life added to the patient, expected years of graft survival, or improvement in the quality of the patient's life?

Integrating these goals into a single formula is a formidable task. I have suggested that, in principle, the medical utility maximizer's goal should be to give an organ to the one who will predictably gain the greatest number of QALYs from the organ. Assuming that the goal can be identified, the next task would be to determine which specific factors—HLA matching, age, diagnosis, availability of alternative treatments—should be taken into account. The ideal formula would be one that includes every factor known to explain some of the variance in the outcome measure we have decided on. Because there are several different outcome goals, we can expect there will continue to be disputes among utilitarians over exactly what the proper formula should be.

Justice

The major problem for the utilitarian solution to the allocation problem is not determining the formula. The real issue is whether such a formula, even if it could be determined, would be fair or just. It is the essence of utilitarianism that it ignores the pattern of the distribution of the good being allocated.[9] Thus we have already seen that utilitarians would be inclined to discriminate against elderly people. They would discriminate against any hard-to-treat group. Data suggest that some racial groups will match to the donor pool better than others and therefore, predictably, will do better. The data also suggest that one gender does better than the other and one socioeconomic group better than another. Before one knows which sociological groups would be advantaged, it would be good to confront the critical question in the abstract.

Knowing that predicted success correlates with race, gender, age, and income level, would it be acceptable to take these sociological facts into account in allocating organs? A good utilitarian would, once it is known that these variables predict success and that it is impossible to identify exactly which people in the various groups will do better.

It turns out that statistically young, white, middle-class males will do best, at least in kidney transplant. We have already seen why age is relevant. Socioeconomic status probably has to do with having an intact support network available to help in recovery and following proper follow-up regimen. It is also relevant to the ability of recipients to comprehend and follow instructions about how to maximize the maintenance of the organ once transplanted. Gender is perhaps related, at least in part, to panel reactive antibodies (PRA), which we shall take up later in the chapter.

The concern of people committed to the moral principle of justice is that the allocation be fair or equitable. Because efficiency and equity sometimes conflict, the most efficient system at maximizing the good resulting from a transplant system will probably not be the fairest. Conversely, the fairest system will probably have to be inefficient. Depending on how one trades off the principles of utility and justice, one will give more or less weight to concerns about distribution.

In the abstract, the focus of any theory of justice is not on the amount of good done but on the pattern of the distribution of the good. Several factors have been proposed as the criteria for the proper pattern of distribution. Most modern theories of justice, however, are egalitarian. They consider a pattern of distribution to be just insofar as it contributes to giving people opportunities for equality of outcome. In health care that often means targeting those who are medically worst off to give them the opportunity, as far as possible, to be as healthy as other people. Because most allocation theories consider both need and utility, the result of defining justice in terms of medical need does not have to lead to an allocation in which members of some group who are terribly sick with incurable diseases command all the resources. The point is merely that, insofar as the principle of justice is concerned, we will strive to give the worst off opportunities to improve their situation.[10] Still identifying exactly what we mean by being medically worst off is a complex task.

At least three factors must be taken into account. I will call them *present need*, *urgency*, and *need over a lifetime*.

Present Need

Existing organ allocation often takes into account the present medical status of the potential recipient. The idea of the principle of justice, interpreted in an egalitarian way, is that all people should have an opportunity to be as well-off as others, as far as possible. That means those who are the sickest or otherwise worst off deserve first consideration. Sometimes those who are the sickest will also benefit the most by receiving a transplant. (If a life is saved from inevitable decline toward death, that is a substantial benefit, as well as saving someone who is plausibly considered to be among the worst off.) If so, the utilitarian would also give these people priority. However, some people are so ill that, although they are the sickest, they will predictably not get as much benefit from a transplant as some who are healthier. They may be so sick that they have a higher chance of dying regardless of treatment or they may simply have a condition that will be only partially ameliorated by the transplant. For example, persons diagnosed HIV positive who are in organ failure may not get as much benefit from transplant as those who are HIV negative who are healthier because the positive patients may die sooner regardless of the transplant.

It is these cases in which the worst off cannot be expected to get as much benefit from a transplant than better off patients that pose the most important moral conflict: the conflict between utility and present need, that is, efficiency and equity. While the utilitarian will favor the healthier patients, someone giving justice priority will want the sickest to get the organs. Someone who affirms both utility and justice will strive to combine both considerations into the allocation formula.

The idea is that the sickest person has the greatest need and, when considering justice, needs to be given priority. This is not a major factor for kidney transplant because these persons can usually be maintained indefinitely on dialysis, but for life-saving organs such as the heart or liver, how sick one is seems like a plausible indicator of need. Hence in the allocation of livers, a patient with fulminant liver failure with a life expectancy without a liver transplant of fewer than seven days is considered Status 1, the highest priority. Certain patients with chronic liver failure who are in the hospital's intensive care unit are Status 2A. Status 2B includes very sick patients such as those requiring hospitalization but not in intensive care. Status 3 patients require continual care but may be at home. The liver allocation formula generally gives higher priority to patients receiving a higher status. This is intended to be a measure of current medical need. This notion of how sick a patient is at the present time has been the definitive notion of need reflected in the national Task Force on Organ Transplantation and UNOS allocation policies. It is not the only way one can think about medical need, however.

Medical Urgency

New York University philosopher Frances Kamm deserves credit for increasing the sophistication of the discussion with regard to ways of thinking about medical need and urgency.[11] She defines urgency as "how soon someone will die without a transplant."[12] The crucial point is that some patients on the waiting list may need a transplant urgently even though they are not presently among the sickest categories of patients.

Among those who are not presently among the worst off, some may still have claims of justice because they are particularly urgent cases—that is, we can predict they will be among the worst off in the future if they are not transplanted soon. We should take into account that some people who are not presently the sickest may eventually become the worst off if they are not treated. A justice-based allocation would give priority to someone who is presently healthy but who will not have another chance to avoid becoming the sickest over someone who is presently sicker but who is stable and will not decline to be as poorly off. Two different kinds of cases of urgent need can be identified.

EXPECTED IMMINENT DECLINE

Consider, for example, a patient with a newly diagnosed primary cancer of the liver. Some centers treat such cancers, if detected early, with a liver transplant. Such persons may not feel terribly ill. They may be at home or even out and about in the community. Thus they may qualify as the rather low Status 3 priority. However, they may decline very rapidly to the point at which a transplant is no longer feasible. They may, in fact, die within months if not transplanted. Such a transplant has an urgency in spite of the fact that the present condition of the patient is that he or she is in relatively good condition. *Urgency*, as I am using the term, classifies transplant candidates on the basis of how long they can be expected to live without the transplant. I would measure this in QALYs, but because we are concerned about identifying who has a claim of justice (rather than a claim based on medical utility) we are not focusing on the expected number of QALYs added by the transplant but rather who has the smallest number of QALYs expected in the future—that is, who is worst off from a "future QALYs" perspective.

Often the patients who are presently the sickest will also have the greatest urgency, but that need not be the case. It seems that if we want to identify those on the waiting list with the greatest medical need, we should seek out those with the smallest number of expected future QALYs without transplant, not necessarily those who are presently the sickest.

LIKELIHOOD OF FINDING A SUITABLE ORGAN IN THE FUTURE

There is a second way in which a patient who is not presently among the sickest might be said to have a particularly urgent need. Some who do not have a rapidly progressing disease such as liver cancer may nevertheless be in urgent need because it can be predicted that there is a lower probability that they will have another chance at getting an organ.

High panel reactive antibodies (PRA). This distinction between those who will decline rapidly and those who are stable but will not have a good chance for an organ in the future is important for understanding why PRA is among the factors in an allocation formula. Some candidates for organ transplant have antibodies in their system from being exposed to foreign tissues previously. They are called *panel reactive antibodies* (PRA). This may be true for people who have received a graft previously. It may also be true of anyone who has received a blood transfusion and for women who have ever been pregnant. These antibodies may react to tissues in the transplant, causing a rejection.

It is possible to measure antibody levels and then cross-match the potential recipient with the specific donor to see if the antibodies are likely to cause a rejection. Anyone with PRAs above 80 percent is considered at particularly acute risk for such rejection. They will not be permitted to receive an organ from a donor who is a positive cross-match. Those with high PRA will thus face a difficult time in finding a suitable cross-match negative donor. Because of this, in kidney transplant they are given four bonus points. The reason is not that people with high PRA can be expected to do particularly well. Rather the concern is that if a cross-match negative organ becomes available, chances are greater that it will be the only suitable organ to become available for a long time. Out of fairness—the likelihood of finding another organ—the high-PRA patient is, therefore, given special consideration.

Blood group. For some organs, such as livers, the recipient must be blood-group compatible with the donor. Hence an O-blood-group recipient can receive an organ only from an O-blood-group donor, whereas an O-group-donor could donate to anyone. By contrast an AB-blood-group donor could donate only to an AB recipient. A-group and B-group donors could donate to their own group or to an AB recipient.

When an O-blood-group organ becomes available it could go to the next person on the waiting list regardless of blood type, but if it went to someone other than an O-group recipient, eventually the supply of O donors will be exhausted and some O recipients will be left without any organs available. Thus there is a sense in which there is greater urgency in transplanting the O recipient. That person will have less of a chance of getting a suitable organ in the future and thus has a shorter life expectancy if not transplanted with the presently available organ. Therefore, to be fair to O recipients, they need to get priority for O-donor organs. Likewise, A-blood-group and B-blood-group recipients should get priority for their blood-group-identical donors (as well as higher priority than those in the AB-blood group for any O-donor organs that cannot be used for O recipients). For this reason, recipients matching the liver donor's blood group get ten points and blood-group-compatible recipients get five points.[13]

There is a possibility that urgency based on short life expectancy will identify recipients who are not presently the sickest. Current serious illness indicated by Status 1 or expected imminent decline could conflict with urgency based on low likelihood of finding another compatible organ in the future. For example, a Status 1 AB-blood-group recipient could be competing with a Status 2 or 3 O-blood-group recipient. Although making all the possible comparisons is beyond the scope of this book, the principle is clear enough: Insofar as justice is concerned, the organ should go to the person who is predictably worse off. If we are focusing on those who can be expected to have the most bleak futures, the goal should be to estimate who, considering present condition, expected imminent decline, and difficulties of finding a future organ, is projected to have the smallest number of QALYs remaining without transplant.[14] Making that calculation for all potential recipients every time an organ becomes available might be too complicated. (The problem would be even greater if we go to some version of a national list, as will be advocated in Chapter 24.) Because relatively healthy O-blood-type candidates (Status 2B and 3, for example) statistically will have some opportunity to get another O organ, the rule that gives Status 1 (and perhaps 2A) candidates of other blood types priority over lower-status O candidates is a workable approximation. Nevertheless, the result will inevitably be a statistically longer waiting time for O-blood candidates. Because liver recipients with long waits increase their risk of dying while waiting, this rule of thumb will necessarily discriminate against those with O blood type. It could be argued that because being Status 1 is, in some sense, a random event and being of O blood type is more genetically determined, need based on blood type should be given more consideration than it presently is.

Need over a Lifetime

There is still a third way that need could be conceptualized. Some persons may not have extraordinary present need or even great urgency in getting transplanted, but may nevertheless be expected to lead lives that we would consider undesirable. If offered these lives, we might say that those leading them are particularly poorly off and that therefore we would not want to "trade places" with them. They can be said to have greater need over their lifetimes.

THE ROLE OF AGE

Consider, for example whether we would view two persons with end-stage liver disease to have lives that are equally desirable if one develops her disease at age 80 and the other develops his at age 30. Even if the two persons were equal in their present need and had equal urgency (i.e., had the same number of predicted future QALYs without treatment), we are likely to have little difficulty concluding that the person getting her disease at 80 has had a much better life, overall, than the one who develops his at age 30. One might plausibly say that the 30-year-old is much needier than the 80-year-old. This is what I refer to as *over-a-lifetime need*.[15] The needier person is the one who will end up with fewer QALYs if not transplanted.

We have seen that utilitarians might insist that younger patients deserve priority over older patients, even when the two are equally sick. The younger person may have a better chance of responding to the surgery and may live longer if the graft is successful. This, obviously, has raised cries of unfairness among the advocates for elderly patients. Although this has the makings of a fight between the efficiency people and the equity people, it turns out that there is also a strong case to be made in the name of justice or equity for giving allocational priority to younger people. It is also possible to make the case that priority for younger people is more fair as well as more efficient.

At present this over-a-lifetime notion of need is almost never taken into account in organ allocation. I have always found this strange. However, rather than incorporate this over-a-lifetime notion of need into the present chapter, I shall devote all of Chapter 22 to this perspective.

However, there are many other allocational factors that some people would take into account that relate to well being over a lifetime and that those committed to justice will handle differently than those focusing on utility.

FIRST VERSUS REPEAT TRANSPLANTS

For example, a variable that raises justice problems is the appearance on the waiting list of some people who have had previous grafts that have failed. Some argue that it is unfair to give these people a second shot at an organ while others are still waiting for their first turn. Moreover, there is evidence that people do not do as well with their second grafts. For kidneys, one-year graft survival is 86.7% for first transplants and 82.4% for those with previous transplants. For livers the difference is even greater—79.1% compared with 55.0%. For hearts the numbers are 84.5% and 66.4%.[16] For reasons of both efficiency and equity, the case has been made that repeat transplant candidates deserve lower priority. On the other hand, there are convincing arguments that repeat candidates do not deserve to be downgraded. In fact, if we are considering how poorly one has done over a whole lifetime, those who are back for a repeat transplant may be thought to have a special claim. These will be explored in Chapter 21.

WAITING TIME

Another factor that is often thought to be relevant to fair allocation is how long one has been waiting. Those who have had need longer can be seen as having had worse lives. If the goal of the allocation system is to be fair to all on the list, we should be concerned if some people must wait inordinately long times for transplants. In some cases, this may be unavoidable. In the case of a kidney transplant, for example, the O-blood-group person who has a high PRA and unusual size requirements may simply require a long time to find a suitable organ. On the other hand, the delay could be caused by the fact that others on the list have a better HLA match or have identical rather than merely compatible blood types. Neither poor HLA match nor compatible rather than identical blood group is a disqualifier for a transplant, however. If a person has been waiting a very long time, we might want to take that long wait into account so that eventually the long wait overrides the HLA or blood-typing considerations. Hence all organ allocations in one way or another take waiting time into account. The kidney formula, for example, awards points for time on the waiting list.

There is a complication. Some of the reasons why people remain on the waiting list a long time are already accounted for by the factors mentioned earlier. One gets four points for a high PRA. If that is what is causing the long wait, is it not already taken into account? Likewise, if being in the O blood group is the reason, the extra points for identical blood group already give one an advantage in the allocation.

It can be argued that no matter what adjustments have been made for these other factors, if someone still has to wait an inordinately long time, he or she has a claim for special consideration. Following the rule that ties go to the person waiting longest seems reasonable. Adding more points merely for the fact that one has been waiting longest seems to be a fair way of taking into account other factors that may not otherwise be accounted for.

GEOGRAPHY

One final factor raises problems of justice. Presently, organs are distributed on a basis by which they go first to those on the waiting list of the local OPO (of which the United States has 62).[17] Then, if no one is available locally, they go next to the region (of which there are 11). Finally, if no one suitable is found at the local or regional level, the organ is allocated nationally. This means that a rather healthy potential recipient locally will get priority over a very critical patient on the regional list and the healthy patient on the regional list will get priority over the very critical patient on the national list. Moreover, some OPOs have relatively small potential for donor organs in comparison with their number of potential recipients, whereas others have a more generous supply of donor organs. Recently, people have asked whether this local priority is fair. A federal regulation mandates that UNOS revise its formula to make it more fair.[18] Some transplant surgeons and UNOS itself have responded, claiming that this may be a less efficient way to allocate organs. The feud between the advocates for efficiency and the advocates for equity will be explored in detail in Chapter 24.

Respect for Persons

The federal mandate for a national organ procurement network requires that the allocation system consider both efficiency and equity, but we saw earlier in this chapter that many ethical theories also include a number of moral principles that I have grouped under the rubric of *respect for persons*. This includes the principles of autonomy, fidelity, and veracity, as well as perhaps the avoidance of killing. It seems clear that these moral principles are also very relevant to a systematic organ allocation theory.

Respect for Persons as a Side Constraint

I have suggested that in organ allocation, the principles grouped under the rubric of respect for persons can often be fully satisfied. This differs from utility and justice, which seem often impossible to satisfy completely. A system that fully maximizes utility or one that is perfectly just seems utopian. On the other hand, one that completely avoids killing people or lying to them or breaking promises is conceivable. It may be that the fact that these respect-for-persons principles can be fully satisfied has led lawmakers to presume they are a prior constraint on the organ allocation system. The philosopher Robert Nozick introduced the term *side constraint* to refer to the demands of respect for freedom.[19] The idea is that certain requirements of morality are prior conditions that constrain whatever policies are adopted. Whatever we do to reconcile the conflict between efficiency and equity, these side constraints must be satisfied. Thus we generally accept the dead donor rule. No one is to be killed to procure an organ, even if that person volunteers for the execution. Likewise, any competent person who wishes to decline a transplant has a right to do so, even if that person would get the most benefit from the organ and would therefore be the first candidate from the point of view of medical utility. By the same reasoning we might conclude that no organ procurement or allocation system should be built on lies or deception— even if the lies or deceptions would increase the overall good that would come from a transplant program. (This insight stands behind my vigorous opposition to presumed consent programs, as discussed in Chapter 10.) Finally, we might conclude that if someone has been promised an organ, he or she has a special claim to it independent of consideration of either utility or justice. We saw earlier in this chapter that many theoreticians hold that, when ethical principles conflict, especially deontological ethical principles, no one principle will always automatically deserve priority. Hence we can imagine a situation in which a promise of an organ could be "trumped" by the realization that it would be grossly unfair to keep the promise. In that case, justice would take priority over promise-keeping. The point, however, is that if a promise has been made, it is morally relevant and, other things being equal, there is duty to keep it. It is unusual that promises will be a crucial factor in the morality of organ allocation, but the case could arise.

The principle of respect for autonomy raises especially important problems for a theory of organ allocation. It deserves special consideration in several contexts.

Free Exchanges among Autonomous Individuals

The moral principle of autonomy holds that people have a right of noninterference with choices they make based on their own life plans as long as those choices do not impose harms on other parties. We saw in Chapter 9 that this raised an important problem for the marketing of organs. The straightforward implication of the principle of autonomy and its correlate of self-determination would be that people should have the right not only to donate their organs but to sell them. We suggested that it is difficult to reject the logic behind this view but that such a policy is open to the charge that markets in organs might be exploitative. It would be if those who would do the buying had it in their power to address the problems in life that would make it rational for people in a desperate situation to sell their organs to meet the basic needs for themselves or their family members.

A similar question arises with regard to organ allocation. We could adopt a policy of permitting people to buy organs—either from individual vendors or from the organ allocation system. The attractiveness of the free-market system to those in modern Western culture cannot be doubted. Those following the logic of Adam Smith believe that there is greater overall utility in a society if the free market is allowed to function. The real issue is whether a free market that would permit buying of organs is also just or fair. Once again, one issue is whether it could be considered exploitative. In the case of individual vendors, if those doing the buying had it within their power to address the concerns of those desperate enough to sell their organs, they would have a moral duty grounded in justice to do so. Presumably, if they have the resources to buy an organ, they might have that ability.

The problem is more complex if the system is the vendor. Here organs would be procured but then sold to the highest bidder. Because the seller would not be in a desperate situation, the buyer would not be in a position to be accused of exploitation. But once again the issue of justice arises. If there is a national procurement network that receives organs by gift from individuals and families that altruistically want to help their fellow citizens, then this public organization would surely have a duty to allocate in a way that gives people a chance to receive organs in proportion to their need rather than on the basis of wealth. Although a private organ system might tolerate a free market in organs, a national public system cannot. Hence in the United States we have a law prohibiting markets in organs.[20]

Directed Donation

A related probe is whether, under the principle of autonomy, those members of the moral community that are motivated to make a gift of their organs can choose to whom they will make the gift. Can they direct the gift to anyone they choose, an individual, an organization, or a social group?

Normally, the ethics of gift giving is that one is permitted to give away anything of one's own to whomever one chooses. The choice of the recipient is up to the donor. But organs raise special problems. In the first place we have seen that individuals have only a "quasi-property right" over their bodies. They can only make a limited range of choices about what they can do with their bodies. Moreover, just as they cannot sell their body parts, they are restricted somewhat in choosing to whom they may make a gift. We have sympathy for someone who wishes to make a gift of an organ to a family member or close friend. The law permits us to make a gift to a named individual.

It also permits us to make a gift to a named hospital or health organization. This is a bit more controversial. The law was written before the emergence of organ procurement organizations. There is the possibility of a conflict between an individual transplant hospital and the OPO if the donation is made to the hospital. The OPO might rightly claim that such a gift circumvents the organ allocation system that has been carefully crafted to make sure organs in the area are allocated efficiently and equitably. Some might claim that after the hospital receives the organ it is bound by its relationship with the OPO to turn the organ over to the OPO for allocation according the standard criteria.

On the other hand, some donors may have long-term ties and loyalty to certain hospitals. They may feel a duty of loyalty to give to that one hospital just as they might feel duty-bound to give to a family member. This occurs so infrequently that it seems that little harm will be done by permitting a hospital to receive such a gift and transplant it in any responsible manner that it sees fit. A hospital that turns the organ over to its OPO for allocation according to preestablished criteria of efficiency and equity would be commended, however.

What is unacceptable is directing the donation by sociological group to unnamed members of a particular ethnic, racial, religious, or gender group. The arguments for this conclusion will be discussed in detail in Chapter 25.

Voluntary Health-Risky Behaviors

There is one final way in which the ethical principle of respect for persons may come into play in a theory of allocation organs. Any society that is committed to the principle of autonomy, which is part of respect for persons, will permit individuals to engage in certain behaviors even though it is known that those behaviors are risky to one's health. These behaviors—smoking, drinking in excess, leading a sedentary lifestyle, and so forth—may increase the likelihood that those engaging in them will need an organ for transplant. In some cases, such as the alcoholic, the person who engages in the behavior and thereby needs a transplant will be competing directly with others who need an organ because of genetic or other reasons beyond their control. The issue is, if we permit people to engage in voluntary, health-risky behavior, do those who do so have an equal claim on organs as those who need an organ through no fault of their own?

The issue is contentious one, hotly debated in both transplant and public circles. The controversy, including four possible policy options, will be discussed in the chapter that follows.

Conclusion

This completes our discussion of a general theory of organ allocation. I began with the premise that any such theory will be dependent on some more general theory of ethics. Holders of specialized moral theories of various religious or secular traditions will logically tease out the implications of their ethics for organ allocation. What is constructed in this book is a theory grounded in the common moral premises of the tradition of Western liberal political philosophy. These are views that seem quite compatible with the mainstream Judeo–Christian ethics of the Western heritage. What has been suggested is an ethic that includes considerations of both utility and justice. My own preference is for an ethic that gives justice a priority over utility, focusing on making those who are worst off among us more equal insofar as possible—that is, giving the sickest the opportunity to recover their health even if that means a less efficient system of allocating organs. I acknowledge, however, that not everyone in our society sees this as the proper relationship between utility and justice. In a democratic society, some political compromise may be necessary. The compromise that has emerged is one in which organs will be allocated on the basis of a formula that gives equal weight to both justice and utility. No allocation formula will be acceptable that is driven exclusively by utility, however, whether that includes social utility or merely medical utility.

Several different approaches would permit operationalizing the notion of giving equal weight to utility and justice. One strategy would be that to incorporate both utility and justice into a common metric, we should give chances for an organ in proportion to need. This would give the worst off the best chance at getting an organ but would refrain from giving them absolute priority. This is an egalitarian variant on Dan Brock's proposal to assign chances in a lottery for organs in proportion to expected benefit, a strategy that would give relatively more, but still not absolute, priority to those with the greatest expected benefit.[21]

There is another strategy for integrating utility and justice that more plausibly would give them equal weight. We could standardize measures of expected medical benefit so that the candidate with the most expected benefit would get a full or maximum number of points for medical benefit. Then all other candidates would be assigned lesser numbers of points in proportion to their expected medical benefit from the particular organ being allocated. (This approximates the assigning of points for kidney allocation based on HLA matching.) Then we could standardize measures of medical need (taking into account present need, urgency, and, as I shall argue in Chapter 22, age) with the most needy person receiving a maximum number of "justice points" and others who are less needy receiving lesser numbers of points in proportion. If we were to give equal weight to (medical) utility and justice, I suggest this would require an equal maximum number of points of each type—that is, an equal maximum number of utility and justice points. The points of each type would then have to be allocated based on empirical evidence of how various factors are related to their target. For example, when considering medical utility in kidney transplant, we would assign HLA points in proportion to how the various antigens influence outcome. Likewise, when it comes to allocating justice points, they would be assigned to such factors as degree of illness, likelihood of being in imminent need, PRA, blood type, and time on the waiting list in proportion to how these variables were believed to be related to being poorly off when considering expected QALYs.

Equal consideration could mean, for example, a maximum of 20 points each for medical utility and justice considerations. As chair of the subcommittee of the UNOS Ethics Committee that recommended the equal-weight notion, that is what I had in mind when I suggested assigning equal weight to these as to moral principles.[22]

I have argued, however, that utility and justice are not the only principles that are at stake. Whatever the proper compromise between utility and justice, the allocation system must be embedded into an arrangement whereby the principles related to respect for persons—autonomy, fidelity, veracity, and avoidance of killing—become side constraints that must never be violated just because it would be more efficient to do so. There may be rare cases in which these respect-for-persons principles have to be balanced against justice. I am open to that in theory. However, I cannot imagine many real-life cases in which that will be necessary.

ENDNOTES

1. National Organ Transplant Act, Public Law No. 98-507 (Oct. 19, 1984), 98 Stat. 2339.

2. The lists of utilities to consider and factors related to justice that follow are taken from the report of the UNOS Ethics Committee Organ Allocation Subcommittee, of which I was the chair and primary drafter. See James F. Burdick, Jeremiah G. Turcotte, and Robert M. Veatch, "General Principles for Allocating Human Organs and Tissues," *Transplantation Proceedings* 24 (5, Oct. 1992): 2227–35.

3. Shana Alexander, "They Decide Who Lives, Who Dies," *Life* 53 (1962): 102–25. Also see Albert R. Jonsen, *The Birth of Bioethics* (New York: Oxford University Press, 1998), pp. 211–13.

4. Richard Zeckhauser and Donald Shepard, "Where Now for Saving Lives?" *Law and Contemporary Problems* 40 (1976): 5–45; Jan P. Acton, "Measuring the Monetary Value of Lifesaving Programs," *Law & Contemporary Problems* 40 (1976): 46–72; Alan Williams, "The Value of QALYs," *Health and Social Service Journal* (July 18, 1985): 3–5; John Cubbon, "The Principle of QALY Maximisation as the Basis for Allocating Health Care Resources," *Journal of Medical Ethics* 17 (1991): 185–88.

5. For the various arguments pertaining to the problem of justice in the use of QALYs see Hastings Center, Institute of Society, Ethics and the Life Sciences, "Values, Ethics, and CBA in Health Care," in *The Implications of Cost-Effectiveness Analysis of Medical Technology* (Washington, DC: Office of Technology Assessment, U.S. Congress, 1980), pp. 168–85; Robert M. Veatch, "Justice and Outcomes Research: The Ethical Limits," *Journal of Clinical Ethics* 4 (3, Fall 1993): 258–61; John Broome, "Good, Fairness and QALYs," in *Philosophy and Medical Welfare*, ed. J. M. Bell and Susan Mendus (Cambridge: Cambridge University Press, 1988), pp. 57–73; Adam Wagstaff, "QALYs and the Equity-Efficiency Trade-Off," *Journal of Health Economics* 10 (1991): 21–41; Klemens Kappel and Peter Sandoe, "QALYs, Age and Fairness," *Bioethics* 6 (1992): 297–316; Ruth Faden and Alain Leplege, "Assessing Quality of Life: Moral Implications for Clinical Practice," *Medical Care* 30 (5, Suppl., 1992): MS166–75; Michael Lockwood, "Quality of Life and Resource Allocation," in *Philosophy and Medical Welfare*, ed. J. M. Bell and Susan Mendus (Cambridge: Cambridge University Press, 1988), pp. 33–55.

6. Graft Survival rates for years 1988–1996 from *UNOS 1997 Annual Report*, Table 26. See also J. K. Connolly, P. A. Dyer, S. Martin, N. R. Parrott, R. C. Pearson, and R. W. Johnson, "Importance of Minimizing HLA–DR Mismatch and Cold Preservation Time in Cadaveric Renal Transplantation," *Transplantation* 61 (5, March 15, 1996): 709–14; Y. C. Shou, and J. M. Cecka, "Effect of HLA Matching on Renal Transplant Survival," *Clinical Transplantation* (1993): 499–510; J. D. Pirsch, R. J. Ploeg, S. Gange, A. M. Allessandro, S. J. Knechtle, H. W. Sollinger, M. Kalayoglu, and F. O. Belzer, "Determinants of Grant Survival after Renal Transplantation," *Transplantation* 61 (11, June 15, 1996): 1581–86; P. I. Terasaki, D. W. Gjertson, J. M. Cecka, and S. Takemoto, "Fit and Match Hypothesis for Kidney Transplantation," *Transplantation* 62 (4, Aug. 27, 1996): 441–45.

7. UNOS Policy 3.5.9.2, from the UNOS Web site at <www.unos.org> (April 15, 1999).

8. A. H. Tejani, E. K. Sullivan, W. E. Harmon, R. N. Fine, E. Kohaut, L. Emmett, and S. R. Alexander, "Pediatric Renal Transplantation—The NAPRTCS Experience," *Clinical Transplantation* (1997): 87–100; R. B. Ettenger, C. Blifeld, H. Prince, D. B. Gradus, S. Cho, N. Sekiya, I. B. Salusky, and R. N. Fine, "The

Pediatric Nephrologist's Dilemma: Growth after Renal Transplantation and Its Interaction with Age as a Possible Immunologic Variable," *Journal of Pediatrics* 111 (6, pt. 2, Dec. 1987): 1022–25; I. D. Davis, T. W. Bunchman, P. C. Grimm, M. R. Benfield, D. M. Briscoe, W. E. Harmon, S. R. Alexander, and E. D. Avner, "Pediatric Renal Transplantation: Indications and Special Considerations. A Position Paper from the Pediatric Committee of the American Society of Transplant Physicians," *Pediatric Transplant* 2 (2, May 1998): 117–29.

9. Utilitarianism, at least since the days of John Stuart Mill, does take into account what is known as decreasing marginal utility. Hence if a utilitarian is allocating money or food or some other good and can choose between someone who already has a lot of the item and someone who has little, the assumption is that often (but not always) giving the resource to the person who has less will produce more utility. Frances Kamm has brought this notion to bear on the question of organ allocation by arguing that the same notion might apply to life. Hence she suggests that one might direct organs to younger transplant candidates on the grounds that the years of life one could add to the younger person would be of greater value than the same number of years added to an older person who has already had many of life's experiences. See Kamm, *Morality, Mortality: Volume I: Death and Whom to Save from It* (New York: Oxford University Press, 1993), p. 237. This is not the concern of those dealing with justice. *Justice*, as used in this book, focuses on the fact that some people have had less well being than others. The goal is on producing greater fairness in the distribution of well being, not on the amount of additional well being a transplant will bring.

10. There is another possible interpretation of the idea of treating people equally. In general, liberal political theory is premised on the egalitarian notion that all human beings are equal in their moral worth—that is, even though they may vary widely in how useful they are to others, they all count equally as human beings who are to be treated as ends in themselves, as moral beings with claims to equality. This could be interpreted as implying not that the worse off have claims to be made more equal to those who are better off but rather that everyone who is in need of a lifesaving intervention has an equal claim to get that intervention. That view was suggested by Dan Brock in "Ethical Issues in Recipient Selection," in *Organ Substitution Technology: Ethical, Legal, and Public Policy Issues,* ed. Deborah Mathieu (Boulder, CO: Westview Press, 1988), p. 93. It has long been recognized that either a strict lottery or the principle of first come–first served would approximate this strict notion of equality. Unfortunately, for organ allocation this would ignore many factors—HLA tissue match, age, organ size, blood type, and geography, as well as degree of urgency. If we could provide equal opportunity while permitting some degree of matching based on these factors, the allocation system could be more efficient while still being fair. In a world in which both effi-

ciency and fairness are taken into account we might be even more inclined to depart from strictly equal claims on organs.

The main problem with allocation on the basis of equal claims for all potential recipients is that it would—in the name of fairness—give the relatively well-off equal claim to that of the sickest. Another interpretation of fairness or justice is the one followed in this book: that all should have equal claim to opportunities for equality of well being. That, in effect, means that the worst off have the strongest claims of justice rather than giving all persons equal claim regardless of how well-off they are.

11. F. M. Kamm, *Morality, Mortality: Volume I: Death and Whom to Save from It*. See esp. pp. 233–65.

12. Ibid., p. 234. Kamm actually distinguishes two types of urgency: urgency^T and urgency^Q. "T" stands for time, referring to how soon someone will die without a transplant, and "Q" stands for quality, indicating how badly off someone will be without a transplant. I have followed the approach of combining length of life and quality of life into a single measure, the quality-adjusted life year or QALY. Hence I will refer to urgency in terms of how soon one will die without transplant measured in QALYs.

13. Information about ABO-incompatible transplantation is limited. See K. Tanabe, K. Takahashi, K. Sonda, T. Tokumoto, N. Ishikawa, T. Kawai, S. Fuchinoue, T. Oshima, T. Yagisawa, H. Nakazawa, N. Goya, S. Koga, H. Kawaguchi, K. Ito, H. Toma, T. Agishi, and K. Ota, "Long-Term Results of ABO-Incompatible Living Kidney Transplantation: A Single-Center Experience," *Transplantation* 65 (2, Jan. 27, 1998): 224–28.

14. Frances Kamm considers potential conflict between blood type and other determinants of urgency such as sensitization. She recommends offering "O material first to an O recipient as urgent^T as other potential recipients, where 'as urgent^T' includes 'as sensitized,' given that sensitized are even more likely to die before another organ is found than O people." F. M. Kamm, *Morality, Mortality: Volume I: Death and Whom to Save from It*, p. 255. In principle she is correct, however, there is a problem. Although sensitization is important for kidney transplant, it is not a factor in liver transplant. On the other hand, blood type is important for livers, but it is not important for kidneys. Hence there is no organ for which PRA (sensitization) and blood type will conflict. There is, however, a potential conflict in liver allocation between urgency status and blood type.

15. Robert M. Veatch, "Distributive Justice and the Allocation of Technological Resources to the Elderly," *Life-Sustaining Technologies and the Elderly: Working Papers, Volume 3: Legal and Ethical Issues, Manpower and Training, and Classification Systems for Decisionmaking* (Washington, DC: U.S. Congress, Office of Technology Assessment, 1987), pp. 87–189; Veatch, "How Age Should Matter: Justice as the

Basis for Limiting Care to the Elderly," in *Facing Limits: Ethics and Health Care for the Elderly*, ed. Gerald R. Winslow and James W. Walters (Boulder, CO: Westview Press, 1993), pp. 211–29. Frances Kamm has more recently given considerable attention to this interpretation of the concept of need, indeed specifying in her work that this should be the primary notion of need. Kamm, *Morality, Mortality: Volume I: Death and Whom to Save from It*, where she says, "I shall use the term 'need' so that it correlates with how much a person will have had by the time he dies" (p. 234).

16. *UNOS 1997 Annual Report*, Tables 26, 30, and 34.

17. A recent modification in this policy gives regional priority to the sickest (Status 1) liver transplant candidates over healthier patients in the local area. This will be discussed in Chapter 24. See UNOS News Release, June 25, 1999, "UNOS Refines Liver Allocation Policy: Broader access for most urgent patients balanced with outcome, other needs," available on the UNOS Web site, <www.UNOS.org> (July 9, 1999).

18. U.S. Department of Health and Human Services, "Organ Procurement and Transplantation Network: Final Rule, 42 CFR Part 121," 63 Fed. Reg. 16296 (April 2, 1998).

19. Robert Nozick, *Anarchy, State, and Utopia* (New York: Basic Books, 1974), p. 29.

20. National Organ Transplant Act, Public Law No. 98-507.

21. Dan Brock, "Ethical Issues in Recipient Selection," p. 97.

22. James F. Burdick, Jeremiah G. Turcotte, and Robert M. Veatch, "General Principles for Allocating Human Organs and Tissues."

TWENTY

VOLUNTARY RISKS AND ALLOCATION: DOES THE ALCOHOLIC DESERVE A NEW LIVER?

AS WE SAW in the previous chapter, one of the implications of the moral principle of autonomy is that people who are substantially autonomous agents should be free to live their own lives even if, on occasion, they make choices that are not in their own best interest. Some of these choices jeopardize their organs and can eventually lead to the need for organ transplants. If justice requires that we give people *opportunities* for medical well-being, should we view these people as having had that opportunity and squandered it? If so, does this mean that people who choose to take such risks deserve lower priority in the organ allocation system? Contrary to fashionable ethics, I argue in this chapter that that *is* the case.

The behaviors involved may include consumption of alcohol, smoking cigarettes, eating fatty foods, and failing to exercise. The jump from these behaviors to the conclusion that people needing livers or lungs or hearts deserve lower priority is, however, a huge one. This chapter looks at the role of purportedly voluntary, risky lifestyle choices in organ allocation. We will focus on alcoholism and liver failure as the primary example, but also consider a range of other possible behaviors that increase the need for organs.

The Theory of Voluntary Health-Risky Behavior

Let us assume for the time being that we can identify certain health-risky behaviors that increase the likelihood that organs will be needed for transplant. How would those who hold the various moral views discussed in the previous chapter use that information in planning an organ allocation system? It turns out that those committed to maximizing aggregate net utility probably will reach different conclusions than those committed to an egalitarian interpretation of the principle for justice.

Utility

In developing the general theory of the ethics of allocation in the last chapter, we distinguished between utilitarians who consider the social impact of giving organs to one recipient or another and those who limit utilitarian judgments to the expected medical benefit of the transplant. We saw that, for one reason or another, almost everyone agrees that the social impact of transplanting one recipient rather than another—the social value of the transplant—is excluded from consideration in the organ allocation. That may be for utilitarian reasons (that the disutilities of determining who is a more worthy recipient outweigh the expected gains by picking the most valuable recipient) or for deontological reasons (that it is unethical to include social worth in the calculation). The utilitarian question that is on the table is which candidate will get the most medical benefit from the organ.

If the concern is who will get the most medical benefit, the history of the medical problem may be irrelevant. In the case of alcoholism, for instance, whether one did in one's liver by consuming alcohol or has cirrhosis from some other cause may turn out to be irrelevant. The utilitarian who is trying to determine the likelihood of medical benefit is interested in the prognosis, not the history. In fact, if one examines the prognosis of a liver transplant as a function of diagnosis, alcoholic cirrhosis patients apparently do quite well—better than some other diagnoses.[1] The utilitarian is concerned about graft survival or patient survival, not whether one voluntarily engaged in some behavior that may have created the need for the transplant.

Some sophisticated utilitarians might not completely accept this analysis, however. They may probe further to ask whether a policy of taking voluntary health-risky behaviors into account might create incentives to discourage the behavior. It could be that one of the consequences of letting voluntary behavior count against getting an organ would be reducing the demand on the organ supply, thus leaving more organs for those needing organs for nonvoluntary reasons as well as improving the health of the risk takers.

That is, of course, a quite speculative claim. In fact, utilitarians who participate actively in the allocation debate have taken the position that a history of voluntary risks such as alcohol consumption should not count in allocation. As we have seen, physicians traditionally think in utilitarian terms. Hippocratic physicians consider benefit to the patient to be the only criterion of moral practice. When physicians take on the more social ethical question of allocation, in great numbers they continued to reason as utilitarians. In the UNOS Ethics Committee Subcommittee on Allocation, when the issue of voluntary health risky behavior was debated, there was a perfect division, with all the physicians taking the utilitarian stance and opposing such considerations and all the nonphysicians taking a more deontological position, seeing some legitimate relevance to the cause of the organ failure in the allocation.[2]

The Deontological View: Concerns of Justice

Still assuming for the moment that some truly voluntary behaviors can be identified that lead to increasing the risk of organ failure leading to transplant, deontologists will see matters differently. They believe strongly in the right of individuals to make autonomous choices according to their own lifestyles. Moreover, they are committed to a principle of justice that is not automatically swayed by the course that will maximize future outcomes. They are more concerned about equality of opportunity of well being. If we are dealing with medicine, that often means medical well being. One logical implication of a commitment to equality of opportunity is that if two people are equally needy because of a medical problem and one has previously had the opportunity to avoid the problem, the one who has not had that opportunity has a stronger claim. On the other hand, if the need is not dependent on behavior that is truly voluntary, one committed to egalitarian justice would insist that persons have an equal claim to the organ even if it turned out to be inefficient to grant access. This means it will be crucial to the deontologist to determine whether the health-risky behaviors are truly voluntary.

VOLUNTARISM VERSUS DETERMINISM

The entire question of voluntary health-risky behaviors is moot if it turns out that we cannot establish whether the behaviors in question are really voluntary. If alcoholism, smoking, and any other behaviors related to organ need are genetically determined or can be traced back to toilet training or some other psychological phenomenon of childhood, then holding the needy patient responsible is nothing more than "blaming the victim."

The literature on voluntary health-risky behavior is filled with this controversy. Left-wing critics of the 1970s tended to claim that behaviors affecting health adversely correlated with socioeconomic status and that they were, in effect, economically determined.[3] Alcoholism, for instance, they saw as a response to socioeconomic oppression and therefore not the alcoholic's fault. Rather it was the fault of the broader, oppressive society. Of course, not all alcoholics are from lower socioeconomic classes, but the claim of these critics was that this was a factor, an important factor, and that making such behaviors a factor in allocating organs would simply transfer the oppression of society further onto people who were suffering because of social causes.

Others interpret these behaviors behaviorally. They viewed them as conditioned responses to stimuli in these people's lives that were trained into them through an environment that is beyond their control. Freudian psychologists might differ with the behaviorists in the details of the causal mechanism, but they share the view that behavior is determined, not chosen. Still others believed that the behavior should not be seen as voluntary because genetics had a significant causal role in the disease. All of the deterministic accounts, whether they involve economic, psychological, or genetic determinism, need to be taken seriously. There is probably some truth to each of them. The issue, however, is whether they provide complete accounts of the behaviors in question. If they do, then the human is totally devoid of freedom of choice. We are creatures of forces outside of us to the point that voluntary behavior choices are impossible.

This is a tragic view of human behavior that, carried to the extreme, makes all ethics impossible. Ethics is the discipline of moral evaluation of human conduct, practices, and character. To the extent that these are determined by economics, psychology, or genetics, such evaluation is meaningless. We simply must continue to operate on the assumption that all human behavior is, to some degree, free and open to human choice. Of course, economics, psychology, and biology are important as well. They set certain limits on our choices. But there must be an element of freedom in behavior if life has any meaning. It is necessary to gamble on the assumption that there is some degree of choice in behavior, at least for adults who are deemed to be substantially autonomous.

The exact proportion of behavioral choices that can be attributed to voluntary choice is probably impossible to determine. It will surely vary from one situation to another and one medical condition to another. It seems, however, that the only assumption that is compatible with human morality is that at least some behaviors have at least some voluntary component and, if we are to treat people with dignity and respect, we will acknowledge that their behavior is significantly voluntary. The corollary of this assumption is that people are to be held responsible for their actions. Whether that has implications for organ allocation policy will require some additional work.

LINEARITY: FAIRNESS IN HOLDING PEOPLE ACCOUNTABLE

If voluntary, health-risky behaviors are relevant to organ allocation, the behaviors will, at minimum, have to meet certain tests. One is that there needs to be a predictable relationship between the amount of the behavior and the degree of risk. This has been referred to as the criterion of *linearity*.[4] The degree of risk should be proportional to the amount of the behavior. It turns out that the health risk of certain key behaviors for organ transplant, including alcohol consumption and smoking, probably meet the linearity criterion.

RESPONSIBILITY RATHER THAN MORAL JUDGMENT

It is important to realize that the position outlined in this chapter is not that behaviors such as alcohol consumption and smoking are morally bad behaviors—vices—and that they are therefore to be given low priority for allocation of organs. It is widely agreed that public health policy will have a very difficult time getting into the business of providing moral evaluations of behaviors. In a pluralistic society it is unlikely that we could reach such agreement in any case. What is at stake is whether people are responsible for their behavior and the impact of that behavior on social policy, including organ allocation.[5] If we are correct that there is a significant voluntary element in certain behaviors, then those engaging in them must be held responsible for them. The critical variable is not whether the behavior is moral or immoral but whether one could have knowledge of the risks involved and voluntarily choose whether to engage in the behavior. To the extent that one knows the risk and chooses to take that risk, in principle, one should be responsible for the consequences.

Thus it is not how evil or sinful the behavior is but rather how serious the impact is on the health care system. In theory, there could be a behavior that we do not consider ethically suspect in the slightest but nevertheless poses a significant risk for needing an organ. Think of mountain climbing: Imagine that it turns out that mountain climbing becomes a significant risk for organ damage, resulting in the need for a transplant. We could probably agree that mountain climbing is a significantly voluntary behavior. We do not think of it as substantially determined by our genetic makeup or our upbringing. We would not consider someone blameworthy simply for climbing a mountain. Nevertheless, it seems that one should be held responsible for the foreseeable consequences.

Consider two people who each engage in voluntary risky behaviors, one of which is quite benign but poses a significant risk of damaging organs and the other of which is generally regarded as morally outrageous but poses essentially no risk. If someone were engaging in the immoral almost risk-free behavior and, through some unexpected freak accident, irreversibly damaged an organ, it would seem wrong to take the behavior into account in organ allocation. On the other hand, the benign but risky behavior would suggest holding the person responsible for the consequences of the behavior, including, perhaps, adjusting the organ allocation formula because of the personal responsibility. The objective is not even to discourage the behavior (as it might be if we were in the business of labeling behaviors as vices and punishing their practitioners). This is simply suggesting that if one is free to engage in these risky behaviors, one must be prepared to take the consequences, even if that should happen to result in a lower position on the organ waiting list.

EXEMPTIONS FOR SOCIALLY NOBLE BEHAVIOR

Although what has been said thus far suggests that it is responsibility rather than moral assessment that is the relevant factor in voluntary health-risky behavior, there is an exception. Some behaviors for which we are responsible are important to society. Society wants to encourage the behavior, not discourage it. A good example might be professional fire fighting. Surely, this is the quintessential socially noble behavior. It is in society's interest that firefighters take chances. Normally, they take these changes knowing the risks and voluntarily choosing to take them. Should a firefighter become injured in such as way that he or she would require an organ transplant—for instance, if a firefighter aspirated hot smoke to the point that lungs were irreversibly damaged in a way that a lung transplant would be necessary—we would not want to penalize the firefighter for taking that risk. Even though the firefighter knew the risk and voluntarily chose to take it, society should see such behavior as noble. If we are debating the question of whether voluntary risk takers should bear the costs of their behavior, the firefighter should be exempt. If we are debating the question of whether voluntary risk takers should have their behavior influence organ allocation, it certainly should not lower the firefighter's claim on an organ. Perhaps it should even raise it.

Alcohol and Liver Transplants

Everything said thus far is meant to be general and theoretical. If behavior can be seen as significantly voluntary and humans should be held responsible for the consequences of their actions, then they may be responsible for the need for an organ resulting from these voluntary behaviors. Furthermore, if justice requires opportunities for equality, then those who voluntarily choose to engage in health-risky behaviors should be seen as having had an opportunity and should be placed in a somewhat subordinate position when it comes to allocating organs. This has nothing to do with whether the behavior is moral or immoral, virtue or vice. It is rather a matter of being responsible for the consequences of one's behavior.

Now it may turn out that even though all this holds in theory, it is of no significance to organ transplant. This will depend on whether there are significant and truly voluntary behaviors in which those who choose to participate can reasonably expect to understand the organ-threatening consequences of their behavior. Because alcoholism and liver transplant are the primary example of this kind of problem, this section of the chapter will look at the question of how plausible it is to treat alcoholism as a voluntary health-risky behavior and whether that should be taken into account in the liver allocation policy.

Empirical Data

There is increasing evidence that alcoholism has a genetic component.[6] In addition, behavioral patterns appear to be learned, so that offspring and siblings may not only inherit tendencies toward alcoholism but also develop alcohol consumption patterns from role models starting at a very early age. Both of these factors are sometimes cited as a basis for claiming that alcoholism is a "disease" rather than a voluntary behavior and that, therefore, alcoholics should not be held responsible for their behavior.

Determining What It Would Take for Alcoholism to Be Considered Nonvoluntary

Given all of these data, it is still not clear what the implications are for allocation policy. We still need to know whether we should view alcoholism as having a significant voluntary component and, if so, whether that should count in deciding organ priorities.

We should begin by asking what it would take to declare alcoholism nonvoluntary. Even if we assume there is a significant genetic component in alcoholism, we need to understand what that could mean. It could mean that alcohol is metabolized differently because of some genetic variant. That could lead to some neurological event that makes alcoholics unable to exercise judgment that would permit them to stop their alcohol consumption, so they tend to end up drunk once they start drinking. But even if all that could be shown to be a true account of why alcoholics get drunk and damage their livers, it does not show that starting a bout of drinking is involuntary. Quite to the contrary, if the genetic factor changes the metabolism once the alcohol is consumed, that would suggest that the effect occurs after the drinking has started. That first drink would, to some extent, be independent of the genetic effects on the metabolism of the alcohol.

Another possibility is that alcoholics become psychologically dependent on alcohol so that even that first drink is beyond their voluntary control. That sounds closer to an involuntary behavior. But there are two problems with that account. First, we have suggested that even those conditions that have a strong psychological component in their causation should nevertheless be seen as under voluntary control to some degree. Can it truly be said that any behavior is psychologically determined to the point that it is totally beyond the influence of the will? It is hard to imagine what evidence one could mount in support of such a claim. Second, even if after a while one becomes so psychologically dependent on alcohol that it is truly nonvoluntary, was the development of the psychological dependence also involuntary? Could the alcoholic have seen the dependence coming and avoided it? If, for example, one realizes that one's parent is an alcoholic, should that be a warning of a potential risk that should lead one voluntarily to take steps to avoid developing the dependence one's self?

The answer is dependent on how that psychological dependence develops. If, for example, it emerges in adolescence before one is substantially autonomous, then perhaps we should say it really is significantly involuntary. On the other hand, if it emerges in adulthood, the ability to see it coming may increase the likelihood that one could have exercised some voluntary constraint before the dependence developed.

Sorting these issues will be very difficult. Some will undoubtedly conclude that we are so uncertain about the casual chains leading to alcoholism that we cannot presume that one could voluntarily control it. That would mean that liver allocation should ignore the history of alcoholism even for one who accepts the general premises of the voluntary health-risk position sketched previously. On the other hand, many of us conclude that even though alcoholism has nonvoluntary components related to genetics, psychology, and social status, it also contains significant opportunity for voluntary decision making. If the alcoholic had the opportunity for any significant choice, he or she should be held responsible for the consequences, including the consequences for liver damage.

This is not meant to be a vindictive policy of punishment for alcoholism. One can be held responsible for the consequences of one's behavior without believing that one should be punished for it. Moreover, it seems that even if there is a voluntary component, there certainly are nonvoluntary elements as well. This should mitigate any claim that there is a dramatic difference in the status of alcoholics compared to others who may need livers.

The Role of a History of Alcoholism in Alcoholism Policy: Four Options

Although the analysis of alcoholism raises many controversial, contentious issues about which there is little agreement, the options for public policy may present decisions that are more manageable. The UNOS Ethics Committee considered four options.[7] Although in the end we could not reach a consensus on these questions, we came closer to a consensus than many expected. Two rather extreme policies were considered and ruled out. Then two more moderate policies were debated.

BAN ALL ALCOHOLICS FROM LIVER TRANSPLANT

The first policy one might consider is to ban all alcoholics from any liver transplants. Stressing the voluntary component along perhaps with manifesting a serious streak of vindictiveness, some have suggested that no organ resources should be used for alcoholics at all. Perhaps exceptions would be made for alcoholics who had never been mentally competent, but adults who are presumed to have made some voluntary choices along the way would simply be could excluded from access.

This proposal probably rests on a moral judgment as much or more than judgments about justice and opportunities for health. In this crude form it is hard to defend. It seems we could agree that, at least in the case in which an organ was available that would otherwise go to waste, the alcoholic should be permitted to receive it.

No one on the UNOS Ethics Committee was willing to accept this view.

TRANSPLANT ALL ALCOHOLICS, EVEN THOSE WITH ACTIVE ALCOHOLISM

A second position was also rejected by the ethics committee. It might be defended by someone who considers the history and cause of the liver failure morally irrelevant. That would be to provide organs to alcoholics, including active alcoholics, without regard to their condition. This proposal, at first, might seem irrational because it might be argued that the active alcoholic would simply do in another liver, repeating the process in an endless cycle. However, development of full-blown cirrhosis takes considerable time. Certainly, even an active alcoholic would have a chance to get many good years from his or her new liver before causing it serious damage.

The active alcoholic might be excluded on the grounds that, as an active alcoholic, he or she would not be able to follow the regimen of immunosuppression and treatment follow-up necessary. That is a legitimate medical reason for excluding the potential recipient, but not all active alcoholics would necessarily fail in their medication routine and follow-up.

TRANSPLANT ALCOHOLICS ONCE THEY HAVE DEMONSTRATED THEY ARE REFORMED

The utilitarians on the UNOS Ethics Committee, including the physicians on the committee, all took a more modest position supporting transplant of alcoholics. They acknowledged that it was inappropriate to transplant alcoholics (perhaps because even if the transplant was a success, it was an inefficient procedure because of the risk of follow-up failure and eventual organ damage). However, as was mentioned previously, they pointed out that the evidence suggests that alcoholics, once they are off alcohol and reformed for a reasonable period of time, do at least as well as other liver transplant patients. Reasoning from these consequences and committed to seeing the history as irrelevant, these utilitarians defended the view that reformed alcoholics should go into the allocation without regard to their alcoholism. They should in no way be penalized once they were sufficiently reformed. There is some dispute about how long the alcoholic should be dry. Suggestions range from six months to a year.

Take into Account the History of Alcoholism as a Modest Negative Factor in Allocation

By contrast the nonphysicians on the UNOS Ethics Committee were more deontological in their approach to the issue. They granted that alcoholism was a complex phenomenon with some causal factors well beyond the control of the alcoholic. At the same time they insisted that, to preserve their dignity as human agents, alcoholics must be viewed as significantly responsible for their behavior, that there is a voluntary element in it. Viewing history as morally significant, they wanted this voluntary behavioral choice to be reflected in the allocation of livers.

The nonphysicians on the committee were not at all inclined to conclude that this should ban alcoholics from the transplant program even in a world in which livers were very scarce. What they concluded was that some small element in the allocation can and should reflect the history of alcoholic cirrhosis. If the liver allocation were based on a point system similar to the kidney allocation, this might suggest a small number of negative points for alcoholic cirrhosis. The number would be set in proportion to how important the voluntary component seemed to be. All agreed that it should be small in comparison to other factors such as medical urgency. If the liver allocation formula continues not to be based on a point system, then there may still be ways that the history of alcoholism could play a small role. For example, until recently livers were allocated primarily on the basis of medical urgency. Among patients in the same category of urgency, ties were broken by time on the waiting list.

In 1999, UNOS changed the liver classification system so that, among patients in urgent need of a liver, chronically ill patients were given a lower priority than those in acute liver failure. (A new category, 2A, was created. All chronically ill patients who previously would have been status 1 were reclassified to 2A.) Since alcoholic cirrhosis is a chronic disease, this had the effect of lowering severely ill alcoholics' priority. This is a step in the right direction, but it was too crude and done for the wrong reasons. It lowered the status of all severely ill chronic patients, including those whose disease was entirely beyond the suspicion of voluntary lifestyle choice. It was probably done from the belief that the chronically ill do not do as well with transplants as those with acute illness. It was done for utilitarian, not deontological reasons.

I support a policy that says that ties should first be broken on the basis of whether one has a diagnosis of alcoholism or other need related to voluntary choice and then by time on the waiting list. This would continue to be subordinate to medical urgency, but, as a tiebreaker, I think it makes sense.

THE RESOLUTION: AGREEING TO DISAGREE

Of all the disputes in which I was involved in six years on the UNOS Ethics Committee, this was the most intractable. In the end the utilitarian physicians and the deontological nonphysicians could reach no further compromise between these two moderate positions. We had to agree to disagree. Our report dealing with the issue simply states the disagreement. What is striking to me in reflecting on those debates was how consistently the physicians insisted that history was irrelevant, that prognosis was all that counted, whereas the nonphysicians considered opportunities foregone as somehow morally relevant. They saw the behavior as complex and not necessarily blameworthy but nevertheless containing enough of a voluntary component that it deserved to be reflected in some small way in the allocation formula.

Other Voluntary Behaviors

Although alcoholism is the most visible example of a possibly voluntary health-risky behavior that could damage organs, other behaviors raise similar questions. The most conspicuous are smoking, which might lead to lung transplant, and poor diet and exercise patterns, which could lead to heart transplant. Voluntarily failing to maintain blood pressure reduction regimen might also be seen as a voluntary health-risky behavior leading to the need for a kidney transplant. To the extent that diabetes is the result of lack of dietary control, it may be another example, this time leading to pancreas transplant. Let us look now at the ways these cases differ from alcoholism and liver transplant.

Smoking and Lung Allocation

It is now well known that smoking can lead to lung damage—lung cancer and emphysema, among other conditions. Should smoking be taken into account in the lung allocation formula?

Lung transplants are much more rare events than either kidney or liver transplants (928 compared with 4,165 livers and 7,768 cadaver kidneys in 1997). Lungs are, thus, less scarce. Moreover, serious cases of lung cancer, at least those with metastases, currently are not treated with transplantation. Nevertheless, some other smoking-related lung diseases may be appropriate for transplant.

The reasoning should be the same as for alcoholism. First, one must determine whether smoking is a significantly voluntary behavior. This is no small task. There are good reasons to believe that tobacco is addicting once one engages in it regularly. In that way it is little different from alcohol, but tobacco may generate more physical dependency than alcohol. Regardless, the same questions raised about alcohol need to be raised about smoking. Was there ever a time when the smoker was not addicted and could voluntarily choose not to smoke? Moreover, we need an account of how so many former smokers have quit, apparently voluntarily. This implies that, at least for some, the smoking was subject to some degree of voluntary choice. On the other hand, many people start smoking at such a young age that they cannot be said to be substantially autonomous decision makers when they start. Moreover, we are now learning that they have been subject to exploitative manipulation by very sophisticated advertising and marketing strategies that, at least until recently, no one could have known enough about to consciously resist.

That suggests a final problem in deciding whether smoking should be a modest negative consideration in allocating organs. Not all who have damaged their lungs are in anything like the same position regarding how much they could be expected to have known when they damaged their lungs. Even if it could be argued that today's adult who begins smoking has been given fair warning, by package warning, school education programs, and enormous publicity about to-bacco industry practices, that was certainly not the case when today's older generation began to smoke. Many may have done their damage well before the risks were understood by the public. This will make it harder to impose any negative consideration for this behavior at all because different people are in different positions regarding their knowledge of risk-taking when they began their smoking.

Diet, Sedentary Lifestyle, and Hearts

An even more complicated dynamic exists when we consider whether those who fail to follow proper diet and exercise regimens should have their behavior taken into account in the allocation of hearts and perhaps other organs that they need. The relationship between these behaviors and organ failure appears to be far more complex than that of alcohol to liver failure and smoking to lung damage. Although almost everyone must have some understanding by now that alcohol and smoking pose risks to livers and lungs, the understanding of the relationship of diet and exercise to heart failure is more incomplete. That is in part because the science is less well understood. The public continues to get mixed messages.[8] Cholesterol and triglycerides apparently have complex relationships with heart disease. The average citizen cannot understand the relationship as easily as with alcohol or tobacco.

It is not even clear whether diet and exercise meet the criterion of linearity. Some people seem to be able to take in a terrible diet and avoid exercise and not have the effects show up in their coronary health. It is not clear whether this is random or relates to poorly understood genetic and metabolic variations. This suggests that, although the public is beginning to grasp that diet and exercise are related to heart disease and other health factors, it is less clear the extent to which they can be held responsible for the outcomes. At least until the dynamics are more clearly understood, it will be hard to separate potential recipients of hearts on the basis of whether they have engaged in health-risky behaviors.

Health-Risky Behavior and Kidneys and Pancreata

The same can be said even more strongly for those who need kidneys because they have failed to maintain blood pressure and those who might need pancreata because they have exacerbated their diabetes with poor diet. In principle, those who accept the general arguments in the first section of this chapter would be willing to let health-risky behaviors count in some small way against those who have damaged their kidneys and pancreata through voluntary choices. Establishing that these people knew the risks they were taking and voluntarily decided to take them will be much harder in this case. Given that even the most bold advocates of taking voluntary health-risky behaviors into account in organ allocation favor only modest, marginal influence on the organ allocation, it is likely that, for these latter conditions, the lack of certainty about the risks will lead to a policy of ignoring these factors when it comes to organ allocation.

ENDNOTES

1. N. De Maria, A. Colantoni, and D. H. Van Thiel, "Liver Transplantation for Alcoholic Liver Disease," *Hepatogastroenterology* 45 (23, 1998): 1364–68; J. Neuberger and H. Tang, "Relapse after Transplantation: European Studies," *Liver Transplantation and Surgery* 3 (3, 1997): 275–79; A. DiMartini, A. Jain, W. Irish, M. G. Fitzgerald, and J. Fung, "Outcome of Liver Transplantation in Critically Ill Patients with Alcoholic Cirrhosis: Survival According to Medical Variables and Sobriety," *Transplantation* 66 (3, 1998): 298–302; and G. F. Stefanini, M. Biselli, G. L. Grazi, E. Iovine, M. R. Moscatello, L. Marsigli, F. G. Foschi, F. Caputo, A. Mazziotti, M. Bernardi, G. Gasbarrini, and A. Cavallari, "Orthotopic Liver Transplantation for Alcoholic Liver Disease: Rates of Survival, Complications and Relapse," *Hepatogastroenterology* 44 (17, 1997): 1356–59.

2. James F. Burdick, Jeremiah G. Turcotte, and Robert M. Veatch, "General Principles for Allocating Human Organs and Tissues," *Transplantation Proceedings* 24 (5, Oct. 1992): 2226–35.

3. Dan E. Beauchamp, "Public Health as Social Justice," *Inquiry* 13 (1976): 3–14.

4. This concept was first developed in my article "Voluntary Risks to Health: The Ethical Issues," *Journal of the American Medical Association* 243 (Jan. 4, 1980): 50–55.

5. The distinction between responsibility and moral judgment was hinted at in my 1980 article and is developed more explicitly and fully in a recent analysis. See Walter Glannon, "Responsibility, Alcoholism, and Liver Transplantation," *Journal of Medicine and Philosophy* 23 (1998): 31–49.

6. L. J. Bierut, S. H. Dinwiddie, H. Begleiter, R. R. Crowe, V. Hesselbrock, J. I. Nurnberger, Jr., B. Porjesz, M. A. Schuckit, and T. Reich, "Familial Transmission of Substance Dependence: Alcohol, Marijuana, Cocaine, and Habitual Smoking: A Report from the Collaborative Study on the Genetics of Alcoholism," *Archives of General Psychiatry* 55 (11, 1998): 982–88; P. M. Conneally and R. S. Sparkes, "Molecular Genetics of Alcoholism and Other Addiction/Compulsive Disorders. General Discussion," *Alcohol* 16 (1, 1998): 85–91; H. J. Edenberg, "Genetics of Alcoholism," *Science* 282 (5392, 1998): 1269; A. M. Goate and H. J. Edenberg, "The Genetics of Alcoholism," *Current Opinion in Genetics and Development* 8 (3, 1998): 282–86; C. Grau, "Genetics of Alcoholism: An International Perspective," *Alcoholism, Clinical and Experimental Research* 20 (8, Suppl., 1996): 78A–81A; S. B. Guze, "The Genetics of Alcoholism: 1997," *Clinical Genetics* 52 (5, 1997): 398–403.

7. James F. Burdick, Jeremiah G. Turcotte, and Robert M. Veatch, "General Principles for Allocating Human Organs and Tissues."

8. I-Min Lee and Ralph S. Paffenberger, "Change in Body Weight and Longevity," *Journal of the American Medical Association* 268 (Oct. 21, 1992): 2045–49.

TWENTY-ONE

MULTIORGAN, SPLIT-ORGAN, AND REPEAT TRANSPLANTS

Daniel Canal's ordeal started when he was 8 years old. The Wheaton, Maryland, boy had been born with a defective small intestine. It was twisted and failed to function properly. It gradually caused damage to his pancreas and liver. Eventually, he was placed on the organ waiting list for a transplant for all three organs at University of Pittsburgh's Children's Hospital, one of only three hospitals in the country that perform this type of multiple-organ transplant. Daniel remained on the waiting list for five years, during which his condition rapidly deteriorated.

In February of 1998 he spoke at a rally in Washington, D.C., about the issue of basing organ transplants on need rather than geography (an issue we will explore in Chapter 24). It was after this speech that his five-year wait gained national attention, and he was then placed on a waiting list at Jackson Children's Hospital in Miami. Only three days after being listed, a donor match was found. After the years of waiting, his response was, "Mom, I don't want to go. . . . I'm scared." His mother prevailed, however, and he was flown to Miami by ambulance plane.

He received his transplant on May 15, 1998, by a team of surgeons led by Andreas Tzakis. The 12-hour operation seemed uneventful, although it was found that Daniel's stomach had deteriorated as well and also needed to be replaced. On May 31, his body had a rare and violent reaction to the small intestine and, because of this rejection, all four organs needed to be replaced. The second transplant occurred on June 2, using donated adult organs, which had to be reduced in size to fit Daniel's body. A hospital spokesperson was quoted as saying, "He's so sick, and we're in such a desperate race against time." They knew the organs were not ideal, but it was an emergency. This transplant failed because the donated liver failed to function properly. The donor was described as "less-than-healthy." On June 20, Daniel received still another set of organs, making 12 in all that he had received.

Doctors worked for 19 hours to transplant organs harvested from a young donor in Puerto Rico. This surgery was deemed successful, as Daniel had no adverse reactions. Four months later he was well enough to have his first solid food in years. This was his request: two pieces of chicken and ten french fries from Burger King. The next spring, he threw out the ceremonial first pitch at a Baltimore Orioles baseball game. His case, however, sparked debate about the fairness of the decision to allocate 12 organs to one person.[1]

One of the most persistent and perplexing problems in organ allocation is what should be done with those who consume more than one of the scarce supply of solid organs. Some people have multiorgan failure, needing both kidney and pancreas, heart and lung, or some other combination of organs. Others have had a previous graft that has now failed so they are in need of another organ. In rare cases, such as Daniel Canal's, patients needing multiple organs find the first transplant fails, thus requiring repeat multiorgan transplants.

Utilitarian allocators do not look favorably on performing multiorgan or repeat transplant.[2] These potential recipients are sick patients. Those needing repeat transplant find that their new grafts do not do as well as the first ones, partly because of the increased risk of antibody reactions. Deontologists who are concerned about fairness and equal opportunity may not look favorably on retransplant cases either, because there is an intuition that fairness requires giving those who have not yet had their first graft a chance before retransplant candidates get seconds.

On the other hand, when these cases are successful, they provide some of the most moving testimonies to the marvels of modern medical technology. Multiorgan recipient Robert Casey returned from his heart–liver transplant to resume his position as governor of Pennsylvania. (His case will be discussed in detail in Chapter 23).

Multiorgan Transplants

Although they are technologically different and pose somewhat different ethical problems, multiorgan transplants and repeat transplants raise some issues in common—problems of a single person making such heavy demand on the common and small organ pool and problems of the fairness issues this demand raises. We will look first at multiorgan transplants, then turn to repeat transplant.

Utilitarian Concerns

It is easy to see why utilitarians are troubled by multiorgan transplants. At their best they save one life and return one person to a normal life when the same organs could have saved two. That makes the utilitarian's mathematics simple. Moreover, for multiorgan transplants the success rate may be lower than it would be for each of the organs transplanted individually. For example, heart–lung recipients have a one-year graft survival of 64.6 percent, whereas heart recipients' rate is 82.6 and lung recipients' rate is 72.5 percent (patient survival rates are almost identical).[3]

Deontological Views

The position of the deontologist is more complex. The primary concern is with the fairness of using two or more organs for one person. The analysis of fairness, however, is complicated.

FAIRNESS AS EQUAL CLAIM ON SCARCE RESOURCES

For the egalitarian, the deontologist whose understanding of justice is arranging social practices so that people have an opportunity for equality, sometimes fairness means that resources are distributed equally.[4] This approach might work for distribution of income in a radically egalitarian society or distribution of food relief in a famine, but it makes no sense to even the most radical egalitarian in the world of health care. Everyone getting the same amount of health care would either mean that those fortunate enough to be healthy would have to needlessly consume or that those with serious ongoing medical needs would have to go without much of what they really need.

One way radical egalitarians respond to this problem is to emphasize an enriched understanding of resources. They might view resources as including not only money and consumer goods but also one's genetic endowment, inherited social position, and fate in the natural and social lotteries of life. This view suggests that, to the radical egalitarian, when we add up the goods that each person possesses we include not only material and economic resources but also the health and talent with which one was endowed. This is sometimes referred to as *assets from the natural lottery*. A radical egalitarian might take the position that the goal of social practices such as organ allocation should be equality of opportunity for resources, taking into account what one has received in the natural lottery as well as what one acquires through the social lottery—that is, through one's family's socioeconomic position, the luck of being born into a favored or disfavored cultural situation, and so forth. This would mean that one endowed with poor health through genetics or culture has a claim on health care resources needed to get even with those who find themselves through natural and social fortune to be healthier. (As we saw in the previous chapter, some critics insist that it is only *opportunities* for health that one is entitled to, so that those who squander their opportunities through voluntary lifestyle choices do not have the same standing as those who were shorted in the natural and so-cial lotteries.)

This interpretation of egalitarianism suggests that if someone was endowed with more than one organ that fails (especially if it is not because of that person's behavior), one has received fewer resources in life's allocation than either those who get a full complement of healthy organs or those who have the misfortune of single-organ failure. If one of the tasks of the social system is to establish practices that continually correct these mal-allocations, then someone who has one organ that has failed is entitled to that one, whereas those who have more than one in failure are entitled to more and those with a full set of functioning organs, none.

Keep in mind that the holder of the justice perspective is not primarily concerned about the inefficiencies of the system. He or she is concerned with establishing a social practice that will make opportunities more equal. In an ideal world in which there are enough organs to go around, everyone would get the number of organs needed to be healthy. In a less than ideal situation in which there is a shortage of organs, all on the waiting list have a claim on the system for an equal chance to get the organs they need. That means whether someone needs one or several organs, he or she has an equal claim.

INTEGRATING CLAIMS BASED ON THE NUMBER OF ORGANS NEEDED
WITH OTHER CLAIMS

There may, of course, be other variables that influence the justice of claims. We have already seen that voluntary health-risky behavior may be one such factor. Those who have had good organs and have engaged in voluntary behaviors that have ruined them may have somewhat less of a claim. In chapters that follow we shall explore whether age, social status, and race are variables affecting the legitimacy of claims. Later in this chapter we shall see if retransplant is such a factor. The point is that the need for multiple organs is not a legitimate factor in deciding one's standing for organs if the justice perspective is taken. For example, consider a situation in which three people are waiting for organs—one needing a heart, one a lung, and one both heart and lung. What should happen if one heart and one lung become available? The utilitarian might easily conclude that transplanting the heart- and lung-only patient is the efficient thing to do. The person taking the justice perspective would, however, be inclined to insist that all three have an equal claim. A drawing might take place to see which of the three wins, with the heart-lung candidate getting the organs if he or she wins. Presumably, if one of the others wins, then the other single-organ transplant candidate would also get his or her needs met.

THE IMPACT OF THE AVAILABILITY OF SUITABLE ORGANS

There is still a further complication. In Chapter 19 we saw that one of the criteria for fair distribution is the likelihood of finding a suitable organ in the future. Because some donors are unable to supply both heart and lungs (because of the medical suitability of the organ or the lack of willingness of the donor to consent), the recipient needing both organs may actually be given a preference. It makes sense to transplant the heart and lungs at the same time.

Even though there are good utilitarian reasons to place single-organ recipients ahead of those needing multiple organs, in fact, we do not adopt that priority. That suggests that policy makers recognize the wisdom of giving more equal access regardless of the number of organs needed and actually give the multiorgan recipient a priority when it is called for by concern for the likelihood of the availability of suitable organs.

THE UNEQUAL DEMAND FOR ORGANS

The criticism of Daniel Canal's use of a total of 12 organs raises one final problem. Not all 12 of the organs Daniel received were equally in demand. Two of the organs—the small intestine and the stomach—are not really scarce resources. Very few such transplants are needed. Only 67 intestinal transplants were performed in 1997. Stomach transplant is so rare that statistics are not even kept. In March of 1999, 445 were awaiting pancreas transplant, making it scarce, but not as scarce as the liver. The only organ in really high demand that Daniel received was the liver. Moreover, the second set of organs transplant received was not medically ideal. It is doubtful whether any of them would have been used on anything other than an emergency basis. That means that Daniel really only received two organs that were in great demand, the two good-quality livers. Daniel's case is rather similar to one in which a patient was a candidate for a second liver after the first had failed. Although some have suggested that repeat transplant candidates deserve lower priority than first-time recipients, such proposals are controversial. No one is advocating a complete prohibition.

Repeat Transplants

Daniel Canal needed not only multiple organs but also repeat transplant. Re-transplant poses a somewhat different set of problems for both utilitarians and deontologists.

Utilitarian Concerns

The fact that some potential transplant recipients have already had grafts that fail is not a direct concern of utilitarians who are trying to maximize medical utility.

THE DIRECT RELEVANCE OF RETRANSPLANT

By the time a graft has failed and the recipient needs a new organ, as long as there is an organ shortage, only a fixed number of transplants can take place. Only one life can be saved with the second organ. Whether it is the same person who has already had a previous graft or is a new candidate makes no direct difference to someone who is not concerned about the distribution of a good, but only the aggregate total. A life is a life. Because utilitarians are not concerned about the distribution of goods but only the aggregate amount of good, especially if we exclude considerations of social worth, it should make no difference to the utilitarian which lives are saved.

RETRANSPLANT AS AN INDICATOR OF GREATER GRAFT FAILURE

Even though utilitarians have no direct concern about the fact that some potential recipients have been transplanted previously, they have an indirect concern. Data reveal that retransplant patients do not do as well as first transplant patients.[5] If graft failure rates are greater with second and succeeding transplants, a utilitarian, who is striving for maximum benefit regardless of how it is distributed, will give priority to those who have not had grafts previously. Other things being equal, the utilitarian will prefer the patient with the better chance of success, which will be the candidate who has not previously had a graft failure. (Of course, other things are often not equal. A true utility maximizer will also take into account the cause of the organ failure, the age of the recipient, and, as we have seen, the race, gender, and socioeconomic status as well, because they all predict likelihood of success. One who is unwilling to take all of these factors into account is probably not a utility maximizer and may come to understand that the slightly poorer success rate of the retransplant candidate is not morally relevant either.)

LONG-TERM IMPLICATIONS OF DOWNGRADING RETRANSPLANTS

Utilitarians may take a more long-term perspective, however. They might ask what the impact would be on a transplant program of giving candidates for retransplant lower priority. Although many in the public do not realize it, not all donor organs are equal. Some organs are what can be called "marginal" (a problem we examined in Chapter 16). They are less desirable because they come from older donors, have medical characteristics that make them more marginal and less desirable, have marginal damage during procurement (such as vessels that were cut too short), have long warm-ischemic times, or come from patients who may be at somewhat higher risk for disease. None of these organs are totally unacceptable or they would not be made available to begin with. However, if recipients and their surgeons knew that they had only one chance at a transplant before being relegated to second status in the allocation process, they would have a strong incentive to decline the marginal organ and hold out for the "perfect" one. From a systems point of view, this is not a good incentive to create. Assuming that some of the marginal organs are only slightly less promising and that it is rational to include them in the donor pool to begin with, we do not want potential recipients declining them if they are otherwise suitable (if not perfect) organs. An incentive to reject these marginal organs will undoubtedly lead to organ waste. Some might be passed along to recipients who are so desperate they will take the chance, but the delays will cause some harm to all organs and complete waste to some. They will show up as "discards." Assuming that the organ had a reasonably good chance of success if taken by the first recipient on the list and that there is an organ shortage that will lead to some deaths of patients while on the waiting list, these are organs that should be transplanted, preferably to the recipient on the waiting list with the highest priority. The reasonable conclusion of the utilitarian might be that the disutilities of giving retransplant candidates lower status outweigh the advantage of giving scarce organs to first-time candidates.

The question of whether downgrading retransplant candidates will lead to greater overall benefit from the transplant system is an empirical question that cannot be answered in the abstract. The answer will depend on the current state of medical science and the relative risk of rejection for first-time and repeat transplants, as well as how much the reduction in status of the retransplant patient will influence the behavior of patients and surgeons.

Deontologists and Retransplant

By way of contrast, deontologists are not as worried about the possibility of a higher failure rate for retransplant or even the incentive to decline marginal organs. Rather they are concerned about treating the potential recipients on the waiting list fairly.

GETTING MORE THAN A FAIR SHARE

Some people may intuitively feel that there is something unfair about giving someone a shot at a second graft when others are still in line for their first. We all have egalitarian instincts about some distributions. No one gets seconds on dessert until everyone has had firsts.

The assumption for desserts, however, is that "need" is not a critical issue. No one can be said to "need" two desserts—or even one. Having received a first portion, the recipient has no particular claim to a second. In the case of organs, however, receiving a graft that fails leaves one in a situation as bad or worse than someone waiting for the first graft. If "fair shares" are proportional to need, then the person with organ failure from the first graft has need that is, in general, equal to the first-time transplant candidates on the list.

RETRANSPLANT AT MOST INDIRECTLY RELEVANT

The UNOS Ethics Committee, when it considered retransplant, came to the reasonable conclusion that when people are in organ failure the crucial issue is not whether one has had a previous graft. The other variables that go into organ allocation—factors such as HLA-match, medical urgency, PRA, or time on the waiting list depending on the organ—are what is morally relevant, not whether one has received a previous graft. Assuming that the candidate for retransplant was not considered personally responsible for the first graft's failure—through refusal to take antirejection medication or otherwise maintain a follow-up regimen—the fact of a previous graft is morally irrelevant to the person concerned with equity in allocation. Just as with the multiorgan problem, retransplant is not directly relevant to organ allocation. At most it will indirectly influence factors considered relevant, such as likelihood of success and likelihood of finding another suitable organ.

Although utilitarians might be perplexed about whether to take need for multiple organs or retransplant into account, deontologists who are committed to equality of opportunity for the resources needed to be healthy will not consider either to be morally relevant. In current policy the deontologists have carried the day. Being a candidate for a repeat transplant does not count against the individual in the allocation of organs. Although the allocation algorithm is more complicated, varying to some degree from one center to another, generally no penalty for being a candidate for multiple organs is recognized.

Splitting Organs

One final issue needs to be taken up in this chapter. It is an issue closely related to multiple and repeat transplant. We now know that just as we can procure a liver or lung lobe from a living donor, we could also divide these organs when procured from cadavers. We, in effect, could decide to give a cadaver liver to one large recipient or two smaller ones. Similar issues potentially arise not only for lungs but for pancreata and for certain kidneys when surgeons must choose between transplanting two small kidneys *en bloc* to one recipient or dividing them so they are transplanted in the more traditional fashion, benefiting two recipients.

The moral analysis is quite similar to that provided for multiple and repeat transplants. From the point of view of the utilitarian, the payoff from dividing cadaver organs, when it is technically feasible to do so, is about double that of transplanting these organs to a single recipient. From the utilitarian's point of view, there is good reason to double the expected benefit when a scarce organ is allocated.

From the point of view of the deontologist, however, such a policy raises serious questions of fairness. If two candidates are on the waiting list, each of whom needs a life-saving organ such as a liver, the principle of justice requires that, other things being equal, they deserve an equal opportunity to receive the organ. Hence among those in the same category for degree of urgency, the same blood type, and so forth, allocation would either have to be made on the basis of time on the waiting list or by some random method such as flipping a coin. From the point of view of the individuals who both want to live, giving advantage to one recipient because he or she is smaller seems unfair.

Justice, at least as we have interpreted it, however, requires opportunities for equality of access to organs. We saw in the previous chapter that a principle of equality of opportunity may still leave open the possibility that some people have had their opportunities and not taken advantage of them. So, for example, if two adults were competing for a liver and one candidate had a much larger body mass (large enough that he would require an entire liver) and the other candidate was sufficiently tiny that a single lobe of the liver would suffice, someone who believed that voluntary lifestyle choices that can contribute to body mass would have to assess whether the candidates' relative size was voluntary and what role these choices played in determining whether they could make do with a lobe rather than a whole organ. If the larger candidate's size were seen as fully within the recipient's control, then, in theory, the larger candidate could be said to have had an opportunity to be of a size at which only a lobe was required. Of course, if large body size is thought to be beyond voluntary control, it would be irrelevant from the deontologist's point of view.

It is rather easy to see how problematic such reasoning is in the case of body size. Those doing the allocating have to determine the extent to which body size is voluntary as opposed to genetically or psychologically determined. The problems seem insurmountable. Even if we decide as a society that certain behaviors (such as alcoholism) are sufficiently voluntary that they should count against a candidate in an organ allocation, it seems impossible to apply this approach to matters of body size. Certainly some large people are large because of factors beyond their control. Deciding which people should be given lower priority on the basis of body size would pose overwhelmingly difficult problems.

If that is the case, then deontologists will be firm in their conclusion that all people with equal need for an organ should have an equal opportunity to obtain one regardless of the fact that some will need an entire organ whereas others will make do with only part of one. This is simply one more case in which we will choose to make our organ allocation formulas somewhat less efficient to make them more fair. The appropriate policy seems to be one in which, when an organ becomes available, it is allocated on the basis of a standardized formula that takes both equity and efficiency into account. If the organ goes to an adult who needs the whole organ, that ends the story. If it goes to an adult who needs only part of an organ, it could be split, with the second portion going to the next available person on the waiting list who could use a split organ.

A related problem exists in deciding whether to allocate an organ to an adult or a child. There may be good moral reasons why children deserve priority independent of the fact that they could use only a part of an organ, thus making the transplant system produce more aggregate benefit. Before determining whether children deserve a liver lobe with priority over an adult who might need the entire organ, we need to examine the role of age in allocation, to which we now turn.

ENDNOTES

1. Based on Lisa Frazier, "Wheaton Family's Dream Comes True: After a Five-Year Wait, 13-Year-Old Gets a Multiple-Organ Transplant," *Washington Post*, May 17, 1998, p. B3; "Wheaton Boy's Transplants Fail," *Washington Post*, June 3, 1998, p. B4; Avram Goldstein, "13-Year-Old Undergoes History-Making Surgery: Boy Gets 3rd Multiple-Organ Transplant," *Washington Post*, June 23, 1998, p. D3; Sue Anne Pressley, "Recovery Leads to Fast-Food Heaven: After Multiple Transplants, Md. Teen Is Finally Able to Eat Again," *Washington Post*, Oct. 11, 1998, pp. B1, 10.

2. Paul T. Menzel, "Rescuing Lives: Can't We Count?" *Hastings Center Report* 24 (1, Jan.–Feb. 1994): 22–23.

3. Available at <www.unos.org>, March 27, 1999, "Kaplan-Meier Graft and Patient Survival Rates at One, Two, Three, and Four Years for U.S. Transplants Performed between October 1987 and December 1997." On the other hand, for kidney and pancreas, the other pair of organs often transplanted together, the graft and patient survival rates do not differ substantially from the transplant of kidney transplanted separately. Compared to the kidney transplanted alone, the one- and three-year patient survival is only slightly lower and the five-year survival is actually higher. The graft survival is also slightly higher at all three time intervals. See UNOS, *1997 Annual Report of the U.S. Scientific Registry for Transplant Recipients and the Organ Procurement and Transplantation Network—Transplant Data: 1988–1996* (Richmond, VA: Author; and Rockville, MD: Division of Transplantation, Office of Special Programs, Health Resources and Services Administration, U.S. Department of Health and Human Services), Tables 26 and 27. Those who receive a pancreas alone do significantly worse (63.5 percent one-year survival) than those receiving a kidney either simultaneously (80.8 percent) or previously (72.8 percent; Table 32).

4. Ronald Dworkin, "What Is Equality? Part 1: Equality of Welfare," *Philosophy and Public Affairs* 10 (Summer 1981): 185–246; Dworkin, "What Is Equality? Part 2: Equality of Resources," *Philosophy and Public Affairs* 10 (Fall 1981): 283–345; Robert M. Veatch, *The Foundations of Justice: Why the Retarded and the Rest of Us Have Claims to Equality* (New York: Oxford University Press, 1986).

5. For the kidney one-year graft survival is 86.7 percent for first transplant and 82.4 percent for retransplant. UNOS, *1997 Annual Report of the U.S. Scientific Registry for Transplant Recipients and the Organ Procurement and Transplantation Network—Transplant Data: 1988–1996.* For livers the comparable numbers are 79.1% and 55.0% (Table 30); for hearts 84.5% and 66.4% (Table 34); for lungs 75.9 and 59.6 (Table 36); and for pancreata 79.6% and 64.9% (Table 32).

TWENTY-TWO

THE ROLE OF AGE IN ALLOCATION

IN CHAPTER 15 we examined the role of age in organ procurement. In that chapter I suggested that it would be both efficient and equitable to use the relation of donor age to recipient age as a factor in allocation. This would encourage a reasonable goal of letting organs of young donors go to young recipients and leaving older organs for older recipients without making this an absolute rule. In this chapter the issue is whether age should play any other legitimate role in the allocating of organs once procured. Independent of whether the age of the donor should create either a categorical exclusion or a bias in favor of similar aged recipients, there is increasing controversy over the role of the age of the recipient in allocating organs. It is widely believed that there are utilities in allocating organs to younger people, but some believe that fairness also is a relevant issue. Many have held that fairness requires giving older persons equal consideration for an organ even if efficiency does not. I shall present a new argument suggesting that justice or fairness actually requires discrimination against the elderly in allocating organs.

The Moral Norms for Allocation

In Chapter 19 I suggested that there are basically three general criteria for allocating any good, including organs: efficiency (incorporating the principle of utility), equity (incorporating the principle of justice), and the right of refusal (which incorporates the principle of autonomy). The U.S. transplant act specifically requires that organ allocation achieve both efficiency and equity.[1] On the question of the role of age in allocation, autonomy plays a very minor role. It supports the right of patients to decline organs if they consider themselves too old to endure the surgery. It also supports the right of patients to refuse organs from donors that they consider to be too old, a piece of information often not provided to potential recipients. I have interpreted autonomy to generate liberty rights—that is, the right to be left alone or to refuse to participate in a transplant.

It would have little, if any, relevance to the systems question of whether to consider age in allocating organs. The principles of utility and justice, however, have more significant implications.

Efficiency (Utility)

As we have seen, most physicians are implicitly committed to a kind of utilitarian perspective. They believe the morally relevant feature of a choice is its consequences. They are often Hippocratic in their concern about consequences. They include only consequences for the patient, but when they are forced into a role in social policy questions, they continue to take the utilitarian perspective, simply shifting to the goal of maximizing aggregate consequences, taking into account all affected parties.

This utilitarian perspective leads to the conclusion that organs should be allocated in the way they will do the most good. Although some try to take into account the social benefits of alternative uses of organs, we have seen that in transplant most people agree to limit their attention to medical benefits. Age can be important in assessing medical benefit.

THE CONSEQUENTIALIST ARGUMENT FOR TAKING AGE INTO ACCOUNT

The most obvious relevance of age in predicting benefit is that an organ, if transplanted into an elderly person, will produce time-limited medical benefit. Even if the graft does not fail, other medical problems will predictably lead to death. Moreover, the elderly are often believed to be more difficult to treat; they are thought to have lower success rates. The 1997 United Network for Organ Sharing (UNOS) data reveal that, indeed, older recipients do not do as well in organ transplant. The one-year graft failure in kidney transplant (controlling for other variables) is 1.238 times as great for 60-year-olds as for recipients at age 40.[2] Even a 50-year-old has graft failure 5 percent greater than someone who is 40 (odds ratio = 1.058). For livers, 50-year-olds do worse than those at age 40, and 60-year-olds do still worse (one-year graft failure odds ratios = 1.112 and 1.313, respectively).[3] The story is similar for hearts. Sixty-five-year-old recipients do much worse than 45-year-olds (one-year graft survival odds ratio = 1.637).

These data clearly do not support the conclusion that transplants into old people are doomed to fail, but these recipients statistically do worse. If one believes that our scarce organ resources should be allocated so they will do the most medical good, a case can be made that old age should count against a patient. At least if medical good is defined as we defined it in Chapter 20 as maximizing the expected number of quality-adjusted life years per organ transplanted, targeting younger recipients will produce more medical good.

THE CONSEQUENTIALIST ARGUMENT AGAINST TAKING AGE INTO ACCOUNT

At this stage of the argument, a sophisticated consequentialist may point out that there are also predictable disutilities of allocating preferentially to younger patients. Some elderly patients may actually do quite well. Moreover, if we know that the organ allocation formula is designed to discriminate against the elderly, those who have elderly relatives will be distressed at the thought that their loved ones will be forced to die for lack of organs. In fact, we ourselves may worry about our future old age, knowing we will not be able to get an organ we might need. These factors should count against excluding the elderly from the organ allocation.

The problem with this counterargument is that although some elderly people may do well, we have seen that statistically they will not do as well and for as long as younger persons would with the same organs. And although we might be distressed at the thought of excluding the elderly, we should also be distressed at least as much at the thought of young persons dying because the available organ went to an older person. On balance, if medical utility were the only morally relevant factor, it would be morally justified, indeed morally required, to discriminate against the elderly. Moreover, it would be physiological age, not mere chronological age, that would be relevant.

Equity (Justice)

The case for nondiscriminatory organ allocation to older persons is often made in terms of equity or justice. It is derived from a more general concern about the injustice of discriminating against the elderly.[4]

THE CASE THAT EQUITY REQUIRES AVOIDING DISCRIMINATION AGAINST ELDERLY PATIENTS

The argument is that even if it is more efficient to give the organs to younger persons, doing so is unfair. The elderly deserve equal treatment. To do otherwise would be ageism—immoral, unfair treatment of the elderly. People who support this view claim that justice requires treating similarly situated people equally and that those who are sickest deserve priority even if it is not always the most efficient use of resources. They claim that all persons who are equally sick, regardless of age, deserve equal treatment.

THE CASE THAT EQUITY REQUIRES DISCRIMINATION AGAINST THE ELDERLY

Although the justice-based argument in favor of equal treatment of the elderly comes easily, recent scholarship on the ethics of age has suggested the picture is more complex. Whether these more complex justice-based arguments in support of allocating organs preferentially to younger people succeed is a matter of considerable current controversy.

It should be apparent that the claim that justice requires giving the elderly who are equally needy equal access to organs depends on what in Chapter 19 we called *present need* or *urgency*. The results turn out to be quite different if we introduce the concept of *over-a-lifetime need*. The arguments are worth examining. At least three different arguments have surfaced suggesting that to be *fair* one should take age into account in allocating organs.

The notion of a natural life span. Daniel Callahan,[5] the former director of the Hastings Center, has gained considerable notoriety for his advocacy of the view that humans have a natural life span and that it is hubris to strive to prolong life indefinitely beyond its natural endpoint with expensive, exotic medical technologies. He would include organ transplants in that group of technologies that merely postpone the inevitable, depriving others of what they need to merely get up to their normal years.

He stresses that those who have completed their life span should still be treated humanely; they should receive pain-relieving medications; compassionate, high-quality care; and simple treatments for acute illness, but he would draw the line at expensive, resource-consuming treatment of chronic illnesses such as those requiring organ transplant. According to Callahan's view, it is not that transplanting the elderly is inefficient, although it may be. It is rather that continuing to pursue more days misunderstands our natural limits and is unfair to others who have not yet reached their natural end.

Even for those such as Callahan who accept the notion of a natural limit to the life span, this approach raises some problems. For one, as a practical matter if we were to incorporate this notion into our organ allocation policy we would need to set a specific, recognizable point when one is no longer eligible for organs. Callahan has variously put this point at age 75[6] and in the late 70s or early 80s.[7] But that is not specific enough to establish a cutoff for entitlement to organs. We would need a specific, sharp line, such as the age-65 cutoff, or Callahan's earlier 75-year limit. This artificial, sharp line would produce a much too dramatic change, so that the day before one's critical birthday one would have a full entitlement, whereas the next day one would have none. That would be arbitrary, hard to enforce, and would have the appearance of being unfair.[8] Moreover, this notion of a natural life span does not seem to provide any theoretical basis for continuing to provide treatment for acute illness, pain relief, and good nursing while expensive treatment for chronic illness is excluded.

The prudential life span account. Norman Daniels,[9] a philosopher from Tufts University, developed a second justice-based argument for allocating health resources based on age that can be adapted to justify organ allocation with priority for younger persons. He points out that allocating resources among different age groups can be reconceptualized as allocation to a single person among different stages of his or her life span. Assuming we live a full life span, we each pass through each of life's stages. It is unrealistic to assume we are entitled to the same kinds of health care resources at the various stages of our lives. What is needed for adolescence is less important for young adults; what is crucial for infancy is not as fitting for old age, when other services may be more essential.

Daniels claims that it is a matter of prudence in how we allocate our resources among the various stages of our lives. As long as all of similar need in a particular stage are treated equally, it is not unfair that our entitlements change from one stage to another.

This account goes a long way toward overcoming the problems not only with utilitarian-based rationing by age but also those growing out of a notion of a natural life span. Still it raises problems. Most critically, Daniels's account does not directly tell us which age groups have claims and what kinds of claims they have. In fact, he suggests that this is a matter of mere prudent judgment rather than there being some intrinsic moral reason to choose one age group over another. On the contrary, there may be sound moral reasons why one *ought* to give moral priority to younger persons.[10] Moreover, this view assumes that all persons pass through all the life stages. In fact, people who are candidates for major organ transplant may not all have an opportunity to live through all life stages if they do not receive transplants. We need an account that explains which age groups have which claims—in particular, which have claims to transplantable organs.

The justice-over-a-lifetime argument. I suggest another approach to allocation by age, one from the perspective of justice that focuses on benefiting the worst off and how we determine who is worst off. It emphasizes that there are two different ways of thinking about who is worst off. The first, which can be called the *slice-of-time perspective*, asks who is worst off at a given moment of time. That is the view taken by those who advocate equal access to organs to those who are equally sick regardless of age. This is the present need view.

But there is a second way to think about who is worst off. I call it the *over-a-lifetime perspective*.[11] Others have referred to it as the *fair innings* argument.[12] It so dominates Frances Kamm's approach[13] that she uses it as the only meaning of need. It asks who is worst off considering people's whole lives. From the moment-in-time perspective, a 40-year-old and a 70-year-old dying of heart failure are equally poorly off, but considering their entire lives who could deny that the one who was healthy enough to make it to 70 is much better off? To be fair, we need to allocate our resources so that the 40-year-old has a chance to make it to 70. From this over-a-lifetime perspective, justice requires that we target organs for these younger persons who are so poorly off that they will not make it to old age without being given special priority. The younger the age of the person needing an organ, the higher the claim. Moreover, in contrast to the utilitarian principle, which would give attention to physiological age, this justice-based perspective would focus on chronological age, something much easier to determine.[14]

Comparing Age-Based Accounts

Thus there are several different accounts of how justice may actually require taking age into account (or at least permit it). Before turning to the question of how age could become a factor in the allocation formula, it is worth comparing the different age-based accounts.

I have already suggested that Daniels's prudential account does not require any particular pattern of distribution based on age. It is a matter of prudential judgment among the social community. The implication is that nothing would be wrong with taking age into account if it were done evenhandedly and if all people of a particular age who were in similar need were treated equally. It would simply be a matter of prudence whether different age groups got different priorities.

By contrast the Callahan life-span-based account would produce entitlements that would look something like the representation in Figure 22.1. All persons below the endpoint of the normal life span would have an equal entitlement, but that would be a greater entitlement than that possessed by those over the critical point. I have already suggested that one practical difficulty with this account is how a public policy could manage the dramatic shift that would occur at some critical moment—say, around 75 years of age—when one day one is fully entitled to an organ and the next day, after "celebrating" the critical birthday, one completely loses it.

By contrast, my view would produce an entitlement to organs that was inversely proportional to age regardless of where one is in the life span. It would provide a smooth, gradual priority inversely related to age rather than producing a precipitous drop off in entitlement at some birthday. It would explain the priority given to children in the kidney allocation formula without relying exclusively on appeals to medical benefit. This is represented in Figure 22.2. With increasing age one would gradually have less and less of a claim to organs. At older ages the curve is almost flat; age would do no more than break ties. At younger ages, however, the differences would be significant.

Entitlement Based on Age
Callahan Approach Based on Lifespan

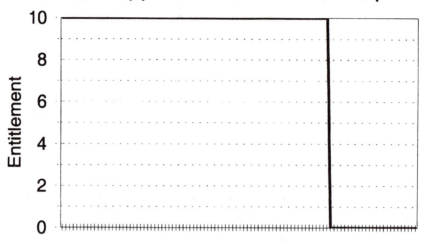

Age (1 to 100 with Lifespan of 75)

FIGURE 22.1

Entitlement Based on Age
Author's Proposal (10 Points/Age)

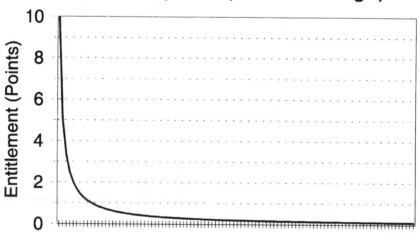

Age (from 1 to 100)

FIGURE 22.2

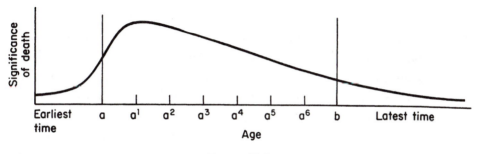

FIGURE 22.3

Kamm has criticized the implications of this view, suggesting that it is implausible that the very young should be seen as more entitled. She produces a figure that I reprint as Figure 22.3. Kamm graphs the "significance of death" against age, but she uses this information to suggest relative entitlement just as the other graphs presented here do. Notice that the curve shows that early years actually produce *ascending* claims. Presumably this means up to some point about at the beginning of adulthood claims increase and then, following the view I have presented, claims gradually decrease. She says[15] there is

> a fairly common feeling that it is less important to save those who have just begun their lives than to save those who are older. So, at least to some, it seems more important to save a 20-year-old rather than a 1-year-old, even if we could provide them both with long lives. (p. 244)

Kamm appears to base this on a comparison between the early years, which she calls "preparatory," and the adult years, which she views as "likely to contain accomplishments." I suspect she is reflecting the biases of a rational philosopher. She cannot bring herself to see that life's value is not always a matter of accomplishments.

I believe she is just wrong. At least if we are concerned about justice in terms of how much of a life one will have, I see no basis for not choosing the simpler decay curve represented in Figure 22.2, at least if the issue is which age has a stronger claim based on being worse off in terms of having had less of a life lived.

A Formula for Taking Age into Account

An allocation that takes an over-a-lifetime approach to allocating organs would incorporate the notion that age is one of the morally relevant factors in allocating organs. The ideal formula would take age into account without making it dominate the allocation.

For systems such as the kidney allocation in the United States that rely on computerized mathematical formulas, we might consider adding a factor made up of a constant divided by age at one's next birthday. In the U.S. formula for kidneys a maximum of seven points is given based on the number of HLA mismatches (excluding zero mismatches, for which there is mandatory sharing that amounts to an absolute priority),[16] four based on PRA,[17] one point for each year on the waiting list plus as much as one point for relative time on the list,[18] and four points for any potential recipient who has previously donated a solid organ or segment of an organ.[19] In addition, children under 11 receive four points and those under 18 three.[20] The impact of age is represented in Figure 22.4.

One problem with the existing point system is that it gives all children up to age 11 the same number of points. On the child's 11th birthday he or she would lose a point. The child at 10 years and 364 days would get a full point priority over the child who was one day older. Even worse, the adolescent transplant candidate would lose three full points when he or she reaches the 18th birthday, a significant drop in standing that surely cannot be accounted for by any evidence that the effectiveness of the transplant in preventing neurological or other impairments changes precipitously on that day.

To illustrate the proposed formula: Using ten as the constant, a newborn up to the age of one year would receive ten extra points, whereas a 10-year-old would receive a single point, and an adolescent who had just passed the 18th

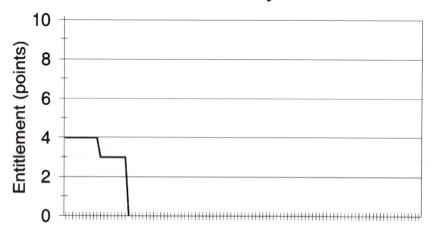

Entitlement Based on Age
Current UNOS Kidney Allocation

Age (4 points under 11, 3 under 18)

FIGURE 22.4

birthday would receive $^{10}/_{18}$ of a point. Older adults would receive smaller fractions of a point. For them, age would normally function merely as a tiebreaker but, all other things being equal, using this formula, a young adult would get preference over an older one, regardless of their ages.

If giving the small child a maximum of ten points based on age seems to give too much weight to age, the constant could be reduced to five or some other smaller number. This would give the child a comparatively smaller advantage. One attractive feature of this formula is that it avoids precipitous changes in the number of points given.

There are justice-based reasons for taking age into account in allocating organs just as there are utilitarian reasons for excluding age as a consideration. Whether they are sufficiently weighty to overcome the presumption that all persons have equal claim regardless of age is a matter for neither philosophers nor transplant surgeons to decide. It is a question that must be answered by policy makers.

Over-a-Lifetime Need versus Present Need

One theoretical perplexity is how using age based on over-a-lifetime notions of need should relate to what in Chapter 19 I called *present need*—that is, how poorly off a person is at the moment the organ or other medical good is allocated. In Chapter 19 I pressed for giving present need considerable importance in the allocation. That meant paying serious attention to time on the waiting list, likely opportunities for future access to an organ (and hence PRA and blood type), and any other factors that are included to attempt to make the system fair. This would also be the basis for incorporating points based on how close the recipient's age matched the donor's age—as suggested in Chapter 15. (We urged trying to bring donor and recipient ages into proximity not only to maximize medical utility but also to make sure that younger recipients would get a fair chance at getting younger organs.)

On the other hand, some medical treatments probably should not be allocated based on over-a-lifetime notions of equality. For example, if an elderly patient who has lived a wonderful life is now in severe pain that could be treated easily with an injection of morphine, almost everyone would agree that the patient should receive the palliative care. This intuition seems sound even though there are young persons whose lives have not been nearly as good who on the basis of an over-a-lifetime view of justice allocation would seem to have a stronger claim to the small funds used to pay for the elderly person's morphine.

Callahan correctly recognizes that there are certain medical interventions that are exempt from his natural life span account. It would be cruel to withhold palliative care from the elderly simply because their natural life span was complete.

Likewise, he would not withhold simple, curative medicines (penicillin for an acute infection) from those above his full life span criterion. Why, then, would he withhold organ transplants and other high-tech, expensive treatments for chronic illness? In spite of the fact that his position—providing palliative care, curative medicine for acute conditions, and good nursing care, but withholding high-technology, expensive interventions for chronic cases—makes good sense, I do not think his notion of completion of a natural life span can account for this difference.

The distinction between present need and over-a-lifetime need provides more of a basis for this separation. There are some services that are appropriately allocated on the basis of present need, whereas others are allocated on the basis of over-a-lifetime need. What is the basis for this? Contemporary personhood theory suggests that continuity of personal identity is important in morality.[21] It has been used, for example, in the definition of death debate.[22] There are some allocational issues for which we think it only fair that one considers well-being over time. For example, if two people sharing a job work equally hard for the same number of hours, one working mornings and the other working afternoons, we would say it is fair that they receive equal compensation. We would say that their contribution was equal in spite of the fact that at no time did they expend equal effort. Over time their contributions could be considered equal. Similar intuitions have been produced for spouses sharing child care or students who rotate clean-up duties. For certain benefits and harms, it is perfectly natural to view lives over time as reflecting continuity of personal identity, so that what counts is net effort or net benefits summed over time.

But for other circumstances, the crisis of the moment is so overpowering that we would consider it irrelevant to take into account the remainder of one's life. For an elderly patient in excruciating pain, it is irrelevant that most of the years of his life have been spent in a relatively well-off condition. Likewise, it seems irrelevant that someone's childhood was good or bad if in old age one has an easily treated acute infection. It does not really even make any difference whether one has had many years before the acute infection or only a few.

For those conditions that seem to be part of one's overall life condition, the over-a-lifetime view is the appropriate assessment. Hence for high-technology, expensive treatments of chronic disease (including transplants) the treatment is merely another stage of a total life experience. Having had many years before the chronic disease is relevant to the assessment of the overall life in a way that it would not be in deciding to spend money, say, on clean sheets for geriatric patients.

The notion of continuity of personal identity is relevant to deciding whether the over-a-lifetime view or the moment-in-time view is appropriate. It is not that the elderly—even the elderly who have completed their "natural life span"—would not benefit from experimental treatment or expensive, high-tech treatment for chronic conditions. It is rather that these, if successful, would just add another phase to an existing life history. In these cases, justice requires using these technologies first for those who have had the worst life histories. By contrast, for crisis interventions for acute pain or illness, the current event is not really appropriately assessed as part of an overall life history. It is an isolated moment of crisis that commands a separate, present-need assessment.[23]

If I am right, then using an age-based factor that is inversely proportional to the age of the potential recipients is a just way to allocate scarce resources. That, however, still leaves the question of how much weight should be given to present need in the overall allocation formula and how much weight should be given to age and other over-a-lifetime considerations. What, for instance, should be done if there are two candidates for a liver: one a 22-year-old who is Status 2B and the other a 66-year-old who is Status 1? On grounds of present need, the older patient has a higher claim. Furthermore, that person would get the clear preference based on today's allocation formula. However, it is not clear to me that this is the correct policy. Surely, the fact that the 66-year-old has already had three times the opportunities for living as the 22-year-old is not irrelevant. The formula I have proposed for kidney allocation in this chapter would give the 22-year-old a slight advantage. I see no reason why that conclusion is not also sound for livers. Yet it is beyond the capacity of this analysis to determine exactly what the relative weights should be for age and medical urgency. If we used the criterion of justice requiring opportunities for equality of quality-adjusted life years, then the younger patient would have a strong claim, even if his healthier status would mean that he could be expected to live several more years without a transplant. It is unlikely he would be a transplant candidate if he had a life expectancy of 44 years without it.

In the case of the kidney allocation, there is relatively little attention given to present need. Urgency (defined as short quality-adjusted life year expectancy without a transplant) is accounted for by considering panel reactive antibodies (PRA) and time on the waiting list, factors that together could account for several points. Adding my proposed points for age would add a maximum of perhaps five points, whereas adults would receive only a fraction of a point. A subjective judgment would have to be made by policy makers to determine the relative importance of present need, over-a-lifetime need, and medical utility. As we have seen, the UNOS Ethics Committee has taken the view that utility and justice—medical benefit and overall need—should count equally. Assuming that is the policy maker's view, then the only remaining question is what the relative weight should be for present and over-a-lifetime need. I would want to give over-a-lifetime need (i.e., age) at least half of the needs-based consideration.[24]

ENDNOTES

1. National Organ Transplant Act, Public Law No. 98-507 98 Stat. 2339 (Oct. 19, 1984).

2. Hung-Mo Lin, H. Myron Kauffman, Maureen A. McBride, Darcy B. Davies, John D. Rosendale, Carol M. Smith, Erick B. Edwards, Patrick Daily, James Kirkin, Charles F. Shield, and Lawrence G. Hunsicker, "Center Specific Graft and Patient Survival Rates: 1997 United Network for Organ Sharing (UNOS) Report," *Journal of the American Medical Association* 280 (Oct. 7, 1998): 1153–60. The story is more complicated. Conditional three-year survival (survival to three years among those surviving the first year) is actually better for 60-year-olds. The authors speculate that this may result from relatively small and selected samples of older recipients—that is, perhaps only very healthy older candidates are actually selected for transplant. Also, recipients younger than 2 years of age do not do as well (one-year graft failure odds ratio = 1.728).

3. Ibid., p. 1157.

4. Larry R. Churchill, "Should We Ration Health Care by Age?" *Journal of the American Geriatrics Society* 36 (1988): 644–47; John F. Kilner, "Age Criteria in Medicine: Are the Medical Justifications Ethical?" *Archives of Internal Medicine* 149 (1989): 2343–46.

5. Daniel Callahan, *Setting Limits: Medical Goals in an Aging Society* (New York: Simon and Schuster, 1987).

6. Daniel Callahan, "Natural Death and Public Policy," in *Life Span: Values and Life-Extending Technologies*, ed. by Robert M. Veatch (San Francisco: Harper and Row, 1979), 162–75.

7. Daniel Callahan, *Setting Limits: Medical Goals in an Aging Society*.

8. F. M. Kamm, *Morality, Mortality: Volume I: Death and Whom to Save from It* (New York: Oxford University Press, 1993), p. 247. I developed this critique of the life-span account in the 1980s, well before Frances Kamm took up the subject. I note, however, that she reaches essentially the same conclusion. In considering a plan similar to Callahan's (but without citing Callahan), that gives equal status to all ages up to some cutoff at the end of the normal life span, she says, "I find this an odd result" (p. 247).

9. Norman Daniels, "Am I My Parents' Keeper?" in *President's Commission for the Study of Ethical Problems in Medicine and Biomedical and Behavioral Research. Securing Access to Health Care*, Vol. 2 (Washington, DC: U.S. Government Printing Office, 1983), pp. 265–91; Daniels, *Am I My Parents' Keeper?: An Essay on Justice*

between the Young and the Old (New York: Oxford University Press, 1988); Daniels, "Am I My Parents' Keeper?" *Midwest Studies in Philosophy* 7 (1982): 517–40.

10. See F. M. Kamm, *Morality, Mortality: Volume I: Death and Whom to Save from It*, p. 247. Again, my view that the preference for the young is morally required rather than a matter of mere prudence converges with Frances Kamm's position, which she appears to have developed independently.

11. Robert M. Veatch, "How Age Should Matter: Justice as the Basis for Limiting Care to the Elderly," in *Facing Limits: Ethics and Health Care for the Elderly*, ed. Gerald R. Winslow and James W. Walters (Boulder, CO: Westview Press, 1993), pp. 211–29; Robert M. Veatch, "Justice and Valuing Lives," *Life Span: Values and Life-Extending Technologies* (San Francisco: Harper and Row, 1979), pp. 197–224; Robert M. Veatch, *The Foundations of Justice: Why the Retarded and the Rest of Us Have Claims to Equality* (New York: Oxford University Press, 1986).

12. John Harris, "Does Justice Require that We Be Ageist?" *Bioethics* 8 (1994): 74–83; Harris, *The Value of Life: An Introduction to Medical Ethics* (London: Routledge & Kegan Paul, 1985), chap. 5; Klemens Kappel and Peter Sandoe, "QALYs, Age and Fairness," *Bioethics* 6 (1992): 297–316; Kappel and Sandoe, "Saving the Young before the Old—A Reply to John Harris," *Bioethics* 8 (1994): 84–92.

13. F. M. Kamm, *Morality, Mortality: Volume I: Death and Whom to Save from It*, p. 234.

14. There is an interesting theoretical problem with giving priority based on chronological age. Consider two candidates for a liver who are in all respects equal (equal in disease and equal in life expectancy without an organ but also standing to gain the same number of years if they get the organ). If their age difference is smaller than the predicted additional years gained from the transplant, then giving the organ to the younger person simply reverses the age-based justice claims. If the candidates are 35 and 38 years of age, respectively, and whoever gets the organ is expected to gain six extra years, then giving it to the 35-year-old will give him a life expectancy of 41 years, thus making the 38-year-old disadvantaged by 3 years. In a purely egalitarian world, this would be as unacceptable as the original inequality.

Kamm (*Morality, Mortality: Volume I: Death and Whom to Save from It*) discusses an ingenious, if purely theoretical, response. She refers to it as "lending organs." If it were technically feasible, we could "lend" the younger patient the organ until he achieves the age of the older competitor and then take it back when the candidates have equal claim, assigning it by some random process such as drawing straws. In fact, precisely this would be feasible for allocating a scarce device such as a hemodialysis machine. We could give the machine to the younger until age parity is established and then allocate randomly. Doing so, of course, comes up against the moral notion that those already receiving a treatment have "dibs" on it until they do not need it any more. That is precisely the moral view that many people take regarding intensive care unit beds. If a patient once occupies the bed, he or she has it until that patient no longer needs it—even if another patient comes along at a later time who could benefit more or who could stake a claim because of a worse-off condition.

Because technically organs cannot be lent (and the disutilities of repeated surgery now preclude the arrangement), this is of no more than theoretical interest. In the meantime, it seems clear that the egalitarian would strive to benefit the person who is worst off (who has the smallest number of expected life years without the organ). The alternative would be to produce an even greater inequality, for example, producing in our example life expectancies of 35 and 43 years, respectively. Assuming we will not give the organ to the 35-year-old and then remove it and discard it after three years, this is the best a strictly egalitarian allocator could do.

15. F. M. Kamm, *Morality, Mortality: Volume I: Death and Whom to Save from It,*

16. UNOS Policy 3.5.2.3., available at <http://www.unos.org/frame_Default.asp?Category=About> (Sept. 22, 1998).

17. UNOS Policy 3.5.9.3., available at <http://www.unos.org/frame_Default.asp?Category=About> (Sept. 22, 1998).

18. UNOS Policy 3.5.9.1.1, available at <http://www.unos.org/frame_Default.asp?Category=About> (Sept. 22, 1998).

19. UNOS Policy 3.5.9.6., available at <http://www.unos.org/frame_Default.asp?Category=About> (Sept. 22, 1998).

20. UNOS Policy 3.5.9.5., available at <http://www.unos.org/frame_Default.asp?Category=About> (Sept. 22, 1998).

21. Derek Parfit, *Reasons and Persons* (Oxford: Clarendon Press, 1984).

22. Michael B. Green and Daniel Wikler, "Brain Death and Personal Identity," *Philosophy and Public Affairs* 9 (2, Winter 1980): 105–33.

23. Kamm (*Morality, Mortality: Volume I: Death and Whom to Save from It,* p. 242) offers a rather similar argument in claiming that such dramatic crisis experiences as torture should not be analyzed in terms of the victim's overall life but should be viewed as an independent momentary event to be judged on its own.

24. If I understand her correctly, Kamm (*Morality, Mortality: Volume I: Death and Whom to Save from It,* p. 252) would give "almost absolute precedence to how much life an individual will have when he or she dies over how urgent the medical need is—that is, how soon one will die if not given a transplant. That, in effect, gives almost absolute priority to young age over the seriousness of the patient's current medical condition. In the terms I have presented, this means Kamm is willing to give strong weight to continuity of opportunities for life and very little weight to the fact that someone is in an immediate crisis. She, like any rational, systematic analyst, is willing to take a very long-term view. I am sympa-

thetic to her perspective but less willing to discount as totally as she the unique moral appeal of the urgency of a moment of crisis. I am not convinced that it is irrational to spend more to save an identifiable life in crisis (the child in the well) than to save a statistical life in a cool hour. I know of no sound theoretical basis for arguing for any particular formula that would establish exactly what the proper ratio should be for considering present need and over-a-lifetime need. I am convinced, however, that for transplants, the over-a-lifetime perspective is legitimate.

TWENTY-THREE

THE ROLE OF STATUS: DID MICKEY MANTLE GET SPECIAL TREATMENT?

THE LIVER TRANSPLANT of former baseball star Mickey Mantle on June 8, 1995, captured more publicity than any transplant in recent memory. We could have encountered his case briefly in Chapter 20 because his liver damage was a result of a long history of alcohol consumption. Many at the time raised the question of whether it was fair for him to receive a liver under those circumstances. It turns out that he also had metastatic cancer, from which he died two months later. It thereby raised the question of whether he was already too sick from the cancer to be entitled to a transplant organ. Finally, the case generated controversy because, even though there were 4,657 people in the United States waiting for a liver and the average wait in the Dallas area where Mantle was hospitalized was 130 days, an organ was found for him the next night after he was listed. Many hinted that they suspected that, because he was a folk hero, he received special treatment, that he was moved to the top of the list, jumping over 4,657 more ordinary, nameless souls who were just as eager to be transplanted. The case provides a context for examining the role of status in organ allocation.

Mickey Mantle: The Real Facts

As a member of the United Network for Sharing Organs (UNOS) Ethics Committee at the time, I was contacted by many members of the press who were eager for me to condemn the organ procurement organization or the national organ network for letting a celebrity get special treatment. As a long-time advocate for the rights of the ordinary patient, I would have been pleased to be able to make such a criticism—if I thought it were true.

I had almost immediate access to the liver allocation formula, which should have been used to allocate any liver that became available, and also the statistics about how many people were on the waiting list. My conclusion was that, once one understood the rules for allocation in place at the time (they have changed slightly since then), it turns out to be very plausible that Mantle got a liver legitimately so soon after he was listed. It raises questions about whether the allocation formula was morally proper, but it is hard to raise the issue of Mantle's status if the organ-procurement organization (OPO) merely gave him an organ by following the same rules that would have applied to everyone else, the rules in place at the time.

The single most important factor is the rule that required that a liver procured first go to anyone on the local OPO waiting list, no matter how sick or how long the person has been waiting. In Mantle's case, he was competing for an organ with others on the waiting list of the Southwest Organ Bank, the OPO serving the Dallas area. Only if no one locally could use the liver are those beyond the local group given access. In that case it went first to those in the region (one of geographical areas in the United States organ transplant system). Finally, if no one in the region could use the organ, it was made available nationally. This three-tier geographical scheme is very controversial. UNOS has been ordered to adjust its allocation formula to alleviate potential unfairness from this geographical priority. This controversy will be the subject of the following chapter. The locals-first priority scheme, however, was what clearly applied to all candidates on the liver waiting list, including Mantle.

The geographical requirement that local candidates get priority meant that Mantle was competing with 140 other people on the waiting list of the Dallas OPO. This reduces the number from 4,657 to 141, considerably reducing the odds. Next the OPO must consider blood type and height and weight characteristics. As we discussed in Chapter 19, priority goes to persons of identical blood type over those with compatible blood. Mantle was of O-blood group, as was the organ donor. In general, 50.9 percent of those on the recipient list are of O-blood group. If that percentage existed in the Dallas waiting list, Mantle was now one of about 70 people competing for the liver based on blood-type criteria. Additional candidates would have been eliminated based on size criteria.

Finally, at the time organs were allocated on the basis of degree of medical urgency. The categories have changed somewhat since the time of the allocation of Mantle's organ, but at the time patients were divided into four groups: Status 1 was for patients in the hospital ICU. Status 2 was for those in the hospital but not in the ICU. Status 3 was for patients who were not hospitalized but were homebound, and Status 4 for others still up and about. The liver allocation rule was governed by what appears to be the principle of justice, that the sickest get first priority. Mickey Mantle was in the hospital but not in the ICU—in what was called Status 2. Thus if there was anyone in the ICU, they should have had priority over Mantle, but Mantle should have had priority over those who were homebound or still healthy enough to be mobile. Moreover, among those in the same category, the tiebreaker is time on the waiting list, so anyone in the hospital in Status 2 longer than Mantle should have received priority as well. For Mantle to be first, there should have been no one in the ICU and no one in the hospital longer than Mantle who had O-blood type and was otherwise available for the organ.

In the Dallas area, 0.45% of the liver waiting list were in Status 1 at the time of Mantle's transplant. That means there should have been about half of one percent of the 70 O-blood-type patients in the ICU. That suggests that, statistically, there should have been zero or one in the ICU with the right blood type and size. The claim that there was none is not surprising.

There are normally about 1.9 percent of the people on the list for livers waiting in Status 2—that is, perhaps one, may be two, people. The claim that Mantle was the only one in the hospital is quite plausible. The claim that Mantle was first in line for an O-blood-type liver in the Dallas area is, thus, consistent with what one might expect, knowing the details of the allocation formula.

Does that imply that Mantle's status played absolutely no role? It is impossible to know for sure. It is clear to anyone who knows how organ procurement organizations function that they feel very strongly about making the allocation system work fairly. There are very strong incentives for them to do this. An OPO that intentionally diverted an organ to someone because of the recipient's status or because the recipient was a favorite patient could be in very serious trouble. Moreover, there are many players on the scene who would have a strong incentive to scream if there were gaming of the system. Surgeons, by their historical Hippocratic conditioning, are militantly committed to their patients. Moreover, they like to do transplants, and their income may be dependent on it. Any surgeons who had O-blood-group patients in a hospital in the Dallas area for longer than a day waiting for a transplant would have known that their patients were bypassed. They would have been morally bound to protest and would have had the self-interest to do so. Moreover, in general, surgeons have the personality to do so. That no surgeons or OPO personnel protested after the enormous publicity given this case reinforces the conclusion that Mantle could reasonably have been the only O-blood-group patient in the hospital in the Dallas area awaiting a liver.

There is still the possibility that Mantle's status gave him some advantage. To one who knows the allocation system, it is apparent that if a surgeon wanted to gain an advantage for her patient, there are some things she could do to help. First, she could put her patient on the waiting list earlier than is medically indicated, realizing that it is likely to be some time before the patient's number comes up in the allocation. By that time her patient might be more nearly ready for the transplant. Also, if the surgeon hospitalizes her patient when he actually could be at home, using the categories in place at the time, she would have moved the patient from Status 3 to Status 2, helping the patient step over almost everyone on the waiting list.

Could that have happened in Mantle's case? In theory, yes, but it would be difficult. There are criteria for listing a patient. There is considerable camaraderie among fellow physicians in a community, as well as considerable competition. Although most might be Hippocratic enough to consider fudging the data for their patients, most would have the integrity and fear of being caught that would incline them to resist. There is no way to prove that Mantle's physician did not list his famous and likable patient sooner than was necessary. He might have at least been moved to hospitalize as soon as was feasible. We have much less control over the individual physician's decision to list a patient than we do once the patient is listed. It is apparent, however, from Mantle's rapid demise that he was a very sick patient. There is no reason to believe he was listed prematurely.

Once the patient is listed, if he were placed in the hospital prematurely, many people—fellow physicians, residents, nurses, and others—would see it. Although we cannot rule out the possibility that Mantle was listed too early or that he was hospitalized before he needed to be, there is no evidence that either of these things happened. The fact that he died so soon after the transplant helps support the conclusion that he was a very sick man.

Was he transplanted when he had a cancer that should have disqualified him? That is another way that Mantle's status could have influenced his care. If the surgeon knew his cancer was metastasized before the surgery, he should not have received the transplant. The surgeon claimed that he did not know about the metastasis in advance. There is no evidence that he did or should have. It is hardly doing a patient a favor to inflict the rigors of transplant surgery on him in the final weeks of his life. If a physician knew his patient had metastatic cancer, it seems unlikely he would have hidden that fact to get him a transplant that would have done nothing to address the underlying cancer problem.

My conclusion is that, even though Mantle was a national hero, there is no evidence his status helped him get an organ. The real issue raised by his case is whether UNOS is right in giving priority to any local patient, no matter how ill, over others in the nation who may be in greater need. Surely there was somebody nationally who was in Status 1 who could have used that organ. That, of course, is in no way a criticism of the Dallas OPO. They seem to have followed the rules in place at the time. In Chapter 24 we will explore the controversy over the change to a national list.

Governor Casey's Case

Governor Robert P. Casey of Pennsylvania, at 61 years of age in 1993, suffered from amyloidosis, a hereditary heart disease that causes the liver to produce a protein that attacks and weakens other organs and adheres to the walls of the heart. He had had a heart attack in 1991 and had undergone quadruple bypass surgery. By 1993 his condition had deteriorated. In the previous four years some 15 patients had undergone liver transplant for amyloidosis, 14 of whom had survived. Many had major improvement. Six patients had undergone a more experimental heart–liver transplant, most of whom had died within a few months.[1]

Casey was placed on the waiting list for a heart–liver transplant at the University of Pittsburgh Medical Center the night of June 12, 1993, and received his transplants in less than a day. It is reported that the median wait at that time for a liver was 67 days and for a heart 198 days. According to Howard M. Nathan, executive director of the Delaware Valley Transplant Program, the OPO for eastern Pennsylvania, southern New Jersey, and Delaware (the neighboring OPO to the Pittsburgh area), in the five years before Casey's transplant, his OPO had overseen 479 heart transplant of which 12 were within 24 hours of listing. It had been involved in 356 liver transplants, 22 of which were less than 24 hours after listing. Six patients were ahead of Casey on the waiting list for a heart and two for a liver.[2] As with the Mantle case, the rapid transplant for this first citizen of the state where his surgery was performed led to suspicions that his prominence as the governor had gotten him special treatment. The fact that this Democratic governor famous for the legal case against abortion bearing his name[3] received the heart and lung of a Black, long-jobless, victim of a drug gang merely makes Casey a more controversial figure.

The allocation rules are not as clear in this case as in Mantle's, in which we saw that even if there were people who had been on the waiting list longer, they could have been excluded because they were the wrong blood type or were not as sick. Casey was reportedly in the sickest category for a heart transplant and the second category for a liver. From the numbers we used for Mantle we can see why so few patients were ahead of the governor. Still, critics were troubled by Casey's rapid access to organs and his apparent priority over those who appeared to be ahead of him.

In this case, the real issue is whether those needing two organs should be taken ahead of those needing only one. We suggested in Chapter 21 that there is good case for such a priority (because it could be a long time before two suitable organs again become available simultaneously). If patients needing two organs are given priority, it is easy to see why Casey was chosen.

UNOS did not have a clear policy dealing with multiorgan allocations for cases involving a heart and liver. Transplant of this combination of organs is extremely rare. However, apparently the University of Pittsburgh Medical Center had such a policy, which gave priority to multiple-organ transplants. John Armitage, director of adult cardiac transplantation at the University of Pittsburgh

Medical Center, was also quoted as saying, "the governor's life was in imminent danger."[4]

Following this episode, the Department of Health and Human Services asked UNOS to clarify its policy on priority for multiorgan transplants. The UNOS board adopted a policy that if a patient is on the waiting lists for both heart and liver, he or she must be ranked first on the waiting list for at least one of the organs. If first on the list for one of the organs, the patient will be offered the other organ or organs at the same time.[5] This does not give actual priority to multiple-organ transplant candidates until they rise to the top of one of the lists. It does ensure, however, that the candidate will get both organs at the same time.

Even if the Pittsburgh program did not follow this policy (written after the transplant) precisely, its procedure of giving priority to multiple-organ transplant candidates for whom both organs were acceptable is not outside the bounds of reason.

It seems that a plausible explanation is available for the governor's rapid transplant, but the situation was ambiguous because the rules were not made clear in advance. It is situations such as these in which the status of the patient can exert an influence. Of course, no organ network can have a rule in place for every possible situation. About all that can be said in this instance is that there was no obvious favoritism shown.

Social Worth versus Social Status

The real issue is would it have been wrong if preference *had* been given in either Mantle's or Casey's case? And if not, why? There are differences in the two cases that are worth examining.

Governor Casey and Social Worth

The governor of a state is in a position of enormous responsibility. Getting him healthy again as quickly as possible not only serves his interests, it serves those of the other citizens of Pennsylvania as well. Can we argue that the common good is so important in his case there was a special priority even if he would not have qualified for such a transplant according to the normal allocation rules?

THE UTILITARIAN POSITION
Classical social utilitarians might be persuaded that someone such as Governor Casey should be given priority status.

Utilitarian acceptance of social worth. We saw in Chapter 19 that they would make allocational decisions by asking the net benefits for all parties affected for the alternatives that are available. That means that they would try to envision the effect on all parties of giving the organs to Casey or to others who are waiting on the basis of what I have called their "social worth." They would take into account all the population affected by restoring the governor to health compared to how they are affected if some other person received the organs.

This, of course, is the assessment of the social worth of the candidates that we indicated in Chapter 19 was excluded by almost everyone in the transplant world. Now, however, we encounter the question of whether there may be special, exceptional cases. On a strictly hypothetical basis, transplant policy makers have asked what should be done if the president of the United States needed an organ. There is a great temptation to say that this would represent a rare exceptional case.

Possible utilitarian case for excluding all social worth judgments. On the other hand, the counterarguments are powerful. First, especially with political leaders, there will be enormous controversy over the amount of good the politician would do if restored to functioning by a transplant. There will always be those who believe the leader is making the wrong decisions and thus doing more harm than good. Trying to reach an agreement on how to estimate the benefits and harms will be as difficult in these cases as in choices between less well-known waiting-list candidates. The quantification of the amount of good done would lead to endless controversy.

Second, even if in principle the quantification problems could be solved for the exceptional case, how would we know when and how often to make the exceptions. Would it be only for the president or would governors qualify as well? What about other politicians? And why only politicians? As I suggested earlier, there may be more disutilities in the utility-calculating enterprise than benefits.

There is a third concern with making these calculations in the exceptional cases. Some utilitarians believe that it is wrong in principle to make these calculations on a case by case basis. They are what is called *rule–utilitarians*.[6] They hold that ethics is a matter of calculating benefits and harms, but these calculations should be done not in the individual case. Rather, they should be done only when choosing the rule under which conduct is to be governed. They will compare the utilities of the rule that "social worth" should be excluded from consideration with two other possible rules: the rule that would routinely take it into account and the rule that would permit it to come into play only in exceptional cases. Taking social worth into account in every case would have the enormous disutility of having to identify the social worth of every candidate on the list, something that would paralyze the transplant program. Taking it into account only in exceptional cases would have the added disutility of the controversies about just who is so socially worthy that the exception should be made.

It is not clear whether a rule–utilitarian would permit exceptions or would, as I suggested earlier, simply rule out all such social value judgments. Perhaps the exceptional case would be ruled out just like the more routine social worth determinations were. At most one could imagine a general policy of excluding social worth considerations but leaving open the possibility of an exception for the extreme case—perhaps one of major international importance. It is at least as plausible to adopt a flat policy of no exceptions.

THE DEONTOLOGISTS AND THE PROBLEM OF JUSTICE

Whether utilitarians would make use of the arguments about the disutility of social worth judgments or adopt a rule-utilitarian stance, most deontologists have their own reasons for resisting social worth as an allocational criterion. Insofar as they include egalitarian justice among their principles, their goal is equality of opportunity. It is hard to imagine how egalitarians would favor making an exception for the governor or anyone else based on social worth.[7] They might use other criteria unrelated to maximizing good consequences (such as promises made or voluntary health-risky behavior discussed in Chapter 20), but not the mere fact that one of the transplant candidates was socially "useful."

The net result seems to be ambivalence if the utilitarian perspective is taken—some arguments in favor of taking social worth into account and some against. However, justice theorists would seem to come down squarely against a social worth exception. One who is committed to considering both utility and justice (efficiency and equity) would thus combine a factor that is quite ambivalent with another that is strongly opposed when it comes to considering social worth. The end result would seem to be clear opposition.

Mantle and Duties of Gratitude

If it is difficult to make the case for an exception to the exclusion of social worth considerations for the governor of a state—indeed, even for the president of a nation—it seems likely that it would be even harder to make the case for a long-retired national sports hero. Whatever social value there might have been in Mantle's career as a baseball player, those days were long-since past. If there was a reason to give Mantle an advantage, it was not because of the good he would have brought to others in the future.

Still, there seems no doubt that some might have been tempted to treat him as someone special. The issue is whether any possible case could be made for that treatment. Although utilitarians and other consequentialists are concerned only about the future, nonconsequentialists, as we have seen so often, consider other dimensions morally important. They consider patterns of distribution; they also consider what has happened in the past.

One of the principles included in some deontological ethics is related to what W. D. Ross calls "duties of gratitude."[8] Ross, and many others, believe that if someone has done something for us in the past, we are in debt to that person. We owe that person something in return. It is the ethic of gift reciprocity;[9] it is captured in the simple gesture of saying thanks but often requires more, perhaps something of monetary or nonmonetary significance. If someone has done a favor, other things being equal, a response is called for that can be thought of as a moral duty.

The idea of a duty of gratitude is used to explain why, when we have an opportunity to do good for others but can do the good for only one, if two potential recipients otherwise have equal claims we may be thought to have a moral duty to pick the one who has previously done something for us.

The idea of a duty of gratitude is not accepted by everyone, but it does explain many of our most basic moral intuitions about repaying favors and showing gratitude. The question, however, is whether it could possibly justify allocating an organ to a national sports hero. Even if we grant that many people received great joy from Mantle's baseball skills, can we express our gratitude by depriving another transplant candidate otherwise equally entitled to an organ? We should at least have to ask whether there are similar or even more substantial duties of gratitude to others on the waiting list.

There are several reasons to suspect that applying the concept of a duty of gratitude to organ allocation will be difficult. First, duties of gratitude normally are understood to apply to close friends or family who have done something very personal that leaves us with a moral sense of owing something in return. It normally does not apply to famous talents who have given us satisfaction in such an impersonal way.

Second, even if the duty of gratitude applies to famous talents, it is not clear that Mantle's "gift" to the public is really one that generates such a duty. We might imagine a public duty of gratitude for national war heroes who have made great sacrifice or for socially noble heros whose works of supererogation are inspiring. Mother Teresa may generate a duty of gratitude, but hardly an athlete who combines luck and natural physical ability to repeatedly accomplish physical feats that are modestly entertaining. National celebrities, at most, might deserve a round of applause—not a life-saving organ at the expense of others.

If Mantle did receive any special consideration, it is more likely that it resulted from some psychological phenomenon other than gratitude. Some people may, out of intimidation or some psychological inadequacy, feel compelled to show deference to status. It is the same feeling that might lead to permitting prestigious, high-status individuals to avoid long waits in lines. It may result from feeling a pride from being associated with the famous. That does not imply that such deference is justified. Surely, there is no possible legitimate reason for giving a folk hero such as Mantle any priority over others on the waiting list just because he is famous or because he accomplished much in his chosen sport. If he got his organ over others on the waiting list because of such factors as blood type and medical urgency, he was deserving (at least according to the then-current allocation rules); if he got it because at one time he could run and hit a baseball, that is not possibly justifiable. Neither social worth to others nor social status can play any legitimate role in organ allocation, at least unless there is an extreme case in which an exception is a matter of international urgency and the rule providing for the exception is articulated publicly in advance.

ENDNOTES

1. This account is based on information in "Controversy about Allocation of Organs for Transplantation: The Case of Governor Casey," *BioLaw Update* (Oct. 1993): U:303–05; Dale Russakoff, "The Heart That Didn't Die," *Washington Post*, Aug. 9, 1993, B1, B6; Paul T. Menzel, "Rescuing Lives: Can't We Count?" *Hastings Center Report* 24 (1, Jan.–Feb. 1994): 22–23; Lisa Belkin, "Fairness Debated in Quick Transplant. [News]," *New York Times*, June 16, 1993, p. A16; Don Colburn, "Gov. Casey's Quick Double Transplant: How Did He Jump to the Top of the Waiting List?", *Washington Post Health* 9 (June 22, 1993): 8–9.

2. Don Colburn, "Gov. Casey's Quick Double Transplant: How Did He Jump to the Top of the Waiting List?", p. 8.

3. *Planned Parenthood of Southeastern Pennsylvania v. Casey*, 112 U.S. 2791 (1992).

4. "Controversy about Allocation of Organs for Transplantation: The Case of Governor Casey."

5. *UNOS Clarifies Multiorgan Allocation Policy*, News Release from UNOS, July 2, 1993, cited in "Controversy about Allocation of Organs for Transplantation: The Case of Governor Casey"; also UNOS Policy 3.9.3., available on at <http://www.unos.org/About/policy_policie3_9.htm>, (Sept. 22, 1998). At the July 31, 1998, UNOS Board of Directors meeting, a change in policy 3.9.3 was proposed so that these same procedures will also be followed for multiple-organ transplants involving the lung as well as the heart and liver, although there are minor technical differences regarding payback if the policy leads to organs being moved beyond the local OPO. These changes took effect late in 1998. Memorandum to UNOS Members and Interested Persons from Douglas A. Heiney regarding UNOS Policy and Bylaw Proposals for Public Comment, Sept. 4, 1998.

6. For a good, if somewhat dated, discussion of the concept, see David Lyons, *Forms and Limits of Utilitarianism* (New York: Oxford University Press, 1965).

7. There is one possibility. Some justice theorists accept the idea of taking into account impacts on other parties while nevertheless rejecting the technique of aggre-

gating the beneficial impacts on these parties. For example, assuming John Rawls's "difference principle" could be applied at this level of specificity (See Chapter 25 for a discussion of this assumption), he would permit practices that consider the benefits to another person of giving a differential advantage to someone who is already well-off. Rawls would permit this provided the other party who was indirectly benefited was among the worst off. For example, if it could be successfully claimed that giving Governor Casey priority for an organ would improve the lot of the worst off citizens of Pennsylvania, then someone who would apply the difference principle at this level of specificity would support the special consideration. Frances Kamm seems to have something like this in mind when she suggests that there may be special exceptions to the policy of excluding consideration of social contribution. She says, "There may be exceptions, for example, for those who can complete projects that have truly exceptional social importance" (p. 260). She goes on, however, to qualify this apparent exception. She would not permit social importance from "aggregation of small gains to each individual in society" (p. 260). This is the mark of a deontologist's concern for giving special advantage based on the claim that doing so will produce greater social good in aggregate. This is seen by Rawlsians and other defenders of the difference principle as morally different from giving a special advantage to help some individual who is even worse off than the one given the advantage. According to them, justice might permit this kind of exception, whereas mere aggregate net benefit would not. In Chapter 25 I will question the legitimacy of even this very limited endorsement of special favoritism. (See F. M. Kamm, *Morality, Mortality: Volume I: Death and Whom to Save from It* [New York: Oxford University Press, 1993], p. 260.)

8. W. D. Ross, *The Right and the Good* (New York: Oxford University Press, 1930), p. 21–23.

9. Richard M. Titmuss, *The Gift Relationship: From Human Blood to Social Policy* (New York: Random House, 1971); M. Mauss, *The Gift; Forms and Functions of Exchange in Archaic Societies*, trans. Ian Cunnison, with an introduction by E. E. Evans-Pritchard (Glencoe, IL: Free Press, 1954).

TWENTY-FOUR

URGENCY VERSUS GEOGRAPHY: THE CONTROVERSY BETWEEN UNOS AND DONNA SHALALA

THE UNITED NETWORK FOR ORGAN SHARING (UNOS) ALLOCATION
rules have traditionally provided that organs should be allocated first locally, then
regionally, and finally nationally so that a relatively healthy local candidate would
get priority over a more distant patient in desperate need. (That is part of the
reason why Mickey Mantle received his liver so quickly, as we saw in the previous
chapter.) The Secretary of the U.S. Department of Health and Human Services,
Donna Shalala (with considerable pressure from the large transplant program of
the University of Pittsburgh), has issued a rule that requires UNOS to abandon
this strict local priority to promote greater equity (with the effect that Pittsburgh
will probably get more organs).[1] In this chapter I will review the current policy
controversy in terms of the equity–efficiency conflict. The penultimate draft of
this chapter was written before UNOS had provided any response to the Secretary
Shalala's rule. In June of 1999, UNOS Board voted to modify its liver allocation
policy by making one simple change.[2] It would place the most urgent regional
patients ahead of the lower urgency status local patients. This exception would
apply only to livers. It seems likely that this adjustment will not satisfy those
who are pressing for something closer to a national list to be more fair to the
sickest patients. We shall see that this adjustment may not satisfy many of the
local transplant programs either.

The Role of Geography in Allocation

As has been discussed previously, when one of the 62 organ procurement organizations (OPOs) in the United States obtains a cadaver organ for transplant it is
allocated first to local patients—that is, to one of the patients in the OPO's local
area. We need to look at this policy by organ.

Kidneys

In the case of the kidney there are only three exceptions: mandatory shares of a zero-antigen mismatched kidney, payback for a zero-antigen mismatch kidney that the OPO has received from another program, and certain very limited voluntary sharing arrangements.[3] This does not mean that each local hospital transplant program retains the organs it procures. Rather, the organ procurement organization, which may work with several transplant centers in a single city or metropolitan area, must allocate the kidney among all those on the waiting list in that OPO's area according to the point system that takes into account degree of human lymphocyte antigen (HLA) mismatch, panel reactive antibodies (PRA), time on the waiting list, the priority for O-blood group,[4] whether the recipient is a minor, and whether the recipient has donated an organ.

If no local transplant center has a suitable candidate for the organ, then it is allocated via the regional list for the region in which the OPO resides, using the same point system. There are 11 regions in the United States. Finally, if no transplant center in that region accepts the kidney, it is then allocated nationally, again using the kidney allocation point system.

Pancreata

Pancreata, which are sometimes transplanted along with a kidney, are allocated using the same geographical priority.[5] The local OPO has discretion in allocating pancreata to its patients needing an isolated pancreas, a kidney–pancreas combination, or a combined solid organ–islet transplant provided there is not a zero-antigen mismatched patient in need of the kidney somewhere on the UNOS waiting list. A zero-antigen mismatch takes priority regardless of location. O-blood group recipients still get priority for suitable (that is, O-blood group) donor organs or tissue. If the pancreas is not placed locally, it is then allocated regionally, and finally nationally. Rules for regional and national allocation establish priorities based on the number of mismatched antigens. Candidates for isolated pancreas transplant with fewer than three mismatches come before candidates needing a combined kidney–pancreas (with O-blood type getting first claim). Then come isolated pancreas candidates with three or more A, B, or DR mismatches. Time on the waiting list is used only to allocate within these groups. If no candidate is available at the regional level, the same ordering is then used at the national level.

Thus the point system used for the isolated kidney is not applied in pancreas allocation. Although some might debate whether this priority squares with the goals of efficiency and equity—whether low mismatches for isolated pancreata should come before combined pancreas–kidney transplants, for instance—the real issue of controversy is why, except for the zero-antigen mismatch case, all local candidates, even those who predictably would get a another chance at a graft, should take precedence over any regional or national candidate, even if that more distant candidate has a good antigen match, has been waiting a long time, and is of the identical blood group.

Other Organs

Until the June 1999 modification for livers, abdominal organ transplants such as the liver and intestine, as well as thoracic organ transplants including heart, lung, and heart–lung combinations, also followed an allocation sequence that placed organs first with local patients, followed by regional, and then national waiting list members. This formula is still in place except for the one modification for livers. The sequence continues in descending order based on medical status and/or points accumulated and finally time accrued on the waiting list. For example, until the change, livers were size-matched through the UNOS match system to acceptable recipients and allocated locally to Status 1 potential recipients in descending point order, then to local Status 2A patients, local Status 2B patients, and local Status 3 patients, all in descending point order. The only modification is that regional Status 1 patients now come in this sequence in front of local Status 2A. Points are accrued based on blood compatibility (ten points for identical blood group and five for compatible group) and time on the waiting list (with a maximum of ten points for the person waiting the longest and then fractions of ten points depending on where the candidate stands on the list). If the liver is not accepted locally (and now regionally in the case of Status 1 patients), it follows a similar sequence for regionally listed patients, and finally national patients.[6]

For thoracic organs (for which no change was made at the June 1999 meeting), points are not accrued for waiting time. Instead, potential recipients are ranked by geographic proximity in terms of miles from the donor hospital, status for heart recipients, blood-type compatibility, and, within each category, by length of time waiting.[7]

The Reasons for the Local Priority

The support for this local priority has been very strong within UNOS and the organ procurement organizations. The question is why? The reasons involve both moral concerns and program self-interest.

Moral Reasons

The most obvious reason for local priority is probably because it is natural for each community to feel it should serve its own members first. If a program is organized to develop an organ donation system that covers a metropolitan area, the members of that community who are being called on to donate organs like to think that they are helping their neighbors. For example, Nancy A. Kay, who is the executive director of the South Carolina Organ Procurement Agency, was quoted as saying, "Our work is based on the giving of South Carolinians. . . . We like to take care of our neighbors here."[8] Oklahoma governor Frank Keating is quoted as complaining that the federal government is trying to "suck organs" from states such as his.[9]

The concern about keeping local organs for local folks has become so great that by 1999 four states (Louisiana, South Carolina, Wisconsin, and Oklahoma) had passed laws requiring locally procured organs to be used within the state if a patient in the state could use them. Other states including Tennessee and Kansas have considered such laws.

Some of these proposals have not been thought through very carefully. Many OPOs, for example, serve metropolitan areas that cross state lines. That means that, under such laws, even locally procured organs could cross a state line. For example, there are three liver transplant programs within the Washington Regional Transplant Consortium (WRTC), two in the District of Columbia and one in Virginia.

A patient in suburban Maryland needing a liver who wanted to go to the nearest liver transplant program would go to either the District of Columbia or Virginia (Howard Hospital and Georgetown Hospital in the District or Fairfax Hospital in Virginia). Passing a law in Maryland requiring that Maryland organs go first to Maryland programs would require the organs go to Baltimore, guaranteeing that they would go outside the area of Maryland residents in the Washington suburbs and away from the three hospitals that would most naturally serve these Maryland residents. Furthermore, the District of Columbia or Virginia could retaliate by insisting that D.C. and Virginia organs be used for their own residents, thus prohibiting suburban Marylanders from getting access. It would also require that organs donated by Virginians within the WRTC area that could not be used by Virginians at Fairfax Hospital would have to be shipped to the Richmond or Virginia Beach OPOs (Virginia's Organ Procurement Agency and LifeNet), where organs would be allocated to hospitals that would not be considered local. This would make them inaccessible for people who are part of the metropolitan area and usually considered neighbors.

Even if one becomes convinced that a local priority makes sense, the allocation should not be based on state lines. Requiring that OPOs retain their priority would serve the goal of keeping local organs for local people much better. This would keep organs within a metropolitan area rather than using state boundaries, which do not reflect metropolitan areas. As we shall see, however, there is a strong moral case to be made for removing the priority for local allocation and going to some version of a national list based on medical urgency.

Increasing Efficiency

Those within the transplant community may give more technical reasons for local priority as well as the notion of loyalty to the local community. They may claim that a system with local priority is more efficient. This could be for several reasons. First, it is believed that delays in implanting organs increase the risk of graft failure. Although a kidney can last 24 hours or more, a heart must be transplanted in about 4 hours. A local allocation not only eliminates travel time or keeps it to a minimum, it also eliminates the delay from having to negotiate communication between OPOs and between the OPOs and UNOS. Local allocation results in a faster, simpler system.

It is difficult to interpret the data supporting the claim that longer waits between procurement and transplant (cold ischemia times) are worse for transplant. They vary for each organ and will change as better preservation techniques are developed. Nevertheless, there does seem to be something to the concern. For kidneys, the mean cold ischemia time (during the January 1988 through April 1994 period for which data are available) was 23 hours. Increasing that time to 33 hours risk of graft failure by 6% (odds ratio of graft failure = 1.062).[10] It is not clear, however, how many transplants would have to be delayed beyond the 23-hour period if the United States went to a national list. Also, it is not clear from the data whether there is a significant advantage in transplanting sooner than the 23-hour mean. Because transportation within the United States is not likely to take more than a few extra hours, the impact on graft survival of a national list probably would be real, but modest.

For livers the picture is somewhat different. The mean cold ischemia time during this period is 11 hours. A delay to 21 hours increases the risk of graft failure by 12% (odds ratio = 1.116),[11] suggesting that a transportation delay might have important consequences. For hearts it might have even more important consequences. The mean cold ischemic time for hearts is 163 minutes, with a delay to 223 minutes increasing the risk of graft failure by 9% (odds ratio = 1.091).[12]

Second, with local organ priority, efficiency might be greater in procuring of organs. People might be more willing to donate in a time of crisis if they know that the organs are likely to be used locally. Moreover, it is widely believed that, with local priority in allocation, hospital personnel may be more inspired to initiate procurement activities (raising the issue with families or, preferably, contacting the OPO so that those skilled in procurement can take over). Also, local transplant surgeons may be more willing to take the lead in developing educational and counseling programs to stimulate organ procurement if they believe there is a good chance that the organs may come to them to do a transplant.

Self-Interest of Transplant Programs

The interest in local priority may not be entirely altruistic. Transplant programs, hospitals, and health professionals involved in transplants all have important self-interests at stake. Transplants are big business for hospitals and surgeons. The estimated first-year charge (in 1996 dollars) for each kidney transplant is $116,100. Charges for other organs range from $141,300 for a kidney–pancreas to $314,500 for a liver.[13] In addition, annual follow-up charges run from $6,900 for a pancreas transplant to $25,100 for a lung. Kidney transplants are estimated to generate annual follow-up charges of $15,900. Keeping the organs locally may mean significant income for both the hospital and the surgeon.

Of course, with local priority other OPOs outside the local area will also have these incentives to keep their organs for themselves. In the long run, on average surgeons will do about the same number of transplants and hospitals will receive about the same income if everyone agrees to share. The only costs of sharing nationally will be modest coordination and transportation costs plus any decrease in donation resulting from donor family awareness that the sharing takes place on a national rather than a metropolitan-area basis.

There may be another self-interest of local transplant programs, however. Surgeons must meet minimal criteria to establish their credentials. Also, centers that function as training programs must perform certain specific minimum numbers of transplants. A program that just barely meets the minimum number risks losing its certification if it exports organs that could have been used locally, at least if it will not import a comparable number. Other than for training, there are no minimal number requirements imposed nationally, but local and state requirements (such as for certificates of need) may impose such minimums.

The shift to any allocation that increases exports could jeopardize the interest not only of the hospitals and surgeons involved but also of the patients. If an area has only one heart transplant program and it is in jeopardy of losing it, then the patients in that community would have to travel elsewhere to get their heart transplants. This is difficult for patients, family members, and friends. Follow-up would be increasingly difficult. Of course, if patients can expect that their program doing a marginal number of transplants is inferior to a large program elsewhere, those patients may have a reason to want to have the local program closed down in favor of the larger, more experienced program anyway.

Determining the relation between program size and quality, however, is difficult. The 1997 "Center-Specific Graft and Patient Survival Rates" report examines these issues. It calculates expected survival rates for each transplant program in the United States for each organ transplanted, adjusting for the risk level of the patients. It then compares actual survival rates, flagging those at which actual survival rates are significantly lower than expected rates. It points out, however, that larger differences between actual and expected rates were nearly always seen in programs that reported relatively few transplants.[14] The report authors point out that this is, in part, a statistical artifact, because large variations in survival rates in small programs can be produced easily. The authors are sensitive to the indignation shown by some small programs when it is assumed that small volume necessarily means poor results. Nevertheless, the 1997 report repeats the conclusion of an earlier study of cardiac transplantation that "the risk of mortality and earlier and intermediate time points is higher in low-volume ... centers,"[15] a finding that the report points out has been demonstrated for other surgical procedures as well. This conclusion is reinforced by a more recent study involving the same researchers. As a result of their 1999 study, they conclude mortality from liver transplantation is significantly lower in centers that perform more than 20 transplants a year.[16] Although some small programs may produce very good results, there are reasons related to both outcomes and economies of scale to question the appropriateness of continuing to fund very low-volume programs.

On balance, many people have an interest in keeping local programs running. That could be part of the explanation of why many people want local organs to be used locally. Still, utilitarians have a hard case to make to defend the claim that more aggregate benefit accrues from sustaining many local programs. It is not clear that the number of organs procured would go down if local programs export organs based on a national allocation. It is also not clear what the impact would be on the survival rates and other measures of patient benefit. If the imports to an OPO equal the exports (as they would on average), the result will be about the same. The utilitarian must rest his or her case on claims about changes in procurement rates, patient benefit from being transplanted nearer to home, and the quality of small programs.

The controversy over the allocation illustrates why small, local programs fear they may suffer a net loss of organs if the United States goes to a national list. The University of Pittsburgh Medical Center's liver transplant program has been, by far, the dominant program in the United States. In 1988, before many cities had developed their programs, the University of Pittsburgh did 406 of the 1,713 liver transplants done in the United States, and Children's Hospital of Pittsburgh, which is affiliated with the Medical Center, did another 99 of them.[17] When it was one of the very few programs, it built its reputation not only as the place to get a liver transplant, but also as the place where surgeons went to train to become liver transplant surgeons. As long as there were few other programs, organs would be sent by other OPOs that could not use them. For example, in 1988, 1,224 of the 1,692 livers transplanted were shipped from one OPO to another, many of them to Pittsburgh. By 1996, 2,770 were kept by OPOs for local use, and the number that was shared (1,243) remained about constant and became a much smaller percentage of the total livers transplanted.[18] By then, the University of Pittsburgh did only 179 of 4,062 liver transplants, and Children's Hospital did only 29.

As those surgical trainees completed their course of training, they gradually moved on to other communities seeking to begin liver transplant programs. In the meantime, however, Pittsburgh retained its reputation as the preeminent liver surgery center in the country. Physicians tended to send their patients to Pittsburgh, especially their sickest ones.

It appears that, in part because of this reputation and its willingness to transplant seriously ill patients, the waiting list in Pittsburgh is particularly long. As people wait longer times, they get sicker. An accumulation of even more seriously ill patients is created. Because there is a local priority for allocation of livers, the small programs across the country that have relatively few patients waiting each get claim on organs to transplant their relatively healthy patients. Their patients get transplanted quicker and healthier while Pittsburgh's waiting list grows because the hospital has to make do with a typically small supply of organs for an atypically large and sick list of patients waiting for surgery.

The Demand for a National List

The result is a cry for a national list for allocating organs, especially life-saving abdominal and thoracic organs, and particularly livers. The concern is, in part, a moral one: As we will see, waiting times vary greatly from one center to another and patients are much sicker at some centers than others. The obvious solution seems to be to go to some version of a national list based on such factors as degree of medical urgency and time on the waiting list. If the current UNOS allocation formulas were maintained as they are, but the priority for local then regional allocation were eliminated, the problem would be solved—so the argument goes.

The Department of Health and Human Services's Mandate

THE MANDATE'S INTENT

That is more or less what Donna Shalala concluded. Urged by intense lobbying from the University of Pittsburgh, she issued an order directing the Organ Procurement and Transplant Network (OPTN), that is, UNOS, to revise organ allocation policies. The order mandates that the allocation fairly and equitably give every citizen access to organ transplantation, requiring the OPTN to create a policy that places medical need as the foremost in criteria. It also called for reducing disparities across the nation by, at least to some extent, taking geography out of the equation. In addition to criteria for allocation based on medical urgency rather than geographic proximity, the rule calls for developing uniform criteria to decide when to place a patient on the waiting list and what status they hold there.[19] The mandate was introduced to reduce waiting times across the entire country, to allow every individual equal opportunity to transplantation no matter where they live or are registered, and to ensure that all criteria are uniform and fair.[20]

In a masterpiece of confused bureaucratic doublespeak, Secretary Shalala and her spokespersons deny they are actually mandating a national list. They claim that the regulation relies on the expertise of transplant professionals to create the policies. Whether these professionals adopt a national list, she says, is their judgment, not the government's.[21]

Although this explanation is technically correct, it is hard to imagine how these transplant professionals could come up with a fair and equitable allocation system that eliminates geographical differences without going to some version of a national list. The June 1999 modification, which is no more than a first step at eliminating the disparities for one organ, moves a step in the direction of a national list.

There may be some way of reducing travel time by making the allocation take distance into account while still preserving the goal of equalizing waiting times. Although it is true that a single national list would not be necessary, some shifting of organs from OPOs and regions with relatively short waiting times to those with relatively long times will be necessary to make the system more fair. A reasonable proposal consistent with the principle of justice described in this book would be to allocate organs to the sickest class of patients (Status 1 in the case of the liver) first locally, then regionally, and finally nationally. Then organs would go locally to patients in the next sickest class followed by those at the regional and national levels. In each case, adjustments might be made to minimize cold ischemia times as long as waiting time within status groups was evened out across the nation. That would eliminate the troublesome cases in which a local patient who is relatively healthy gets priority over a patient with much more urgent need at a more distant site. There is probably no need to move organs across the country to meet secondary allocation criteria (such as time on the waiting list) when a local patient equally needy could use the organ with shorter ischemia time and less transportation expense.[22] It is probably possible to arrange an allocation so that organs would move shorter distances while still accomplishing the goal of minimizing differences in waiting times.

This funniness of Secretary Shalala's deference to the transplant professionals results from a confusion in the minds of both health professionals and lay people about the proper division of labor between technical experts and policymakers. UNOS executives and politicians alike seem to believe that the formation of the policy that should govern allocation of organs should be in the hands of professionals rather than politicians.

There are, of course, technical questions requiring scientific knowledge that are relevant to deciding how to allocate organs—questions of organ deterioration during cold ischemia, relative graft and patient survival for patients at various stages of their illness, and so forth. But in the end, the real issues in the debate over a local or more national allocation are moral. Assuming there may be some losses in efficiency in reducing disparities (and going to something like a national list), deciding whether to trade off efficiency to make the allocation more fair is fundamentally not a technical medical question. It is a question of the relative moral priority of efficiency and equity (of maximizing aggregate utility and distributing the utility equitably). I have suggested that my personal moral theory would give priority to equity over efficiency but that I recognize that there is no consensus in favor of that view. I continue to support the compromise developed in the UNOS Ethics Committee during the time when I served as chair of its Organ Allocation Subcommittee. That compromise, as described in Chapter 19, endorsed giving efficiency and equity equal weight. That suggests a modified national list that may not be perfectly equitable (at least if something close to equal waiting times can be developed that is significantly more efficient), but it will at least be considerably more equitable than the present system.

There is no reason to believe that the transplant professionals administering UNOS or serving on its board have any special expertise in making these moral policy choices. In fact, as we have seen, there is good reason to believe they make them in an atypical way, influenced by the particular moral perspective of health professionals. The intellectual mistake of assuming that those who are expert on the technical aspects of a technology are also experts on the moral and other evaluative questions I long ago called the *generalization of expertise*. I called it one of the primary fallacies of modern technological society.[23] Although it is obviously necessary to rely on the enormous technical skills of such professionals for the data on which specific allocation protocols will have to be based, it is a serious mistake for the society to cede to those experts the responsibility for making policies such as those on which the society will allocate organs. The choices are fundamentally moral and philosophical. They cannot be made on the basis of technical knowledge alone.

The crucial choices involve how a society should affirm that it is a moral community of equals and how much it should sacrifice maximum efficiency in adding years of life in order to add them more equitably. That is fundamentally not a question for transplant professionals; it is a choice all members of a society must make. Rather than engaging in the fiction of denying she is mandating a national list, Secretary Shalala should proudly insist that the issues she is addressing are matters for public policy that must be decided by the community, not left to technical experts. The project must be one of having the society examine the moral arguments for and against some version of a national list, leaving to transplant professionals only the task of setting the operational rules for fulfilling society's moral policy choice.

The Arguments in Defense

Although many of the defenders of the local priority claim that there are benefits from the priority from making donors more willing to donate, from maintaining the quality of organs by keeping ischemia times brief, and from supporting local transplant centers so that patients will be able be transplanted close to home, defenders of the national list also can point to benefits that they believe would accrue by going to the national list.

MORAL REASONS BEHIND THE MANDATE

Utilities of a national list. For one, they argue that some small programs are marginal in quality as well as quantity. They suggest that some of them going out of business might mean that patients would get transplanted from programs with more experience and the efficiencies of larger scale operations.

For example, John Fung, a transplant surgeon at the University of Pittsburgh and an advocate of a national list, claimed in the testimony at the Department of Health and Human Services Hearings of December 1996:

> Recent analysis by . . . UNOS, and verified by the Cleveland Claim . . .
> data, revealed that the volume of liver, heart and pancreas transplants per-
> formed by a center is directly correlated with survival outcome, and on the
> whole low volume centers have significantly lower survival than high vol-
> ume centers, in spite of what we heard before. This was highlighted at a re-
> cent consensus conference on indications for liver transplantation held in
> 1993 that stated, "The competence of liver transplantation teams, which var-
> ies widely from center to center, depends largely on the number of opera-
> tions carried out. Thus there should be a yearly minimum to ensure uniform
> quality." Unfortunately, patients are enticed to the centers with shorter wait-
> ing times and lower waiting list deaths with less emphasis on the quality of
> the programs.[24]

These claims are controversial. Some small centers have produced results as good or better than larger volume programs. The general pattern of better results from higher-volume centers, however, seems to be documented in the literature.[25]

Second, they point to benefits that would come from getting organs to sick patients who may die soon if they do not get transplanted. They suggest that, in the case of livers, for example, small programs that have few patients on a waiting list may get organs from the local priority policy that end up going to Status 3 patients who are still up and around and relatively healthy. They suggest that these patients could wait for their organs with little loss. If those organs go to sicker Status 1 or 2 patients in other areas, the good they receive could exceed the harms to the Status 3 patients in the area in which the organ is procured.

Of course, this is an empirical claim. It could turn out that giving the organs to the sicker patients not only jeopardizes the organs by delaying implant time but also gets the organs to patients whose illness is so severe that they may be less likely to survive even with the transplant. This could mean that the expected number of years of life from an organ may be greater giving it to the healthier patient. Thus deciding whether more or less benefit will emerge from a national list will depend on some complex empirical questions for which we really do not know the answers. According to computer models cited by the government, however, as many as 300 lives a year could be saved with an allocation giving greater priority to sicker patients.[26]

Equity rather than efficiency. The real claim of defenders of the national list often has nothing to do with increasing expected benefits. They are concerned instead with increasing the equity of the organ transplant system. They say it is patently unfair to have a national organ transplant system maintained by federal funds in which patients in one OPO have average waiting times for life-saving organs that are much greater than those in another OPO. Secretary Shalala illustrates the claim of unfairness in waiting times in her letter to Congress of June 1, 1998:

> For example, the median waiting times for the two major liver transplant centers in Kentucky were vastly different—38 days at one center, 226 at the other. Similarly, in Louisiana, the median waiting time at one center was reported to be 18 days, while at another, it was 262 days. In Michigan, the numbers were 161 days and 401 days. Although these numbers do not tell the whole story, they certainly reflect that unacceptable disparities in waiting times exist, even within States. I believe that basic fairness to patients demands that these disparities be substantially reduced and that the transplant community should ultimately develop the means to this end.[27]

To be sure, people can transfer their registration to another center that has a shorter expected waiting time for an organ. They can even register at more than one transplant center, thus having two or even three chances at getting an organ and shortening the expected waiting time. Shifting to another center is not easy, however. It would have to be in another metropolitan area (because other transplant programs in the same area would involve the same waiting list with the same poor odds). Getting registered in another community would mean moving to that area or at least traveling there often enough to establish a medical relationship. When transplanted not only would the patient have to travel to the new community; family members who are to become the support system would as well. All of this takes money, time, and mobility—commodities available more readily to wealthier patients. Registering in more than one center likewise takes extensive resources. Many insurance programs would not fund the repeat testing and medical workups. Shifting to a program with a shorter waiting list or double-listing are options more likely to be available to wealthy patients.

The bottom line is that local priority makes the transplant program inequitable. People who are equally sick, who have equal entitlement to a transplant, and who are equally good candidates will have significantly different probabilities for getting an organ. Because many people die while on the waiting list, a delay in getting an organ equals an increased risk of death. The moral principle of justice requires that people who are equally situated are entitled be treated equally. This is referred to by theorists as the "formal" criterion of justice, the most general and widely accepted element of the concept of justice.

Defenders of the egalitarian version of the principle of justice go further. They not only claim that equals deserve equal treatment but also go on to state which group deserves the priority: the worst off. They are offended by a system that is designed to let a relatively healthy person—such as a Status 3 liver transplant candidate—get an organ over a much more critical Status 1 patient just because the healthier patient happens to live in an area that has a large supply of donated organs compared to the demand for those organs. Such an arrangement leaves the acutely ill patient in fulminant liver failure to die simply because he or she happens to live in a location in which the supply of organs is disproportionate to the number needing them.

Both supply and demand can be determined by utterly arbitrary variables. The supply will be contingent on such factors as the socioeconomic status of the residents of the community, the quality of the highway construction, and the religious persuasion of the community members. The demand may be great simply because a high-quality transplant center attracts many out-of-towners to register, increasing the competition for the organs. Defenders of the egalitarian version of the principle of justice claim that the inequities in waiting times for people with equal severity of illness is the essence of an unfair system. If we have a national organ system, they say that waiting times must be evened out and that the sickest patients deserve first claim (even if it turns out to decrease the efficiency of the system).

Political/economic reasons. It also cannot be denied that the movement for a national list has economic and political dimensions. Shalala did not simply dream up the idea of mandating that UNOS change its organ allocation system to make waiting times more equal. Groups with an interest in that outcome worked very hard to see that the issue was brought to her attention and that she see the arguments for making the change.

The University of Pittsburgh was instrumental in organizing testimony in favor of allocations that overturned the locals-first priority. Of the 106 individuals scheduled to testify at the December 1996 hearings, which provided the background for the issuing of the departmental rule, at least 20 were associated with the University of Pittsburgh, including surgeon John Fung; Mark A. Joensen, Ph.D., from CONSAD Research Corporation in Pittsburgh (which is associated with the university); at least ten University of Pittsburgh transplant recipients; four transplant candidates; two relatives of deceased University of Pittsburgh transplant recipients; one relative of current candidate; and an attorney with ties to university-affiliated organizations and Pittsburgh's organ procurement organization. In addition, Pittsburgh was instrumental in encouraging others to testify. (I know because I was telephoned by personnel associated with the University of Pittsburgh urging me to testify.) Even though I agreed with their position, I was unable to testify due to a schedule conflict.

The University of Pittsburgh Medical Center news bureau issued press releases showing that many liver transplant candidates, including all those from 15 states without an active transplant program, cross state lines to receive transplants from programs not necessarily near where they live.[28] One patient opposed to the changes even claimed in her testimony that she had heard that the federal intervention was triggered by President Bill Clinton being pressured by a request of a personal friend with business connections to the University of Pittsburgh Medical Center.[29] It is clear that the University of Pittsburgh has an economic interest in increasing its transplants.

Of course, other, smaller centers also have economic interests in keeping organs locally, and the lobbying on behalf of those centers was also intense. Of the people testifying at the December 1996 hearings, substantial numbers collectively spoke for centers with an economic interest in maintaining the status quo. The point is not that Pittsburgh's efforts were inappropriate or merely self-serving. This would not be the first time in which someone advocating their self-interest simultaneously reached what turned out to be the morally correct decision.

Other Advocates for a More Nationally Oriented List

At the same time others beyond Pittsburgh have concluded that some version of a national list is morally equitable and the right thing to do. Clive Callender, the head of the transplant program at Howard University in Washington, D.C., and an outspoken defender of greater equity in organ allocation, is one of the few leaders of UNOS other than those from Pittsburgh who support the DHHS call for a more fair national allocation system.[30] He has long been aware that sometimes the most efficient allocation system is not the fairest. He has, for example, criticized excessive emphasis on HLA tissue-typing in kidney transplant, pointing out that tissue-typing works to the disadvantage of Black patients and other minorities whose HLA antigens do not match the donor pool as well as the Caucasian majority.

The Ethics of the Conflict over Geography

It could be that the final outcome of the conflict between urgency and geography will be settled by the political and economic forces involved. They are enormous. In a book on the ethics of transplant, however, it is appropriate to look at the ethics of the conflict.

The Inconclusiveness of the Utility Argument

Utilitarians may come out of this conflict perplexed. The defenders of local priority have couched their arguments in utilitarian terms: shorter ischemia times, better quality organs, more willingness to donate, and preservation of local programs with more convenient care for local patients. However, we have seen that defenders of the national list can mount utilitarian arguments as well: more lives saved with modest burdens on patients in OPOs with short waiting lists who lose organs to sicker patients elsewhere. The defenders of local priority counter by suggesting that a national list will simply force local patients in areas with short waiting lists to wait until they are as sick and as hard to treat as those who would get the new priority claims on organs.

It is not immediately obvious which side wins the utilitarian debate. We may not have all the data we need. Moreover, utilitarian disputes have a way of depending on nonempirical questions such as how we quantify outcomes. This debate may hinge on such nebulous, hard-to-quantify issues as how bad it is to make a very sick person travel to another town to get multiple-listed and transplanted. It is not only the mortality rate that is at stake; it is the quality of life of patients as they are on the waiting list.

Perhaps the defenders of the existing local priority win the utilitarian argument, but it seems to me to be a complicated, close call. The utilitarian analysis is about a draw.

The Clear Implications of the Justice Argument

On the other hand, the justice analysis, especially if it is carried out from an egalitarian perspective that I defended in Chapter 19 seems overwhelming. There are gross inequities in making people who in all morally relevant respects are equal wait radically different lengths of time for desperately needed organs. There are even greater inequities in directing organs to healthier patients over those who are desperately ill (Status 3 rather than Status 2 or 1 in the case of liver transplant) simply because of the morally irrelevant variable of where one happens to live.

If justice takes priority over utility, as I have consistently claimed in this book, something resembling a national list seems to be a moral necessity. But even if one makes the rather common move in moral theory (and in the UNOS Ethics Committee) to claim that conflicts between utility and justice must be resolved by considering the weightiness of each principle and balancing the competing claims, the national list seems to carry the day. The utilitarian calculation leads to a standoff, whereas the principle of justice is weighted strongly on the side of some version of a national list (or at least one in which enough organs cross local area boundaries to offset existing inequities).

Only a pure, uncompromising utilitarian seems to be left perplexed. He or she is pulled between the claims of the smaller programs that have been pointing to the purported benefits of the local priority and the claims of the advocates of a national list who point to new benefits to be expected from the change to a national perspective. It is not clear where the pure utilitarian will come out. It is clear, however, that adopting the pure utilitarian position requires the belief that justice is irrelevant as a moral principle.[31] I argued in Chapter 19 that accepting the utilitarian principle of utility-maximizing has horrendous implications that are so offensive to the moral senses that they have to be rejected.

Even if one is unwilling to accept this as a moral conclusion, one is still confronted with the legal reality that in the United States the federal law requires taking into account both equity and efficiency—that is, justice and utility. When one principle (utility), with implications so evenly balanced that it is hard to tell which allocation it supports, is balanced against another that overwhelmingly supports one of the allocation options, then that option, on balance, has to carry the day. Anyone committed to giving justice and utility equal consideration has to support a single national list. Anyone who gives justice priority over utility must be even more convinced of that conclusion.

The Nation as a Moral Community

There is another dimension of the controversy that must be confronted that leads to the same conclusion. Defenders of local lists, especially shortsighted politicians in those states that are passing laws prohibiting the export of organs when they can be used within the state, adopt the moral position that the residents in the local area constitute a moral community that has a prior claim on citizen loyalty before "outsiders" deserve any benefit. Only in cases in which none of the in-group can be benefited will export outside the group be accepted.

This is a troublesome view about the nature of the moral community. First, there is an obvious problem of whether people are supposed to be loyal to the citizens of their state or the citizens of their metropolitan area (their OPO) when they donate their life-saving organs. More seriously, we must ask why it is that we ought to feel morally bound to be loyal to human beings of our particular state or metropolitan area over those of other parts of the country. Is there some reason why we need to be so parochial in our identification with the needs of our fellow humans that a stranger a few score miles from us counts more morally than one a few hundred or thousand miles away?

In the United States the organ procurement and transplant program is a national program. In the case of kidneys, it is funded almost entirely by Medicare. For other organs, some of the funding is national—the organs funded by Medicare, CHAMPUS, and other public insurance systems. Even most private health insurance systems have a national perspective. The transplant program is established by Congress. It is administered nationally. It is hard to see how nearby transplant candidates have a moral claim over those in more distant communities.

There is something to be said for the provision in the Uniform Anatomical Gift Act that permits donation of an organ to a member of one's own family who is in need. That law also permits donation to friends, to a hospital with which one has had an ongoing relationship, or to a transplant surgeon who one knows. It is widely accepted that there are special duties of loyalty to one's family and friends. A mother with very limited resources confronted with her own child in need and a stranger child in equal need will undoubtedly pick her own child for favored treatment. We would be shocked if she did not. Family bonds of loyalty are strong and command priority over strangers.

It is hard to see why the same should be said for one's state or metropolitan area, why the people in that geographical area have any claim of loyalty over others, equally needy, in some other state or metropolitan area. Cultural maturity requires recognizing the irrationality of preference based solely on geographical proximity.

In the case of a state such as Louisiana or Oklahoma that has attempted to pass a law restricting export of organs, the parochial restriction may not even be in the citizen's self-interest. Without examining the data, it is hard to know whether Louisiana is a net importer or exporter of organs. Ethics requires the principle of reciprocity. If it is morally correct for Louisianans to restrict export, it must also be acceptable for other states to restrict shipment of organs *into* Louisiana. If Louisiana happens to be a net importer at the present time, they will lose in their efforts to be ethnocentric.[32] Even if restriction turns out to be a winning policy—that is, if they happen to be exporters once a national list is adopted based on principles of fairness and equal treatment—morality cannot support such irrational preference for one's "own kind" over outsiders.

Some of the most vicious wars of history have been fought between peoples who think they can discover some basis for a difference between themselves and the residents of a neighboring community. Although science and reason would find no significant difference between the groups, prejudice and ethnocentrism provide some basis for giving preference to one's own group. At its worst, the National Socialists thought that membership in the Aryan race was so superior that being a Jew or a Gypsy justified extermination. In America's own history, racial prejudice led to similar horrendous offense. The difference between being a Louisianan in heart failure and being a Mississippian similarly in heart failure is really not all that great. Taking a moral point of view, there can be no basis for each state giving its own citizens priority over the citizens of the other, especially in a national program in which all are asked to participate as equals.

A full-blown ethic of organ transplantation would press on to ask similar questions about the morality of giving priority to the citizens of one's own country over those of another. That question raises complexities, no doubt. It would be particularly problematic to hold that morality requires sharing organs with nations that themselves have resisted developing organ procurement programs. (On the other hand, it seems strange to hold those citizens who need organs responsible for their nation's objections to organ procurement, at least if the one needing the organ was not opposed to a procurement program.) For purposes of the present discussion, the least we can conclude is that residents of the United States form a moral community with a single organ transplant practice. There can be no reason why organs should be restricted solely on the basis of geographical proximity between the donor and the recipient except in those cases in which medical necessity prohibits transport of the organ in a way that would maintain viability. Even then, the moral claim of all potential recipients similarly situated with regard to medical urgency, blood type, and time on the waiting list is the same. That means we have to have a single national list for allocating organs modified only in ways that increase efficiency without significantly sacrificing equity.

Determining Whether the UNOS Response Is Adequate

Given the strength of the case for modifying the original locals-first allocation system, is the June 1999 UNOS response to Donna Shalala adequate? It retains the status quo with one exception: It places Status 1 regional patients for livers ahead of Status 2A local patients.

Certainly this modest amendment does nothing to address the question of national equity for any organ other than the liver. We have seen that hearts pose a special problem of being able to tolerate only much shorter cold ischemia times. Nevertheless, it seems that even hearts may not be immune from some allocational adjustments across OPO boundaries to make the allocation more equitable. For other organs, such as kidneys, a more national allocation system is even easier to defend.

But even with regard to livers the modification poses serious questions. The questions are made more serious by an earlier modification in the allocation system. Some time before adopting the new geographical priorities, UNOS reassessed its Status 1 category. It had included patients with acute fulminant liver failure as well as those with chronic failure as long as they were ill enough to be in intensive care. The adjustment removed chronic patients from the Status 1 category, making them Status 2A. This had the effect of placing an acute failure patient in front of a large group of chronic patients, including many suffering from alcoholic cirrhosis. This move, which itself was controversial, gave alcoholics (as well as others with chronic conditions) a lower priority.

Although controversial by itself, the June 1999 adjustment that places regional Status 1 patients above local Status 2A patients made the lowering of chronic disease patient priority even more controversial. It meant that an alcoholic at death's door has a lower priority than an acute illness patient who is equally sick. Moving regional acute patients in front of local chronic patients means that seriously ill chronic patients (alcoholics and others) pay the entire price for responding to the DHHS demand for moving away from an absolute local priority.

There is another complication. Insofar as Pittsburgh will be a major beneficiary of the adjustment, it is not just that alcoholics and other chronic patients who are desperately ill will pay the price, it is also exclusively Region 2 alcoholics and other chronic patients who are desperately ill who will pay. If Pittsburgh is a repository of a large number of acute patients who are very sick, they will be helped (as they should be), but they will be helped only by Region 2 alcoholics and chronic patients. Similar patients in other regions will be exempt from contributing (although they will, of course, contribute to responding to any regional liver movements in their own region). It is possible that Pittsburgh's acute patients could consume all the Region 2 livers that are not used locally for acutely ill Status 1 patients. Because that group makes up a very small portion of the total group of liver transplant candidates, it is possible that Region 2 liver transplant centers other than Pittsburgh will be in jeopardy.

During the last half of 1999 important policy developments came quickly. In July, the Institute of Medicine released its congressionally mandated report that walked a middle course between DHHS and UNOS.[33] It claimed the present allocation was working reasonably well but that there was room for improvement. It differentiated disparities in waiting time for less sick patients, which it acknowledged were great, from the more even times for those in greatest need. These were findings that were to be cited by UNOS. However, the Institute of Medicine report also concluded that donation rates would not decline if organs were distributed over a larger area and encouraged the federal government to take a more active role in overseeing transplantation, conclusions that would support the DHHS agenda. Most critically, it concluded that the transplantation system would be "significantly enhanced" if organs were shared over larger areas than they are at present.

The Institute of Medicine report was followed in the fall of 1999 by Republican-supported efforts to pass a law that would have stripped DHHS of its authority to control transplant policy. The law, which was pushed by some transplant centers and surgeons, was approved by the House Commerce Committee but did not gain approval by the full house. In October, soon after the House Commerce Committee action, DHHS clarified its regulations to make clear that it was not mandating a literal national list. The October statement did, however, continue to insist that organs should be distributed over as broad a geographical area as feasible.

The new DHHS mandate went into effect on March 16, 2000. In February, UNOS issued an extensive "memorandum" outlining its response.[34] The most visible feature remained the elevation of regional status I patients above lower-status patients at the local level. The question remains whether this rather modest response will be sufficient.

The only answer seems to be that much more is needed. This reaction must reassess whether intensive care chronic patients really deserve lower priority than equally sick acute patients. It must assess why the highest-status patients do not have priority claim over lower-status patients nationally as well as regionally. It must determine whether Region 2 patients will end up carrying the major burden for the adjustment and, if so, making sure that organs are moved across regions to equalize waiting times for equally sick patients. For those who take justice seriously—at least giving it equal consideration with medical utility—the UNOS response of June 1999 does not seem to go very far in the direction of equalizing waiting times. It may be that some compromises are in order so that medical utility is taken into account as well, but transferring livers from Region 2 Status 2A alcoholic patients to other Region 2 Status 1 acute liver failure patients does not seem to solve the problem. Even if similar moves take place in other regions, we will still have local and regional inequities.

ENDNOTES

1. U.S. Department of Health and Human Services, "Organ Procurement and Transplantation Network: Final Rule, 42 CFR Part 121," 63 Fed. Reg. 16296 (April 2, 1998).
2. United Network for Organ Sharing, "UNOS Refines Liver Allocation Policy: Broader Access for Most Urgent Patients Balanced with Outcome, Other Needs," News Release, June 25, 1999, available at <http://www.unos.org> (July 12, 1999).
3. UNOS Policy 3.5.5.1., available at <http://www.unos.org/frame_Default.asp? Category=About> (Sept. 22, 1998).
4. As we discussed in Chapter 19, O-blood-group recipients can only receive organs from donors with the same type blood, whereas O donors can donate to any recipient. If O-group recipients did not get priority, some O-donor organs would go to recipients based on other factors in the allocation. This would eventually leave O recipients stranded on the waiting list from the shortage of O-type organs available. As it is, O-type recipients have atypically long waits for organs. As of 1994, the last year for which full data are available, the median waiting time for a kidney was 824 days, whereas for O-blood group recipients the median was 1,007 days. AB-group recipients', the "universal recipients," median wait is 637 days, because they can accept any otherwise suitable organ. (A-group recipients have an even shorter waiting time—median = 544 days—whereas B-group recipients have the longest waiting times (median = 1,329), suggesting that fairness might require a reexamination of the allocation formula to give more advantage to those in the B group and less to those in the A group as well as giving absolute priority to O-group recipients for any organs they can receive. "OPTN Waiting List and Removal Files as of September 2, 1997," UNOS Table 47, available at <http://www.unos.org/frame_Default.asp?Category=Search> (Oct. 7, 1998).
5. UNOS Policy 3.8, available at <http://www.unos.org/frame_Default.asp?Category =About> (Sept. 22, 1998).
6. UNOS Policy 3.6, available at <http://www.unos.org/frame_Default.asp?Category =About> (Sept. 22, 1998). This system has changed slightly since the liver allocation to Mickey Mantle described in Chapter 23. Under the new classification system, Status 1 is reserved for patients with fulminant liver failure and a life

expectancy without transplant of fewer than seven days. The change in the formula generally gives patients with acute liver failure priority over those with chronic disease.

7. UNOS Policy 3.7, available at <http://www.unos.org/frame_Default.asp?Category=About> (Sept. 22, 1998).

8. "States Want to Keep Residents' Donated Organs: Supporters Say Local Patients Would Benefit," *CNN Interactive*, July 14, 1998, as posted at <http://cnn.com/HEALTH/9807/14/keeping.organs.ap/index.html>.

9. Ibid.

10. Hung-Mo Lin, H. Myron Kauffman, Maureen A. McBride, Darcy B. Davies, John D. Rosendale, Carol M. Smith, Erick B. Edwards, Patrick Daily, James Kirkin, Charles F. Shield, and Lawrence G. Hunsicker, "Center Specific Graft and Patient Survival Rates: 1997 United Network for Organ Sharing (UNOS) Report," *Journal of the American Medical Association* 280 (Oct. 7, 1998): 1153–60.

11. Ibid., p. 1157.

12. Ibid., p. 1158.

13. UNOS Internet data available at <http://www.unos.org/cinetpub/wwwroot/patients/financ%5Fcosts.htm> (Dec. 1, 1998).

14. Hung-Mo Lin, H. Myron Kauffman, Maureen A. McBride, Darcy B. Davies, John D. Rosendale, Carol M. Smith, Erick B. Edwards, Patrick Daily, James Kirkin, Charles F. Shield, and Lawrence G. Hunsicker, "Center Specific Graft and Patient Survival Rates: 1997 United Network for Organ Sharing (UNOS) Report," p. 1158.

15. Ibid., p. 1160, quoting J. D. Hosenpud, T. J. Breen. E. R. Edwards, "The Effect of Transplant Center Volume on Cardiac Transplant Outcome," *Journal of the American Medical Association* 271 (1994): 1844–49.

16. Erick B. Edwards, John P. Roberts, Maureen A. McBride, James A. Schulak, and Lawrence G. Hunsicker, "The Effects of the Volume of Procedures at Transplantation Centers on Mortality after Liver Transplantation," *New England Journal of Medicine* 341 (1999): 2049–53.

17. "Transplant Recipient Characteristics 1988–1996, Liver Recipients," UNOS Annual Report for 1997, Table 21, available at <www.unos.org>.

18. UNOS Scientific Registry data as of Sept. 4, 1997, from the UNOS Annual Report for 1997, Table 76, "Disposition of Organs Recovered from Cadaveric Donors: Liver Donors," available at <www.unos.org>.

19. Some other provisions of the regulation include a basic definition of the makeup of the OPTN, the procedure for the DHHS to review OPTN policies, better availability to center-specific data about transplant centers, and authority to approve the OPTN waiting list registration fee.

20. U.S. Department of Health and Human Services, "Organ Procurement and Transplantation Network: Final Rule, 42 CFR Part 121."

21. "Statement of Donna Shalala, Secretary U.S. Department of Health and Human Services before the Senate Subcommittee on Labor, HHS and Education on Appropriations," Sept. 10, 1998. Posted on the department Web site at <http://www.hhs.gov./progorg/asl/testify/t090910a.txt> (April 1, 1999). Shalala said,

> UNOS has claimed that the rule creates a single national waiting list for patients that would result in more patients' deaths and longer waits for all patients across the country. This claim is completely false. As I have said, the rule asks UNOS to develop the allocation policy. There is no requirement for a national waiting list anywhere in the rule. The rule calls for fairness. How the fairness is achieved in terms of allocation policy is primarily up to UNOS.

21. This proposal is similar to the one offered by Clive Callender, the head of the transplant program at Howard University Medical School, one of the world's leading transplant authorities and an outspoken voice for greater equity in organ allocation. In testimony in the Dec. 1996 DHHS public hearings, he proposed a four-stage allocation for liver patients, with patients on the local list who are Status 1 and 2 getting first priority then Status 1 and 2 patients nationally, followed by Status 3 and 4 patients locally, and finally Status 3 and 4 patients nationally. He essentially combines Statuses 1 and 2 as well as 3 and 4 and eliminates the regional level. My proposal is in the same spirit.

23. Robert M. Veatch, "Generalization of Expertise: Scientific Expertise and Value Judgments," *Hastings Center Studies* 1 (2, 1973): 29–40.

24. Testimony of Jung Fung, M.D., Hearings of the Department of Health and Human Services, Bethesda, MD, Dec. 10–12, 1996. Text available at <http://www.hrsa.dhhs.gov/osp/dot/group1.htm#Fung>.

25. Jeffrey D. Hosenpud, Timothy J. Breen, Erick B. Edwards, O. Patrick Daily, and Lawrence G. Hunsicker, "The Effect of Transplant Center Volume on Cardiac Transplant Outcome. A Report of the United Network for Organ Sharing Scientific Registry," *Journal of the American Medical Association* 271 (June 15, 1994): 1844–49; Hung-Mo Lin, H. Myron Kauffman, Maureen A. McBride, Darcy B. Davies, John D. Rosendale, Carol M. Smith, Erick B. Edwards, Patrick Daily, James Kirkin, Charles F. Shield, and Lawrence G. Hunsicker, "Center Specific Graft and Patient Survival Rates: 1997 United Network for Organ Sharing (UNOS) Report"; G. L. Laffel, A. I. Barnett, S. Finkelstein, and M. P. Kaye, "The Relation between Experience and Outcome in Heart Transplantation," *New England Journal of Medicine* 327 (17, Oct. 22, 1992): 1220–25; S. H. Belle, K. M. Detre, and K. C. Beringer, "The Relationship between Outcome of Liver Transplantation and Experience in New Centers," *Liver Transplantation and Surgery* 1 (6, Nov. 1995). 347–53; Y. W. Cho and J. M. Cecka, "Organ Procurement Organization and Transplant Center Effects on Cadaver Renal Transplant Outcomes," *Clinical Trans-*

plants (1996): 427–41; D. W. Gjertson, "Center-Dependent Transplantation Factors: An Analysis of Renal Allografts Reported to the United Network for Organ Sharing Registry," *Clinical Transplants* (1993): 445–68; cf. D. W. Gjertson, "Update: Center Effects," *Clinical Transplants* (1990): 375–83; R. W. Evans, F. B. Dong, and D. L. Manninen, "The Center Effect in Heart Transplantation," *Clinical Transplantation* (1991): 45–59; K. Ogura and J. M. Cecka, "Center Effects in Renal Transplantation," *Clinical Transplants* (1991): 245–56.

26. Paul Thompson, "Transplant Tribulation: The Government Wants a New System for Doling out Donated Organs. Oh, What a Ruckus It's Causing!" *Time* 152 (14, Oct. 5, 1998): 56.

27. Donna Shalala's Letter to Congress June 1, 1998.

28. "Data Analysis Supports Idea of Broad Sharing of Donor Livers," UPMC News Bureau Release, Nov. 18, 1997, available at <http://www.upmc.edu/NewsBureau/ consad.htm> (Dec. 4, 1998).

29. Testimony of Sandra Walker, Dec. 12, 1996, available at <http://158.72.83.3/osp/ dot/liver.htm> (Dec. 4, 1998).

30. Statement of Clive Callender, M.D., Howard University Medical School, Hearings of the Department of Health and Human Services, Bethesda, MD, Dec. 10–12, 1996. Text available at <http://www.hrsa.dhhs.gov/osp/dot/grou13.htm>.

31. Utilitarians may not accept this claim without a fight. They may point to the British utilitarian John Stuart Mill, who devoted chapter 5 of his *Utilitarianism* to pointing out that even a utilitarian will recognize that more equality in the distribution of benefits is likely to lead to more aggregate benefit because usually giving a resource to a person who is poorly off will produce more good than giving it to one who is well-off. This is normally the case with food or money, for instance. Giving food to someone who is starving does much more good than giving the same amount of food to someone who is already satiated. Giving $100 to a pauper may produce more good than giving it to a millionaire. This is the economist's notion of "decreasing marginal utility." Transplantation (and many other medical allocation problems), however, are interesting precisely because it is not obvious that giving the medical resource to the sicker person will do more good than giving it to the healthier one. In some cases, allocation will reflect decreasing marginal utility just like it does in many economic problems. In some cases, however, giving the resource to the worse off persons will actually do less good. They may already be so ill that they will predictably get less benefit from the resource than those who are healthier. There may be no decreasing but rather increasing marginal utility. In that case, the utilitarian who is honest will accept the implications and defend the proposition that utility requires directing resources away from the worse off. Those in the worst off category, unfortunately, will simply lose out. They will die from lack of an organ. Utilitarians will insist they did not set out in-

tentionally to exclude the person so sick he or she is inefficient to treat. They will, in all honesty, say that it simply turns out when the numbers are crunched that more overall good is achieved if the organs go to those who are healthier.

32. Determining whether a state is a net importer or exporter is more difficult than it may appear. We cannot simply count the organs imported to the state's OPOs and the number exported. As we have seen, many OPOs cross state lines, so it is not easy to track whether an organ procured in one state is moved to a part of the OPO in another state. Moreover, patients do not always get transplanted in the state in which they live. For example, Louisiana residents who have become listed for a transplant in another state would have their interests jeopardized by a rule requiring Louisiana organs to stay in Louisiana.

33. Institute of Medicine, Committee on Organ Procurement and Transplantation Policy, *Organ Procurement and Transplantation: Assessing Current Policies and the Potential Impact of the DHHS Final Rule*. (Washington, DC: National Academy Press, 1999).

34. Douglas A. Heiney, Director, Department of Membership, UNOS, "Memorandum: Proposed Liver Allocation Policy Development Plan for Public Comment." (Richmond, VA: UNOS, Feb. 15, 2000).

Twenty-Five

Directed Donation of Organs for Transplant: Egalitarian and Maximin Approaches*

MUCH OF THIS volume has been an exercise in what could be called practical or applied ethics. I have examined various problems in defining death, organ procurement, and organ allocation using general categories in ethical theory: utilitarian and deontological approaches to deciding what is morally correct action, various theories of justice, the relation of the principle of autonomy to utility, and the like. One final problem remains to be addressed, which turns out to show that ethical analysis is not always a "one-way" movement from ethical theory to application.

A concrete problem in transplantation policy called *directed donation* has arisen in the past few years. Directed donation involves the attempt by individuals or their surrogates to donate organs to specific individuals or groups. Although the possibility of donating organs to a specific individual who needs an organ— a family member or friend—has been recognized since the beginning of organ transplant, recently some people have attempted to direct organs to a specific social group: to a group defined by race, religion, ethnicity, gender, or sexual orientation, for example. This chapter examines how organ transplant programs should respond to such attempts. The goal is not merely to spell out our current national policy regarding this socially directed donation but also to tease out its surprisingly radical implications for some major questions in ethical theory—in particular, the theory of justice and what it means to have a just or fair social practice. The implication is that by careful consideration of our considered moral intuitions about a specific policy we will not only have a better understanding

*I am grateful to Catherine Ehlen, an intern at the Kennedy Institute of Ethics, for her research assistance and to the members of the Kennedy Institute of Ethics lunch seminar, especially David DeGrazia, for their comments on an earlier draft of this chapter.

of the morally correct practice, but we may be able to advance more fundamental work in ethical theory, a development that could have implications well beyond transplantation. The suggestion is that practical ethics may turn out to be a two-way street. Not only do we move from ethical theory to practical problem solving, but we may also move the other way, from clear considered moral judgments to a more sophisticated and precise ethical theory.

The Problem in Theory

In the field of ethical theory the past two decades have seen a resurgence in relatively egalitarian theories of justice. When John Rawls's A *Theory of Justice* (1971) emerged as a dominant force in the contemporary discussion, his view was described as an egalitarian challenge to utilitarian theories of allocation. In comparison to classical utilitarian allocation, the Rawlsian principles would tend to create practices that would improve the lot of the least well-off and thereby make people more equal. Nevertheless, in this chapter I argue that it is a mistake to label the Rawlsian justice principles a true egalitarian system of justice and suggest that justice is better understood in stricter or more radical egalitarian rather than Rawlsian terms. I will use a fascinating debate within the ethics of organ allocation—the so-called directed donation controversy—to show why this is so.

Why Rawlsian Justice Can Be Inegalitarian

Rawls's principles of justice give first priority to the equal right to the most extensive total system of equal basic liberties and then distribute other primary goods (such as income, wealth, power, and opportunities) to maximize the position of the least advantaged.[1] (Hence there is an effort to maximize the minimum, and the notion is often referred to as a "maximin.") It should be clear that maximizing the position of the worst off groups need not lead to greater equality—even if there is some tendency for that to happen. The interesting case is the one in which the best way to improve the lot of the worst off is actually to increase inequality between those who are worst off and their better off counterparts. For example, it may be that large manufacturing corporations can make their lowest-paid employees better off (in terms of their overall well being including, of course, salary) by raising rather than lowering the salary of their highest-paid officials. In fact, to inspire the greatest dedication to improving the welfare of the worst off employees, the salaries of the executives may need to be raised by more than the increase seen in the income of the lower paid workers. As long as total productivity is not a zero-sum game, it is possible to improve the lot of the worst off by rewarding in even larger amounts the better off. If so, this approach to increasing the position of the least advantaged would actually increase inequality at the same time.

It need not work that way. If, for the moment, we assume that Rawls's principles can be applied at this level of specificity, such pay raises for the elite would be justified by maximin theory only if there were no other way of improving the lot of the worst off as much. But, according to a Rawlsian maximin theory of justice, if a practice can only improve the lot of the least well-off by increasing inequality between the best and worst off groups, then increasing the inequality is not only permitted, it is required.[2] That is hardly a true egalitarian approach. If it is egalitarian at all, it is only by the accident of circumstance. For purposes of this discussion I will consider a principle of justice to be a *true* or *strict* egalitarian principle if it holds that opportunities for equality per se are called for, whereas a principle of justice that affirms allocations that redound to the benefit of the worst off groups (even if such policies actually increase inequality) will be termed *relatively egalitarian*.

The Inegalitarian Maximin: Hypothetical Examples

Although the inegalitarian implications of maximin theory have been understood by theorists for quite some time, there have been relatively few practical policy problems in which the theoretical inegalitarianism of the maximin principle made much difference.[3] The best examples seemed quite hypothetical.

For example, consider a hypothetical airplane crash in which there were many victims needing attention. If a small number of egalitarian rescuers reach the scene with only modest emergency rescue skills, they would presumably either seek out the worst off or offer their limited services randomly without regard to the social utility of the lives being saved. In such a situation it is hard to imagine what egalitarianism would lead to other than one of these choices.

Consider, however, the possibility that it could be immediately established that one of the victims was an emergency room physician with advanced life-support skills who was at less immediate risk but who would need rescuers' attention before she could assist (perhaps because she was trapped in a way in which she was not in danger but from which she would have to be extricated to assist). It could be argued that everyone would be better off (or at least in a statistical sense everyone would have a better chance at being better off) if the rescuers gave the first attention to the relatively well-off physician who, if rescued, could go on to help others on the scene. Giving the physician (arguably one who is already in a relatively advantaged position either considering her fate in the accident or considering her overall well-being as a high-income professional) the first priority support is hardly egalitarian. One who believed in true equality as the only morally controlling principle would hardly be able to support such a preference; at least it could not be supported in the name of equality. From the maximin difference principle, however (if it is to be applied at this level of specificity), the priority to the physician is easily supported even though the physician gets a special advantage. What justifies the special favoritism for the physician is not the sum total of the good she can do but the fact that the worst off will be better off if they forgo their claim to being rescued first. On the other hand, the true egalitarian would not be persuaded that this inequality is automatically justified. At least the true egalitarian would not be persuaded that it is just. (The possibility that it is justified but not just is an interesting alternative, which I shall take up later.)

This is the kind of hypothetical that illustrates that occasionally there can be a difference between the relatively egalitarian maximin approach and true egalitarianism. Although this example may, at least at first, lead one to favor the less egalitarian position (a view that I shall suggest is inappropriate for transplantation and many other settings), it at least illustrates that the maximin cannot always be equated with a full egalitarianism.

This is the kind of hypothetical example that one might use in a classroom exercise to try to show that the maximin theorist and the true egalitarian would reach substantively different conclusions on certain kinds of moral problems. There are other somewhat more plausible examples. To the embarrassment of some Rawlsians, the trickle-down economics of the Reagan administration might also be cited as a policy that could be supported by the maximin difference principle (as well as utilitarian reasoning), depending on the actual effects of the policy. Utilitarian reasoning would support trickle-down if the aggregate net benefit were increased (even if some other arrangement that produced a smaller gain in utility would increase the welfare of the worst off more). By contrast the maximin would support trickle-down only if it were the way to maximize the position of the worst off. In either the utilitarian or the maximin case, the result can be inegalitarian—an actual increase in the gap between the best and worst off groups.

Directed Donation: A New Example

Until now these examples have been the best available to try to understand the difference between maximin and true egalitarian interpretations of the principle of justice. Now a dispute has emerged within the field of organ transplantation that seems to test the difference between maximin and true egalitarian understandings of justice. As we have seen in earlier chapters, normally if organs are donated, they go to the individual selected by an allocation formula that, depending on the organ, takes into account such factors as human lymphocyte antigen (HLA) tissue histocompatibility, time on the waiting list for organs, blood type, degree of medical urgency, and so forth. In the United States, the selection is made by computer independent of the wishes or knowledge of the family of the deceased. It can be claimed that the computer allocation is procedurally fair. Once the patient is listed in the system, it is virtually impossible for a patient or a physician to manipulate the system for a special advantage.[4] The computer does not take into account race, gender, socioeconomic status, or other social classification.[5] In this sense the computer allocation could be considered fair and impartial.

When Thomas Simons, a resident of Florida, died as a result of being shot in a $5 robbery, he became a potential source of organs for transplant. Members of the family were approached by the organ procurement officials. The family made an unusual request. He had been a sympathizer of the Ku Klux Klan. Three Klan cards were found in his wallet. His family offered his organs, but stipulated on the donation form, "donation to White recipients only."[6] Similar requests for "directed donation" have been reported that direct organ donation to members of a specified race, religion, gender, sexual orientation, or disease group. Some have considered directed donation in favor of a specific hospital or surgeon, for or against people with liver disease as a result of alcoholism, and so on.

Those within the transplant community are unanimously unsympathetic to directed donation. They support the allocation by formula because it is likely to provide organs that have a good chance of survival and/or allocates organs fairly. When families persist, however, the question arises about whether the directed donation should be accepted with the limits set by the donors rather than intentionally losing a set of organs that have the potential of saving several humans' lives and improving the quality of lives of others. The organ procurement agency in the Simons case agreed to the family's conditions on the donation. That decision has generated considerable controversy.

The Ethics Committee of the United Network for Organ Sharing (UNOS) has, without opposition, adopted the position that donation directed to a particular social group (race, religion, or gender) is morally unacceptable. Florida, since the Simons's case, has passed legislation making directed donation illegal in that state.[7] The Washington Regional Transplant Consortium, the group responsible for producing and allocating organs in the Washington, D.C., metropolitan area, has banned donations directed by social group. But some people, including a number of transplant surgeons and advocates for groups who presently do not get organs in proportion to their numbers in the recipient pool, have argued that it is wasteful to refuse life-saving organs even if they come with discriminatory conditions. They have proposed that the society tolerate the directed donation in cases in which the family members, after personnel from the organ procurement organizations (OPO) attempt to persuade them to the contrary, persist in making a donation with discriminatory limits attached.

Even though the UNOS Ethics Committee adopted its position without opposition, there continues to be a moral division of opinion in UNOS, in the transplant community, and among donor families over what is the morally preferable policy. At first it appears that the surgeons and others who favor tolerating directed donation do so on utilitarian grounds. If some plausible assumptions are made, it appears that more lives will be saved and more years of organ graft survival expected with a policy that tolerates directed donation than one that simply wastes the organs that are donated conditionally. Surgeons are known often to be moral consequentialists. They might hold that they should choose the policy on donation that will maximize the aggregate net benefit from the organs that are available. If they did, they would be utilitarians.

Opponents of directed donation, when asked, offer an array of reasons for their opposition. Occasionally a sophisticated utilitarian may oppose directed donation, claiming that the overall transplant enterprise could be jeopardized if a dramatic directed donation case such as that of the Ku Klux Klan member or donation limited to a gay recipient turned the public against the organ transplant system.

However, based on my experience with the UNOS Ethics Committee and as the chair of a local OPO Task Force on Directed Donation, as well as the existing literature opposing directed donation[8] and the Florida law[9] that has made donation directed to a sociological group illegal, many opponents, when asked why they oppose directed donation, will respond with the statement that it is unfair, inequitable, or unjust. The policy is one that would take the computer-generated priority list of recipients and pluck a recipient out of the middle, based solely on factors such as race, gender, or religion to give that person a life-saving advantage. In general, the dispute has the appearance of a feud between utilitarians who tolerate directed donation and egalitarians committed to the principle of justice who oppose it even at the expense of losing some valuable organs. This would be yet another example of a commitment to justice sacrificing efficiency for equity.

The analysis, however, must be more complex. Utilitarian aggregate-net-benefit maximization is not the only plausible defense of a policy that accepts or tolerates directed donation. The Rawlsian maximin difference principle, to the extent that it can be applied at this level of specificity, also provides a basis for supporting directed donation. After showing that the maximin has the potential of supporting directed donation, I will use that fact together with the widely held view that directed donation is morally unacceptable to argue that there is a lack of coherence, a lack of reflective equilibrium. To the extent that one is convinced that directed donation is unacceptable, then something must be wrong with the maximin.[10]

Organ allocation in the United States is made on the basis of a formally developed list of priority formulated on the basis of what is the fairest and most efficient criteria.[11] With directed donation one person is given what is easily seen as an unfair and undeserved life-saving advantage.[12] He or she is taken from the middle of the ranked priority list and given an extremely scarce and valuable good—a human organ. It is unequal treatment based on morally irrelevant considerations—race, gender, or religion. But this is a very special kind of advantage. It is realistic to say that no one is disadvantaged by the privileged position of the designated recipient. In fact, those above him or her on the waiting list are left exactly where they were before the directed donation, assuming that the alternative to discriminatory allocation is letting the organs go to waste.

The intriguing thing about directed donation is that everyone below the privileged recipient is actually made better off because of the discrimination. They all move up one on the waiting list.[13] This is a pure example of a case in which tolerating the unequal treatment of one person by permitting discrimination based on race or religion is to the advantage of everyone who is worse off (lower on the list) and to the disadvantage of no one.

The maximin principle holds that inequalities are justified when (and only when) they are to the benefit of the least well-off. Because the worst off are made somewhat better off if they are discriminated against, the maximin principle seems to support directed donation. The moral basis of that support converges with the utilitarian's basis, although the claim is a different one. The maximin supports directed donation because it benefits the worst off, not because it maximizes the aggregate good of the transplant enterprise. This seems to be a real-life case in which a maximin version of the principle of justice leads to a significantly different conclusion from a true egalitarian version.

The Inadequate Case for the Maximin

Rawls is very much aware of the difference between the maximin and what I call *true egalitarianism*. He suggests the rather strange notion that egalitarianism "admits to degrees," so that in some forms of egalitarianism disparities are permitted.[14] Thus, according to this view, some equalities are more equal than others. In a critical section of A *Theory of Justice* he addresses the reasons for supporting the maximin difference principle version over the idea that justice requires allocating resources to produce opportunities for equality of well-being as far as possible.[15]

Rawls's Grounding of Strict Egalitarianism in Envy

Rawls apparently views the principle of true egalitarianism—of striving for opportunities for equality of outcomes—as grounded in envy. He begins the analysis with the plausible presumption that envy is to be "avoided and feared" and that the principles of justice should not be influenced by this trait.[16] He is quite committed to showing that his principles of justice need not be based in envy but in the process posits that strict egalitarianism can only be founded on it. Note in the following passage his movement, without argument, from the claim that strict egalitarianism "conceivably" derives from envy to the view that this strict egalitarianism would be adopted only on the basis of this psychological propensity. He begins by attempting to defend the maximin version of equality from the foundation in envy differentiating his version from strict egalitarianism in the process.

> To be sure, there may be forms of equality that do spring from envy. Strict egalitarianism, the doctrine which insists upon an equal distribution of all primary goods, *conceivably* derives from this propensity. What this means is that this conception of equality would be adopted in the original position only if the parties are assumed to be sufficiently envious [italics added].[17]

Of course, Rawls is correct that envy could be the basis for a striving for greater equality, whether he has in mind the strict or the maximin version. But is there any basis for his statement that strict egalitarianism would be adopted only if the parties are sufficiently envious?

He posits that rational people are not envious. He can think of no reason why rational people behind a veil of ignorance (i.e., if they did not know their own position in society[18]) see moral significance in pursuing equality per se. It is only getting the worst off as well-off as possible that has moral significance. Often this can be achieved by transferring assets from the well-off to those who are worse off, which would shrink the gap between the two groups, but it is not the shrinking of the gap itself that is morally significant, it is the raising of the floor (even if the only way to do so is to increase the gap between the haves and the have nots).

Problems Grounding Strict Egalitarianism in Envy
There are some serious problems with the position that grounds strict or true egalitarianism in envy, however.

MANY WELL-OFF PEOPLE FAVOR EGALITARIANISM
For one, it seems to assume that it is only those who are the have-nots (or think from the perspective of the have-nots) who would favor strict egalitarianism. In fact, it is often the elites, the well-off, who have a moral sense of justice that supports greater equality, other things being equal. Thus, for example, many of

the most vocal defenders of a strict egalitarian prohibition on directed donation of organs come from the groups (e.g., the White liberal intelligentsia) who are precisely the ones who would be most favored by certain directed donations.

From behind a Rawlsian veil of ignorance rational self-interested contractors might imagine themselves among the worst off and favor equality of outcomes as a result. That might reflect envy (but not necessarily so). Rawls posits that his contractors should be conceptualized as free of envy. Without envy, he claims, no one would favor equality as an interpretation of the principle of justice. They would favor inequalities when necessary to benefit the worst off groups. What this interpretation cannot explain is why those in the most favored groups (such as White liberals) also favor strict egalitarianism.

This grounding of support for equality in envy must be challenged. What is at stake is our understanding of what Rawls calls the "sense of justice." According to him those contracting behind the veil of ignorance imagining their interests if they happened to be among the well-off would never favor equality from the framework of the advantaged; they would only support boosting the floor out of empathy for the worst off. Yet many who have cultivated a sense of justice who are well-off in fact feel discomfort when they contemplate inequality. It is surely not envy that would lead them to favor equality.

Of course, it is not acceptable to assume that this discomfort is automatically evidence for the existence of some moral force grounded in equality. The discomfort could result from other psychological phenomena, such as long-held cultural belief that inequalities were ethically suspect or were disapproved of for other reasons. For example, if it were only the worst off who experienced this discomfort, Rawls's explanation based on envy might provide an adequate account.

A "SENSE OF JUSTICE" MAY PERCEIVE OPPORTUNITIES FOR EQUALITY TO BE INHERENTLY RIGHT-MAKING

However, the widely experienced discomfort throughout all sectors of the population casts doubt on the envy hypothesis. One possibility is that a properly cultivated sense of justice would see moral rightness in equality as well as in improving the lot of the worst off.

What is missing from the Rawlsian sense of justice is any notion of community solidarity. Some have such an empathy for their fellow humans that they have a moral sense of revulsion at a lack of opportunities for equality regardless of whether they are among the best or worst off. For example, parents, contemplating the life outcomes for their children, may not be content with the utilitarian arrangement that would maximize the sum total of net well being for all their children by making one do particularly poorly. They might not even favor a maximin arrangement whereby inequalities among their children would be accepted provided they served the interests of the worst off. They might hope for some similar amount of well being for each. They might, in fact, purposely arrange their resources so as not to maximize either the aggregate total well-being or the well being of the worst off but rather to give each child a fair opportunity for equality of well being. This orientation seems particularly plausible when the improvement in the lot of the worst off would be small and the inequalities large. Rawls's account does not seem to be able to account for this aspect of the sense of justice.

Likewise, persons who have a well-developed sense of justice complete with sympathy for their fellow humans might see moral rightness in arrangements that provide opportunities for equality of well being. They might consider it morally right-making to arrange resources to accomplish this end (other things being equal).

Egalitarian Justice as a Prima Facie Principle

Thus there is an alternative that is a much more simple and straightforward conception of the principle of justice: View justice as a right-making characteristic of actions that strives for equality of well-being. Doing so seems much more straightforwardly an understanding of the notion of equality that drives egalitarian notions of justice than the maximin.

There are, of course, problems with this more strictly egalitarian approach to justice. The most obvious is that strictly egalitarian justice would require giving a resource such as an organ to the worst off even if the advantage to that person was tiny compared to the advantage that could be obtained from it by others. It would seem to require, for example, giving a liver to the worst off person even if that person could gain only a few days while some other better off patient could gain years.

One response of the egalitarian is to point out that when the advantage to the worst off person is so minimal, that person might simply waive his or her right of access. In the case of organ transplant, it would not plausibly be in the candidate's interest to undergo major, painful, risky surgery to gain only a day or two of life. That candidate would rationally decline the organ even if he or she were entitled to it by the consideration of justice.

Some people might go further. They might say that this worst off person who could gain only a minimal benefit is not even morally entitled to the resource (and so should not be given the opportunity to refuse it).[19] There are also other lines of argument open to those who would sometimes conclude that following the rule of always giving the organ to the worst off person is implausible.

Justice as One among Many Prima Facie Principles

Justice is not plausibly going to turn out to be the only moral principle, not even in cases of distribution of benefits and burdens. Other principles may pull simultaneously in other directions by identifying other characteristics of actions that independently make them right. We have seen that current American law requires attention to both efficiency and equity, utility and justice. The UNOS Ethics Committee adopted a policy that gives these two principles equal weight. This makes true egalitarianism (merely) a prima facie principle—that is, a principle that expresses one characteristic of actions that will tend to make them morally right but that may have to be balanced against other considerations such as the amount of good done. A morally right distribution of resources would have to take into account other moral principles, including beneficence and autonomy. Rawls, in fact, at some points makes a similar point,[20] but for some reason conceptualizes justice in such a way that considerations of maximizing benefit (for the worst off) are packed into the principle of justice.

Justice as Opportunity for Equality

The alternative is to conceptualize justice more purely as dealing with matters of equality, leaving to the task of resolution of conflict among principles the problem of reconciling conflicts between justice and beneficence or justice and autonomy.[21]

True egalitarians face a serious problem at this point, however. It is clear that one easy way to make everybody equal in well-being would be to reduce everyone to the level of the worst off. Everyone with zero well-being (everybody dead) would be pure equality. Surely that cannot be the goal of any moral system. There is after all something to be said for tolerating at least moderate differences in salary if they are necessary to make those receiving the lowest salaries get salaries that are as high as possible. No one favors a medical policy that would reduce everyone to the level of health that is the best that can be achieved for the incurably ill or disabled. Is not the more plausible interpretation the maximin in which the goal is the get the worst off as well-off as possible while not reducing the well-being of the better off unless it serves the interest of the worst off?

At the least, surely it is better for everyone to be equal at a high level rather than equal at a low level of well-being. That intuition can be explained by the maximin principle but not true egalitarianism taken by itself.

Explanations of Tolerance of Inequality: Sacrificing Justice for Other Principles

There are alternative explanations, however.

THE MAXIMIN AS A RULE TO RESOLVE CONFLICTS BETWEEN JUSTICE AND BENEFICENCE

First, the maximin might be seen as a moral rule that integrates two prima facie principles: justice (in the true egalitarian sense) and beneficence. A full normative moral theory includes several moral principles in addition to justice. Rawls held as much.[22] One of these principles is surely beneficence. How one integrates the claims of (true egalitarian) justice and beneficence is a matter that must be addressed in a moral theory of resolution of conflict among principles.

One hypothesis worth pursuing is that the Rawlsian maximin is, in fact, not a moral principle at all but a proposal for a moral rule that integrates the conflicting claims of the principles of justice and beneficence in situations dealing with allocation of scarce primary goods. It would hold that, when the goals of maximizing benefit and minimizing inequality come into conflict, one should resolve the conflict by striving for equality unless inequalities redound to the benefit of the least well-off. This would incorporate beneficence as a reason to override (egalitarian) justice when (and only when) it increases beneficence to the worst off.

This view of resource allocation involving conflict between egalitarian justice and beneficence easily explains why we would prefer equality at a high level over equality at a low level. Beneficence presses us toward higher levels of well-being. When that can be achieved without sacrificing equality, then beneficence pulls us, without opposition, in favor of the higher level. There is no conflict between the principles.

This suggests that justice should be interpreted in its egalitarian version as a prima facie principle that on occasion conflicts with a prima facie principle of beneficence. The maximin is a rule for deviating from justice rather than being a principle of justice itself. It is a *specification* of the principles.[23]

Whether the maximin is the best possible rule for resolving conflict between beneficence and justice is controversial. In some cases it seems to lead to quite plausible conclusions (such as the hypothetical example of the airline accident), but in other cases it does not. I suggest that there are other priority rules that better explain our considered moral judgments.

The directed donation example poses a real challenge to the maximin rule interpreted this way. If the maximin rule applies, it seems likely that directed donation would have to be accepted. Yet many people find directed donation intolerable. The UNOS Ethics Committee, after considerable contemplation, concluded without opposition that directed donation was ethically unacceptable. Likewise, government attorneys have held that such a practice would violate current civil rights laws. These commentators have concluded that their considered moral judgment is firm against the practice of directed donation. If the maximin rule is the correct reconciliation of the conflict between justice and beneficence, then why should directed donation generate such resistance?

LEXICALLY RANKING JUSTICE OVER BENEFICENCE WHILE BALANCING IT AGAINST OTHER PRINCIPLES

One possible conclusion is that the maximin rule is not the correct rule, at least in all cases. In some cases it appears that holding out for a right to an opportunity for equality is preferable to tolerating inequalities merely to improve somewhat the lot of the worst off. Directed donation may be one such case. If so, directed donation would not be made acceptable merely because it raises the worst off one notch on the waiting list.

A more plausible rule for reconciliation of conflict may be that egalitarian justice is lexically ranked over beneficence, that is, equality is always a more weighty claim when only those two principles come into conflict. (This is the reconciliation between these two principles that I outlined in Chapter 2.) If other prima facie principles can constrain egalitarian justice (even though beneficence cannot), then it may be possible to explain certain social acceptance of inegalitarian outcomes without permitting beneficence to compete with justice. Other principles, such as respect for autonomy and promise-keeping, may provide a more limited and more plausible basis for overriding egalitarian justice on occasion without opening the flood gates to permit beneficence to offset it.

If inequalities are to be tolerated in the name of the maximin, it seems to make a difference whether it is the worst off who are making the case for the toleration of the inequality or if it is those who will be given unique, unjustified advantage. Rawls himself acknowledges as much,[24] but the defenders of the Rawlsian version of the maximin cannot explain this sense that it makes a difference who proposes tolerating the inequality. Those who favor a lexical ranking of egalitarian justice can easily explain it. If the worst off have a claim to equality ranked above the principle of beneficence, then they could have the right grounded in autonomy to waive that claim. If they waive it, then there would be no moral imperative to pursue equality. If the advantages gained are great in comparison to the amount of inequality created, then they could plausibly exercise their autonomy to waive their right to equal treatment. Beneficence would then run free to permit maximizing the well-being of the worst off by increasing inequality. If the worst off do not exercise their waiver, then the unequal advantage created by directed donation would not be acceptable.

Likewise, promises made could provide a counter claim to justice in a way that does not permit beneficence to run amuck. Consider, for example, a case in which a fair health care system promised certain benefits, such as transplantable organs, to certain groups of people. For example, the present allocation promises children a special advantage in obtaining kidneys over their older colleagues on the waiting list. If persons are promised an advantage they may have some moral claim to it, even if fulfilling the promise will tend to produce inequality.[25]

The True Egalitarian Alternative

I have used the directed-donation example to suggest that the maximin is not a formulation of a basic principle but rather is a rule for resolving conflict between the principle of justice and beneficence (interpreted as requiring maximization of aggregate net well-being). If so, then a different priority rule could give a different resolution of this conflict if one lexically ranked the other principles over beneficence. If justice (taken as requiring true egalitarianism) is lexically ranked over beneficence, then only if the requirements of justice are waived by the least well-off or if other prima facie principles (beyond beneficence) override justice could directed donation be morally acceptable. Because in many cases the least well-off are not in a position to exercise such a waiver and in other cases it would be procedurally very difficult for them to do so, a general practice of banning directed donation in favor of a policy of refusing the organs that can only be obtained by agreeing to discriminate becomes a plausible way to respond as a matter of public policy. A good case can be made that the UNOS Ethics Committee and the local organ procurement organizations that have opposed donation directed by social group are expressing a decision grounded in the priority of true egalitarian interpretations of the principle of justice. They see this as the appropriate resolution of a potential conflict between true egalitarian justice and the maximin.

Conclusion

The case of directed donation of organs poses a special problem not only to utilitarians but also to maximin justice theorists who claim to be "relatively egalitarian." Directed donation of organs that otherwise would go to waste not only plausibly maximizes the aggregate net utility of an organ allocation system, it also tends to be to the advantage of the worst off persons while being to the disadvantage of no one. If so, directed donation satisfies not only utilitarian but also maximin criteria. Anyone who retains a considered moral judgment opposing directed donation must either have some clever way of showing that directed donation will not satisfy utilitarian or maximin criteria or must conclude that the utilitarian and maximin allocation principles are unacceptable.

One plausible conclusion is that directed donation simply treats people unequally and that, per se, is prima facie unethical, even if it maximizes the position of the least well-off. Directed donation challenges the currently dominant maximin interpretation of the principle of justice forcing us to consider a prima facie true egalitarian interpretation as an alternative.

Does the Maximin Apply at this Level of Specificity?

A critical question for Rawls scholars is whether it is legitimate to apply the Rawlsian principles of justice at this level of social policy. Rawls insists that his principles are designed to be used at the level of the basic structure of a society.[26] He has in mind abstract formation of norms such as those found in the constitution of a state and acts of the legislature. He does not envision the principles being taken directly to moral choices about individual acts such as how to allocate pieces of a birthday cake, but he does see the principles reflected in societal policies.

Two Reasons to Believe the Maximin Applies

Some Rawls scholars might argue that directed donation is not at a general or basic enough level for the two principles to be applied directly. This raises difficult questions. Two replies are in order.

Applying the Maximin to Specific Issues by Rawls's Followers

First, even if it is correct that Rawls himself would not approve of applying the principles of justice directly to the question of allocation of organs by directed donation, many others directly or indirectly influenced by Rawls would. They see the maximin interpretation of justice as a way for society to allocate any scarce resource. For that reason alone it is critical to get clear on the difference between maximin and true egalitarian versions of justice at this level of policy formation.

The Case that Rawls Would View Organ Allocation as a Practice

Second, a case can be made that Rawls would, in fact, extend his principles to basic social practices such as establishing a health care system or even an organ allocation system. What is at stake in the directed donation controversy is not an allocation choice made for the individual case. The controversy concerns national policy. Rawls is quite vague about exactly how far down in the level of policy making the principles should reach.[27] For him the basic structure includes such institutions as the family, the organization of the economy, and legally recognized forms of private property.[28] It also includes "those operations that continually adjust and compensate for the inevitable tendencies away from background fairness. . . . " such as inheritance taxation.[29] He claims the principles of justice apply to the main public principles and policies that regulate social and economic inequalities.[30] It is not a long stretch to view the health care system or the organ allocation system as part of the basic structure. A case can be made that it should be included, in which case the two principles should provide the moral foundation for what is a just allocation from a Rawlsian perspective. At least the principles should shape constitutional and statutory requirements that could make a directed donation policy unconstitutional or illegal. Even if one concludes that Rawls would not include organ allocation policy as part of the basic structure, what is said in this argument would apply to those under his influence who go beyond Rawls in making such an application to more specific policies. Rawls's principles concern the distribution of the primary social goods, which include the fundamental bases of self-respect, which (arguably) include access to needed health care. To the extent that the organ allocation system is part of the national health policy serving this function, the case can be made that the national organ allocation policy must satisfy the principles.

Three More Egalitarian Interpretations of Rawls

If the full Rawlsian theory were applied to organ allocation policy, there is still some controversy over exactly how it should be applied. The most obvious interpretation would be that health care should be considered a primary social good, a good that facilitates whatever more specific goods one pursues, whose allocation is governed by the principle of equality of liberty and the difference principle (the maximin). The claim that inequalities in access to organs as a result of directed donation is tolerable would appear to be supported. But there are at least three other ways in which some Rawls scholars attempt to apply the two principles to health care. Although each relies on a different argument, the net result of each is to argue that health care access should be distributed not based on the maximin but according to need. This could suggest that even if one were allocating organs according to Rawlsian principles, it would be unacceptable to rely on the maximin to justify directed donations.

Equal Health Care Access Is Needed for Equal Liberty (Ronald Green)

Ronald Green[31] sees implications for health care not in the maximin portion of the second principle but in the first principle—the principle that "Each person is to have an equal right to the most extensive total system of equal basic liberties compatible with a similar system of liberty for all."[32] Green claims that a certain level of health is on a par with basic civil liberties.[33] This might be understood as claiming that health is a minimal necessary condition to participate in this system of liberties and that it is thus a requirement of the first principle. If, however, people have a right to equal basic liberties and a certain minimal health status is a necessary condition for liberties, it would appear that an attempt should be made to distribute opportunities for that minimal health status equally, not based on the maximin. If this is correct, then even if Rawls would apply the two principles to health care and specifically to organ allocation, access to health care should be distributed to give people an equal opportunity for the minimal level of health necessary for equality of liberty. Discrimination in allocating organs by social group rather than by health care need would appear to be unacceptable. The result would be that the maximin is not relevant to health care, at least up to the point necessary to enjoy equal basic liberties. Even a full-blown Rawlsian would allocate health services (up to this level) according to true egalitarianism, and possessing a functioning major internal organ would certainly appear to be included in that required minimum.

That follows, however, only if the first principle requires equal liberty for all within the system. One little known feature of Rawls's *Theory of Justice* is that in it he does not always insist that the system of liberties be arranged so that all have an equal system of liberties. Although most of his summary statements have that implication, in many places he explicitly acknowledges that liberties may be unequal provided the inequality contributes to greater liberty for all. Rawls, in effect, provides a maximin for liberty analogous to the maximin for other primary social goods in the second principle. Liberties can never be unequal to promote a greater amount of the other primary social goods for the worst off, but they can be unequal to provide the maximum liberty for the ones with the least liberty.

> An inequality in the basic structure must always be justified to those in the disadvantaged position. This holds whatever the primary social good and especially for liberty. . . . If liberty is unequal, the freedom of those with the lesser liberty must be better secured. . . . A less than equal liberty must be acceptable to those citizens with the lesser liberty.[34]

Thus if certain health interventions are necessary for liberty and liberty can be distributed unequally to secure maximum liberty for those with the least liberty, it would seem to follow for a Rawlsian willing to apply the principles to organ allocation that inequalities resulting from directed donation can be tolerated when they redound to the benefit of the persons with the worst health (and therefore potentially the most risk to losing liberty). This conclusion applies even if health care is to be allocated by the first principle. If there were ever a case in which unequal right of access to a health status could be said to serve one's liberty, it would have to be when the unequal access increases the probability of keeping one alive.

Equal Health Care Access Is Needed for Equal Opportunity (Norman Daniels)

There is a second way in which health care is attached to the principles. Its best known proponent is Norman Daniels.[35] He sees implications for health care allocation in neither the maximin position of the second principle nor the basic system of liberties of the first. Rather he finds them in requirement for fair equality of opportunity, which is the second portion of the second principle (lexically ranked after protection of equality of access to a system of basic liberties and before the maximin[36]). The fair equality of opportunity principle seems to require equality of opportunity for offices and positions. Daniels argues that a certain health status is necessary to have that fair equality of opportunity. So any health service needed to provide an opportunity for normal species-typical functioning could, arguably, fall under this provision. Once again, if anything is needed for equality of opportunity, it would seem to be this health status.[37] If fair equality of opportunity requires an equal right of access to this health status, then perhaps life-saving organs must be allocated with equal opportunity, not according to the maximin.

However, we must again face the question of whether Rawls would permit the maximin to operate within the allocation of fair opportunity just as we have argued he would with the allocation of liberties. There are several hints that Rawls, in fact, would do so. He discusses fair equality of opportunity much less extensively, but if he would permit a maximin within liberty and a maximin for the other primary social goods and he opposes equality for equality's sake, it seems he would permit fair inequality of opportunity when such inequality maximized the opportunity of those with the least opportunity. Permitting inequality in organ allocation through directed donation would appear to limit opportunity in a way that all, including the one with the least opportunity, might consider fair. Thus he might well favor a maximin for opportunity. What would then be important is not equality of opportunity but fair opportunity or an arrangement that maximized the opportunity of the one with the least opportunity for offices and positions.

Equal Health Care Access Is Needed for Adequate Self-Respect or Self-Esteem (David DeGrazia)

There is a still a third way of grounding a right to health care that may avoid treating it as a primary social good to be allocated directly by the maximin in

Rawls's second principle. David DeGrazia[38] has argued that health care is linked to self-respect or self-esteem, which he sees as providing a basis for a limited right to health care. The implications could be interpreted in one of two ways. If the fundamental bases of self-respect and self-esteem are primary social goods on a par with the other primary social goods, then they would be distributed according to the difference principle—that is, inequalities would be acceptable provided the inequalities redound to the benefit of the least well-off. We have already suggested this as a possibility. Self-respect and self-esteem would then support differences of the sort we envision with directed donation.

The other possibility is that self-respect and self-esteem have a special status among the primary social goods. Rawls identifies self-respect as a primary social good, and one that is the most important.[39] Rawls sees it as being of primary importance because of its connection to basic liberties. DeGrazia[40] also appears to link self-respect to liberties.[41] By connecting health care to self-respect and self-esteem DeGrazia potentially has leverage to give health care special status above other goods. To the extent that liberties are to be distributed equally and independent of the difference-principle portion of the second principle, DeGrazia could make a case for a right of access equal to one's health care needs (at least up to the level needed to appreciate the basic liberties), which in turn would serve self-respect and thereby liberties. But if we are correct that even the first principle is subject to its own maximin, then it is possible that health care would not always have to be distributed to produce equality of health status. Inequalities would be permitted to the extent that there can exist inequalities in liberties.

If this discussion is correct, we are addressing both those who claim that the Rawlsian difference principle should apply to allocating something like life-saving organs (even if Rawls himself would not) and those who believe that life-saving organs fall under Rawls's notion of the basic structure—whether they see the basis for allocating these organs under the first principle or either part of the second principle. In either case, Rawlsians would appear to endorse a social practice that applies the maximin to the allocation of organs. They would support inequalities in allocation that would result from socially directed donation as long as those worst off would have their position improved. Those large numbers of people who reach considered moral judgments opposing socially directed dona-tion—the UNOS Ethics Committee, the government civil rights attorneys, the Washington Regional Transplant Consortium board, and many others who con-sider racial and other discrimination by social categories in matters of life and death intolerable—must abandon the maximin account of the principle of justice. An analysis of a very practical, concrete problem in organ transplantation may turn out to stimulate not only a more moral organ allocation but also a revision in basic ethical theory about what is just in a society.[42]

ENDNOTES

1. John Rawls, *A Theory of Justice* (Cambridge, MA: Harvard University Press, 1971), p. 302; cf. p. 62.

2. I am aware that Rawls would apply the principles to the establishment of basic practices in a society and not directly to specific public policy decisions (see John Rawls, *A Theory of Justice*, pp. 195 ff.). Others, however, have seen fit to apply the principles to a more specific stage of decisions. I will discuss this problem in detail in an appendix to this chapter addressed to those who have a particular concern about the problem of whether Rawls and Rawlsian approaches can be applied to specific policy decisions.

3. This is, of course, because the maximin tends to be egalitarian. Often the best way to improve the lot of the worst off is by taking something from those who have more and transferring it to those on the bottom. Improving the lot of the worst off thereby also makes people more equal. It is only in the special cases in which increases in inequality would be necessary to improve the lot of the worst off that a difference between stricter egalitarianism and the maximin will be encountered.

4. If manipulation occurs it is much more likely to come at the stage when the patient is listed, a possibility discussed in Chapter 23. A manipulative surgeon, for example, could list a patient before an organ is actually needed, anticipating that by the time the patient's turn comes up, the patient will really need the organ. Physicians treating patients in liver failure might, for example, place their patients in the hospital when not really necessary. As we saw in the discussion of Mickey Mantle's case in Chapter 23, patients in the hospital have a higher priority than those at home. Although I found no evidence of any manipulation of the allocation in the case of Mickey Mantle, if it happened it almost certainly would have had to have come before the listing.

5. Of course, income, socioeconomic status, and other social variables can play a role in deciding who gets on the waiting list for organs. I know of no one who would claim access to the list is totally impartial or fair. That does not take away from the claim that the stage in the allocation in which organs are allocated among those on the list is fair. There is also concern that some of the factors that are used in the allocation formula—HLA and panel reactive antibodies (PRA), for example—are indirectly related to race or gender.

6. Jeff Testerman, "Should Donors Say Who Gets Organs?" *St. Petersburg Times*, Jan. 9, 1994.

7. FLA. STAT. ANN. tit. XLII (1994); "Estates and Trusts," ch. 732, *Probate Code: Intestate Succession and Wills*, pt. X, Anatomical Gifts, § 732.914.

8. Wayne B. Arnason, "Directed Donation: The Relevance of Race," *Hastings Center Report* (Nov.–Dec. 1991): 13–19; Mark D. Fox, "Directed Organ Donation: Donor Autonomy and Community Values," in *Organ and Tissue Donation: Ethical, Legal, and Policy Issues*, ed. Bethany Spielman (Carbondale: Southern Illinois University Press, 1996), pp. 43–50, 163.

9. FLA. STAT. ANN. (1994).

10. This is a version of Rawls's own method of reflective equilibrium. When one's moral intuitions about a particular case and one's principle are incompatible, then one or the other must give. In this case we are arguing that, for those who, on reflection, are not willing to modify their considered moral judgment that directed donation is wrong, then the maximin must give way provided one can show that the maximin would support directed donation.

11. This combination of fairness and efficiency is mandated by the U.S. National Organ Transplant Act of 1984. The specification of the exact formula is a task assigned to the board of directors of UNOS. That body must reconcile the potentially conflicting moral principles of justice (equity) and utility maximization (efficiency). For kidneys, for example, a formula is endorsed that takes into account both equity criteria (such as time on the waiting list) and efficiency measures (such as extent of histocompatibility). As a matter of social policy the rank-ordering of potential candidates is the morally most acceptable list the board can develop.

12. It might be argued that donation of organs is an example of gift-giving, which is normally immune from the moral requirement of fairness. Gifts are, by their very nature, undeserved and unfair. This, however, simply calls into question the use of gift-giving and donation metaphors to refer to a national organ allocation system. In fact, current national policy specifically authorizes specific donation of organs to named individuals, such as family members or loved ones in need of organs. Such donation to named individuals appears to be conceptually outside the national organ allocation system. When donation is not made to a named individual, however, the organ is placed into a national allocation system that is quite analogous to allocating other national resources held in common. The "gift" is made to the society, which is then allocated according to statutory and administrative policies legally mandated to be equitable and efficient. The organ is removed from the mode of gift-giving and placed into a system in which recipients have rights, specifically a right to fair treatment by the allocation system.

13. Technical matters make this analysis still more complex. The waiting list for kidney transplants is generated anew for each donor. The ranking is based not only on time on the waiting list but such factors as HLA tissue compatibility and

PRAs (a measure of exposure to foreign tissues). For the potential recipient, these factors vary for each donor, so someone who ranked below the candidate favored by the directed donation on one allocation could rank above him or her on the next. Still, for any pool of candidates waiting for an organ, certain persons could be described as statistically among the worst off. One who has unusual HLA antigens and a high percentage of PRA is statistically going to have to wait a long time for an organ. A group of worst off persons on the waiting list can be identified either on a specific waiting list or on a statistical basis independent of any given organ. The point made in this instance—that directed donation improves the position of the worst off persons—holds whether we identify the worst off on a particular list or identify the worst off on the waiting list statistically.

14. John Rawls, A *Theory of Justice*, p. 538.

15. Ibid., pp. 534–41.

16. Ibid., p. 530.

17. Ibid., pp. 538–39.

18. The concept of the "veil of ignorance" is a device used by Rawls as a way of recognizing that most people believe that ethics requires impartiality. Rawls says that if one wants to know the general principles that govern social practices, one should imagine what rational people would agree to as the general principles if they did not know their individual position in the social system—that is, if they were behind a veil of ignorance. This fictional device has the effect of forcing people to try to imagine what people would accept if they could exclude their personal self-interest based on their knowledge of their own gender, income level, age, ethnicity, and the like. Rawls is not claiming that principles were actually created at any real, historical time before people knew their personal positions. His contract is hypothetical, but it provides a mental exercise for people to try to imagine what would be reasonable from an impartial point of view—that is, a point of view that ignores personal perspectives.

19. F. M. Kamm, *Morality, Mortality: Volume I: Death and Whom to Save from It* (New York: Oxford University Press, 1993), p. 270, see also p. 293. Although Kamm is considering a maximin rather than a strictly egalitarian view, she proposes excluding consideration of minimal gains to the worst off. She says "we could minimally change a strict maximin theory in the following way: Only when what would be gained by the worst off is a gain that makes a real value significant different to him should we forgo giving the better-off person a much greater gain." She calls this the "Modified Maximin Rule."

20. John Rawls, A *Theory of Justice*, pp. 9, 16, 17, 110, 276.

21. Robert M. Veatch, "Resolving Conflicts among Principles: Ranking, Balancing, and Specifying," *Kennedy Institute of Ethics Journal* 5 (3, Sept., 1995): 199–218.

22. John Rawls, A *Theory of Justice*, pp. 9, 16, 17, 110, 276.

23. Henry S. Richardson, "Specifying Norms as a Way to Resolve Concrete Ethical Problems," *Philosophy and Public Affairs* 19 (1990): 279–310.

24. John Rawls, *A Theory of Justice*, p. 231.

25. There are other possible reasons for explaining the priority for children. Both utilitarian and egalitarian reasons have been proposed. Giving children a priority for kidneys is utilitarian on two grounds: (1) If a child gets the kidney, other things being equal, predictably he or she will get more years from the organ, and (2) neurological side effects of end-stage renal disease in children are more devastating, thus making the benefit to children greater even if the graft survives the same number of years. An egalitarian argument has been made for the priority to children that is a version of the "fair innings" argument. According to it, someone who is in kidney failure early in life is worse off from an over-a-lifetime perspective than someone whose failure comes later. In this sense children can be said to be worse off, and therefore a priority for them could be supported on egalitarian grounds and maximin grounds. Giving them organs makes them more equal to other people and it improves the lot of the worst off. The point, however, is that even if one did not accept these utilitarian, maximin, and egalitarian arguments for the priority for children, the mere fact that they have been promised priority is a prima facie moral reason why they have a special claim. For a fuller discussion of the role of age in rationing see Robert M. Veatch, "How Age Should Matter: Justice as the Basis for Limiting Care to the Elderly," in *Facing Limits: Ethics and Health Care for the Elderly*, ed. Gerald R. Winslow and James W. Walters (Boulder, CO: Westview Press), pp. 211–29.

26. John Rawls, *A Theory of Justice*, pp. 196–99; Rawls, *Political Liberalism* (New York: Columbia University Press, 1993), pp. 257–88.

27. John Rawls, *A Theory of Justice*, pp. 55–56. *Political Liberalism*, pp. 266–68.

28. Ibid., p. 258.

29. Ibid., p. 268.

30. Ibid., p. 282.

31. Ronald M. Green, "Health Care and Justice in Contract Theory Perspective," in *Ethics and Health Policy*, ed. Robert M. Veatch and Roy Branson. (Cambridge: Ballinger Publishing Co., 1976), pp. 111–26; Ronald M. Green, "The Priority of Health Care," *Journal of Medicine and Philosophy* 8 (1983): 373–80.

32. John Rawls, *A Theory of Justice*, p. 302.

33. Ronald M. Green, "The Priority of Health Care," 373–74.

34. John Rawls, *A Theory of Justice*, pp. 231, 244, 250. Also see pp. 207, 214, 542. As I understand Rawls, this toleration of inequalities of liberty applies not only to those societies before establishing more or less just institutions but also to those that are beyond that point.

35. Norman Daniels, *Just Health Care* (Cambridge: Cambridge University Press, 1985).

36. John Rawls, *A Theory of Justice*, p. 303.

37. Education is another condition necessary for equality of opportunity. A similar analysis would seem to apply.

38. David DeGrazia, "Grounding a Right to Health Care in Self-Respect and Self-Esteem," *Public Affairs Quarterly* 5 (Oct. 1995): 301–18.

39. John Rawls, *A Theory of Justice*, p. 440.

40. David DeGrazia, "Grounding a Right to Health Care in Self-Respect and Self-Esteem," 301–18.

41. This is not to say that DeGrazia links self-respect exclusively to liberty. He also mentions effects on ability to use one's fair share of income or wealth.

❖ INDEX